THE INTERVENTIONAL CARDIAC CATHETERIZATION HANDBOOK

T0195529

THE INTERVENTIONAL CARDIAC CATHETERIZATION HANDBOOK

5th Edition

Edited by

Michael J. Lim, MD, FACC, FAHA, FSCAI
Chief, Cardiac Catheterization Lab
Professor, Cardiology
Hackensack University Medical Center
Hackensack, NJ

Paul Sorajja, MD
Director
Center for Valve and Structural Heart Disease
Minneapolis Heart Institute Abbott Northwestern Hospital
Minneapolis, MN

Morton J. Kern, MD, MSCAI, FAHA, FACC
Professor of Medicine
Cardiology
University California Irvine
Orange, CA;
Chief Cardiology
Long Beach Veterans Health Care System
Long Beach, CA

ELSEVIER

Elsevier
1600 John F. Kennedy Blvd.
Ste 1800
Philadelphia, PA 19103-2899

THE INTERVENTIONAL CARDIAC
CATHETERIZATION HANDBOOK, FIFTH EDITION   ISBN: 978-0-323-79066-6

Notice

Practitioners and researchers must always rely on their own experience
and knowledge in evaluating and using any information, methods,
compounds or experiments described herein. Because of rapid
advances in the medical sciences, in particular, independent verification
of diagnoses and drug dosages should be made. To the fullest extent
of the law, no responsibility is assumed by Elsevier, authors, editors, or
contributors for any injury and/or damage to persons or property as a
matter of products liability, negligence or otherwise, or from any use or
operation of any methods, products, instructions, or ideas contained in
the material herein.

Previous editions copyrighted 2018, 2013, 2004, 1996.

Senior Content Development Manager: Somodatta Roy Choudhury
Senior Acquisitions Editor: Melanie Tucker
Senior Content Development Specialist: Malvika Shah
Publishing Services Manager: Shereen Jameel
Project Manager: Vishnu T. Jiji
Design Direction: Brian Salisbury

Working together
to grow libraries in
developing countries

Printed in India

www.elsevier.com • www.bookaid.org

Last digit is the print number: 9 8 7 6 5 4 3 2

To those in my life who have supported
me and helped along the way:
My parents, Dorothy and Jess Lim;
my beautiful children, Parker and Taylor;
and my love – Kerri.

Michael J. Lim

I dedicate this to my loving parents,
Kent and Mon Sorajja, my two
incredible daughters, Natali and Amalin,
and my loving wife, Abbie.

Paul Sorajja

I thank my wife, Margaret, and daughter,
Anna Rose, for giving me purpose
beyond measure. They are the true
systole of my life.

Morton J. Kern

Contributors

Youseff Ayatt, MD
Interventional Cardiologist
Advocate Medical Group
Chicago, IL

Subhash Banerjee, MD
Professor
Department of Medicine
UT Southwestern Medical Center
Dallas, TX

Mir Babar Basir, DO
Director of Acute Mechanical Circulatory Support
Cardiology
Henry Ford Hospital
Detroit, MI

Yonatan Bitton-Faiwiszewski, MD, FACC, FSCAI
Vascular Interventional Cardiologist
Adventist Health
St Helena, CA

Emmanouil S. Brilakis, MD, PhD
Director
Center for Complex Coronary Interventions
Minneapolis Heart Institute
Minneapolis, MN

M. Nicholas Burke, MD
Senior Consulting Cardiologist
Interventional Cardiology
Minneapolis Heart Institute
Minneapolis, MN

Yiannis S. Chatzizisis, MD, PhD, FAHA, FACC, FESC
Professor of Medicine
Director, Cardiac Catheterization Laboratory
University of Nebraska Medical Center
Omaha, NE

Douglas E. Drachman, MD, FACC, FSCAI
Director of Education, Cardiology Division
Teresa G. and Ferdinand F. Martignetti Endowed Chair for
Cardiovascular Medicine
Cardiac and Vascular Invasive Services
Massachusetts General Hospital
Boston, MA

Matthew T. Finn, MD, MSc
Assistant Professor of Medicine
Cardiology
Columbia University
New York, NY

Allison Barbara Hall, MD, FRCPC
Clinical Assistant Professor of Medicine
Faculty of Medicine
Memorial University of Newfoundland, St. John's
Newfoundland
Canada
Cardiologist/Interventional Cardiologist
Cardiology
Eastern Health/Cardiology Consultants, St. John's
Newfoundland
Canada

Beau M. Hawkins, MD
Associate Professor of Medicine
Cardiovascular Section
University of Oklahoma Health Sciences Center
Oklahoma City, OK

Tarek Helmy, MD, FACC, FSCAI
Chief, Division of Cardiovascular Disease
Co-Director of the Heart & Vascular Institute
Professor of Medicine
LSU Shreveport School of Medicine
Shreveport, LA

Morton J. Kern, MD, MSCAI, FAHA, FACC
Professor of Medicine
Cardiology
University California Irvine
Orange, CA
Chief Cardiology
Long Beach Veterans Health Care System
Long Beach, CA

Abdul Ahad Khan, MD
Interventional Cardiology Fellow
LSU Shreveport School of Medicine
Shreveport, LA

Andrew J. P. Klein, MD, FACC, FSVM, FSCAI
Interventional Cardiology, Vascular and Endovascular Medicine
Cardiology
Piedmont Heart Institute
Atlanta, GA

Dhaval Kolte, MD, PhD, FACC, FSCAI
Structural Interventional Cardiologist
Corrigan Minehan Heart Center
Massachusetts General Hospital
Instructor in Medicine
Harvard Medical School
Boston, MA

Alejandro Lemor, MD
Divison of Cardiology
Henry Ford Hospital
Detroit, MI

Michael J. Lim, MD, FACC, FAHA, FSCAI
Chief, Cardiac Catheterization Lab
Professor, Cardiology
Hackensack University Medical Center
Hackensack, NJ

Yves R. Louvard, MD
Institut Cardio Vasculaire Paris Sud
Interventional Cardiology
Hôpital Jacques Cartier
Massy
France

Sahil A. Parikh, MD
Associate Professor of Medicine
Director of Endovascular Services
Columbia University Irving Medical Center
New York, NY

H. Kiran Kumar Reddy, MD, MPH
Interventional and Structural Cardiology
UMass Memorial Medical Center
Division of Cardiology
Worcester, MA

Partha Sardar, MD
Interventional Cardiology
Ochsner Clinic Foundation
New Orleans, LA

Sanjum S. Sethi MD, MPH
Assistant Professor of Medicine
Columbia Interventional Cardiovascular Care
Columbia University Irving Medical Center
New York, NY

Arnold H. Seto, MD, MPA
Cath Lab Director
Long Beach Veterans Affairs Medical Center
Long Beach, CA
Director of Interventional Cardiology Research
University of California, Irvine Medical Center
Orange, CA

Adhir Shroff, MD, MPH
Professor of Medicine
University of Illinois–Chicago
Chicago, IL

Paul Sorajja, MD
Director
Center for Valve and Structural Heart Disease
Minneapolis Heart Institute Abbott Northwestern Hospital
Minneapolis, MN

Jose D. Tafur, MD
Interventional Cardiology
Ochsner Clinic Foundation
New Orleans, LA

Megan Toole, MD
Assistant Professor of Medicine
University of Missisippi
Jackson, MS

Christopher J. White, MD
Chairman and Professor of Medicine
Department of Medicine and Cardiology
Ochsner Clinical School
Medical Director of Value Based Care
Ochsner Medical Center
New Orleans, LA

Preface

It is a pleasure to provide to those working in the field of interventional cardiology a practical and yet detailed handbook to guide both the novice and the advanced practitioner toward best practices. Since the American Board of Internal Medicine certified the subspecialty almost 20 years ago, it is common knowledge that an operator needs an in-depth understanding of the extensive array of techniques to apply them appropriately and solidify the unique skill sets that will make cardiovascular interventions successful. It is our fervent wish that this book will help the interventional cardiologist and the entire heart team in their mastery and acquisition of both the complex skills and knowledge base.

Beyond providing the foundational information of percutaneous coronary intervention (PCI), this edition is noted for addressing the most recent, advanced techniques used to implant coronary and peripheral stents, repair injured vessels, and treat structural heart defects. It highlights the management of the critically ill patients in the cath lab before and during their interventions. *PCI* is, in part, a team sport; that is, it involves the entire lab team members who *should all have a thorough understanding* of the indications, contraindications, and guidelines for percutaneous coronary and structural interventions, coronary bypass graft, and valve surgery, and concomitant medical therapy for an individual patient coming into the lab. The patient's conditions and findings must also be integrated into tailored decisions for a specific patient, given a large variety of clinical factors and comorbidities.

The 5th edition of *The Interventional Cardiac Catheterization Handbook* continues to provide critical instructional information to those beginning their journey into interventional cardiology. It is understood that the practice of interventions cannot proceed without the prior mastery of techniques and methods employed for diagnostic catheterization and specially described in *The Cardiac Catheterization Handbook,* 7th edition. Excellence in intervention begins with excellence in diagnostic catheterization. As with all "handbooks," the material covered here cannot include every aspect of interventional cardiology. For those interested in more detailed information and studies supporting the approaches for the treatment we discuss, we refer you to the larger textbooks in the field.

The contents of the *ICCH,* 5th edition, have been brought up to date as much as possible. The basic chapters on understanding what PCI does, how to achieve best vascular access, and useful approaches to angiography now reflect current thinking regarding radial access, drug-eluting stents, and lesion assessment before, during, and after the procedure, always emphasizing the methods that increase safety whenever possible. Optimal angiographic views for coronary intervention, use of different contrast media, and identification of patients at high risk are fundamental reading for all students and physicians embarking on this path.

The *ICCH,* 5th edition, presents more focused specific chapters emphasizing the unique nature of several well-studied angiographic subsets undergoing complex PCI, such as bifurcation lesions, left main stenosis, chronic total occlusions, saphenous vein graft interventions and peripheral vascular disease, as well as a chapter on PCI-related complications. Each chapter presents the topic in a concise and practical way by experts in the field.

Chapter 12, "Complications of PCI," highlights the fact that no area of cardiology has a greater need for the latest in information than PCI. To minimize unanticipated complications, the planning and execution of PCI require an in-depth understanding of the options, limitations, and alternative methods of proceeding if the initial approach fails.

As all learners know, it is impossible for reading alone to substitute for experience, but the knowledge gained by hands-on exposure to the different types of guiding catheters, guidewires, balloon catheters, stents, intravascular ultrasound imaging, and other nonballoon interventional devices is greatly enhanced by reviewing the descriptions, pitfalls, and anticipated technical problems that may occur during the procedures.

The most critical step in performing an intervention begins well before introducing a stent. That step involves the cognitive review of patient-specific symptoms, precatheterization data from lab and noninvasive testing, prior catheterization data that a patient has undergone, and focusing on the indication and intent of the upcoming procedure. The use of intravascular ultrasound imaging and translesional physiology as well as other tools that present adjunctive data to the coronary angiogram are essential in matching the outcomes of the procedure for the benefit of the patient.

We thank our colleagues and cardiology fellows in training who contributed their valuable time, knowledge, and effort to make this book possible. Finally, this book would have no value were it not for our belief that the knowledge gained will aid the ever-present desire of the cath lab physicians, nurses, techs, and fellows to help their patients through what may be a life or death procedure. We are humbled and at the same buoyed by our mutual goals to care for our patients through better knowledge in the cath lab.

Michael J. Lim
Paul Sorajja
Morton J. Kern

Contents

Section I – Coronary Interventions

Section II – Noncoronary Vascular Intervention

Video Contents

The Basics of Percutaneous Coronary Interventions

MORTON J. KERN

KEY POINTS

- Percutaneous coronary intervention (PCI) procedures in today's cath lab require assimilating numerous details regarding a patient's clinical history, testing before catheterization with anatomic information provided from the diagnostic angiogram.

- PCI requires an understanding of anticoagulation therapy, guide catheters, guidewires, balloons, coronary physiology, and intravascular imaging procedures, before and after stent implantation.

- Appropriate selection of patients and coronary lesions for PCI, weighing the risk of complications against long-term clinical benefits remains the key to quality coronary interventional procedures.

Introduction

On September 16, 1977, Andreas Grüentzig performed the first human percutaneous transluminal coronary angioplasty (PTCA) in Zurich, Switzerland. Until then, coronary artery bypass surgery was the only alternative to medicine for the treatment of coronary artery disease (CAD). Since that time, PTCA has rapidly evolved into more sophisticated techniques involving predominantly stenting and other nonballoon devices and is now called *percutaneous coronary intervention (PCI)*. PCI is a highly successful method of coronary revascularization with more than 1.5 million procedures done in the United States annually. Because of significant technical advances in treating chronic total occlusions (CTOs), mechanical left ventricular (LV) support, and novel atherectomy devices, to name just a few, PCI operators have taken on more complex patients and lesions than the initial PTCA substrate of discrete single- and double-vessel coronary stenoses. It is now routine to see many PCI centers treating cases of complex multivessel CAD, including significant left main stenosis. High-risk PCI, including the treatment of patients with depressed LV function, requires a Heart Team approach, much like that convened before many structural heart disease interventions.

PCI encompasses various mechanical approaches to addressing coronary stenoses, such as balloons, stents, cutters, lasers, grinders, aspirators, filters, and other tools. The term *percutaneous transluminal coronary angioplasty* or PTCA may be used when describing balloon catheter techniques and older studies related to use of the original balloon catheter first employed by Grüentzig. Percutaneous coronary and structural heart disease interventional techniques are commonly performed after diagnostic angiography for patients with ischemic and structural heart disease. Table 1.1 lists diagnostic and therapeutic interventional procedures performed in the catheterization laboratory.

This chapter, an expansion of the chapter from *Kern's Cardiac Catheterization Handbook*, 7e (2019), will present the basic method and mechanisms of coronary angioplasty and stenting, as well as many of the fundamental techniques associated with the practice of interventional cardiology. An overview of the various devices of PCI used for specific applications is provided in Table 1.2. The interventions used for peripheral vascular and structural heart disease will be discussed in their corresponding chapters herein.

Table 1.1

Diagnostic and Therapeutic Procedures in Cardiac Catheterization Laboratory	
Diagnostic Procedures	**Therapeutic Procedures**
Coronary angiography	Percutaneous coronary interventions (balloon, stents, rotoblator, etc.)
Ventriculography	Valvuloplasty, TAVR, mitral clip
Hemodynamics	ASD, PFO, PDA, VSD Shunt closure
Shunt detection	Thrombolysis, thromboaspiration
Aortic and peripheral angio	Coil embolization
Pulmonary angio	Pericardiocentesis, window
Coronary hemodynamics	
Endomyocardial biopsy	

Angio, Angiography; *ASD,* atrial septal defect; *PDA,* patent ductus arteriosus; *PFO,* patent foramen ovale; *Rx,* treatment, *TAVR,* transaortic valve replacement; *VSD,* ventricular septal defect.

Table 1.2

Niche Applications of Percutaneous Coronary Intervention Devices

Lesion Type	Stent	CB	RA	Thr Asp	Special Devices
Type A	+++	+	±	−	−
Complex	++	++	++	−	Guideliners
Ostial	++	++	+	−	−
Diffuse	+	−	++	−	−
CTO	++	−	±	−	Special equip[a]
Ca^{++}	±	++	+++	−	(orbital ath, IV lithotripsy)
SVG focal	+++	±	±	−	Filters,
SVG diffuse	+	±	−	−	−
SVG thrombotic	±	−	−	++	Filters,
Dissection	+++	−	±	±	imaging catheters
Acute occlusion	++	−	−	±	−
Thrombosis	+	−	−	+++	−
Perforation	±	−	−	−	Covered stent
Device embol	−	−	−	−	Snares, forceps

+++, highly applicable; ++, somewhat helpful; +, applicable; ±, marginal depending on status; −, not applicable.
[a]Specialized equipment includes unique guidewires, balloons with reentry ports, and transport catheters for antegrade or retrograde access.

Ca^{++}, Calcified; CB; cutting balloon; CTO, chronic total occlusion; embol, emboli; RA, rotational or orbital atherectomy; SVG, saphenous vein graft; Thr Asp, thrombus aspiration.

PCI Overview

The technique of PCI is an extension of the basic methods used for diagnostic cardiac catheterization and coronary angiography. Obviously, one should master the basic techniques, concepts, and knowledge of diagnostic cardiac catheterization before moving into the specialty of interventional cardiology.

After the required clinical evaluation to establish an appropriate indication for revascularization, PCI is often performed either as a separate procedure or as an add-on, ad hoc procedure after the diagnostic study.

Fig. 1.1 shows how a stent is implanted during PCI. In brief, a guiding catheter is seated in the coronary ostium. A thin, steerable angioplasty guidewire is introduced through the guide catheter to the coronary artery, crossing the stenosis and positioned in the distal aspect of the artery. A balloon angioplasty

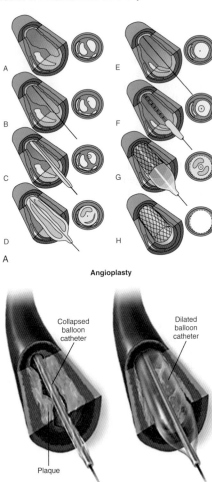

Figure 1.1   **Panel A:** How angioplasty and stenting are performed. **A,** The artery is filled with atherosclerotic material, compromising the lumen. A cross-section of the artery is shown on the right side. **B,** A guidewire is positioned past the stenoses through the lumen. **C,** A balloon catheter is advanced over the guidewire. **D,** The balloon is inflated. **E,** The balloon is deflated and withdrawn. **F,** The balloon catheter is exchanged for a stent (on a balloon). **G,** The stent is expanded. **H,** The expanded stent remains in place after the deflated balloon is withdrawn. **Panel B:** Close-up cross-sectional representation of a coronary stenosis and balloon catheter deployed across the stenosis (*left*) and inflated (*right*). (Reproduced from the American Heart Association, Your PTCA, Our Guide to Percutaneous Transluminal Coronary Angioplasty, 2001.)

catheter, which is considerably smaller than the guiding catheter, is inserted through the guiding catheter, tracking over the guidewire, and is then positioned, spanning the narrowed stenotic area. After correct positioning within the stenosis, the balloon catheter is inflated; repeat inflations are often required. The inflation and deflation of the balloon in the blocked artery restores blood flow to the deprived myocardium supplied by the stenosed artery. After balloon dilation, a stent is implanted in the same fashion as balloon dilation. Full stent deployment is should be confirmed with intravascular imaging (e.g., intravascular ultrasound [IVUS]). After successful stent implantation, patients may be discharged the same day or may need to stay overnight in the hospital to be discharged the following morning. Patients can usually resume their normal routine within days.

Decision Points in the PCI Procedure

For all catheterization procedures, but particularly PCI, the type of vascular access is one of the most important decisions. The techniques for the placement of an arterial sheath through the arm (radial, ulnar, or distal radial artery) or leg (femoral artery) are described in detail in Chapter 2, Vascular Access. In contrast to diagnostic catheters, PCI requires larger lumen, specialized "guiding" catheters, and often larger vascular access sheaths. The risk of access site bleeding must be carefully considered for the individual patient. The bleeding risk for radial artery access is significantly lower than femoral access. Currently, the most common guide catheter and sheath size is 6F. Larger-sized (>7F) PCI equipment often requires femoral access.

After vascular access, the next decision is selecting an effective guide catheter that will remain well seated in the coronary ostium and support the passage of a balloon catheter and stent. The operator will then review the angiographic vessel anatomy and select an angioplasty guidewire and balloon dilation catheter. Both the guidewire and the guide catheter have specific characteristics to manage difficult guide support and negotiate vessel tortuosity and complex lesions.

The choice of an angioplasty balloon to dilate the target lesion is based on the diameter of the unaffected reference segment of the target vessel and the length of the stenosis. Specialized balloons to score or cut the lesion are available. Calcified lesions may require additional treatment with grinding burr catheters (called rotablation or rotational atherectomy or most recently, an intrvascular lithotripsy balloon system, Shockwave) before stent placement (see Chapter 6).

After the initial balloon dilation of the stenosis, the next decision is which stent to use. There are several manufacturers and types of stents but the most common are balloon expandable, thin metal mesh-like designs, which are selected based on characteristics of the stent as a scaffold, the type of drug coating, diameter of the artery, and length of the stenosis to be treated. The stent is positioned in the dilated stenosis and deployed by balloon inflation. Optimal stent implantation after high-pressure inflations with a noncompliant (NC) balloon is confirmed not only by angiographic images of the stent but also by specialized imaging catheters (intravascular ultra sound [IVUS] or optical coherence tomography [OCT]) to see appropriate vessel/stent matching and full stent strut expansion and apposition (contact without space against the wall), features required to give the best short- and long-term results (see Chapter 5).

The last decision point is the type of arterial hemostasis to be used after sheath removal. Radial artery access uses a pressure band. Femoral artery access hemostasis can be achieved with one of several different vascular closure devices. For uncomplicated PCI, same-day discharge is now routine. Decisions for timing of discharge depend on the clinical situation and potential of a late complication. The patient commonly returns to work shortly (<2 days) thereafter.

Indications, Contraindications, and Complications of PCI

The American Heart Association (AHA), American College of Cardiology (ACC), and Society for Cardiac Angiography and Interventions (SCAI) PCI Updated Guidelines of 2015 provide recommendations for the performance of PCI. Specific anatomic and clinical features for each patient should be considered for the likelihood of success; failure; and risk for complications, morbidity, mortality, and restenosis. Restenosis and incomplete revascularization must also be weighed against the outcome anticipated for coronary artery bypass grafting (CABG). The indications, contraindications, and complications of PCI are listed in Table 1.3. There are no absolute contraindications to emergency life-saving interventions except for patient refusal and malfunctioning equipment. There are several anatomic factors that are associated with poor stent outcomes and may be considered relative contraindications. These include:

- Small coronary vessels of less than 2.5 mm
- Vessels with poor distal runoff or severe diffuse disease
- Vessels supplying poorly functional or nonfunctional myocardium
- Extensive and heavily calcified vessels

Table 1.3

Indications, Contraindications, and Complications of Percutaneous Coronary Intervention (PCI)

Indications for PCI

1. Angina pectoris causing sufficient symptoms despite optimal medical therapy
2. Mild angina pectoris with objective evidence of ischemia (abnormal stress testing or physiology) and high-grade lesion (>70% diameter narrowing) of a vessel supplying a large area of myocardium
3. Unstable angina or non-ST-elevation myocardial infarction (STEMI)
4. STEMI as primary therapy or in patients who have persistent or recurrent ischemia after failed thrombolytic therapy
5. Angina pectoris after coronary artery bypass grafting (CABG)
6. Restenosis after successful PCI
7. Left ventricular dysfunction with objective evidence of viability of a vessel supplying the myocardium
8. Arrhythmia secondary to ischemia

Contraindications for PCI

1. Unsuitable coronary anatomy
2. Extremely high-risk coronary anatomy in which closure of vessel would result in patient death
3. Contraindication to CABG (however, some patients have PCI as their only alternative to revascularization)
4. Bleeding diathesis
5. Patient noncompliance with dual antiplatelet therapy and unwillingness to follow post-PCI instructions
6. Multiple in-stent restenosis
7. Patients who cannot give informed consent

Complications Associated With PCI

1. Death (<1%)
2. Myocardial infarction (MI; <3%–5%)
3. Stent thrombosis (approximately 1%)
4. Emergency CABG (<1%)
5. Abrupt vessel closure (0.8%)
6. Coronary artery perforation (<1%)
7. All the complications that can occur during cardiac catheterization, including access site bleeding, pseudoaneurysm, atrioventricular (AV) fistula, ischemic vascular complications, stroke, allergic reaction to contrast media, and renal failure

Complex or High-Risk PCI

Stenting for patients with complex and high-risk anatomy or clinical presentations should be carefully considered. Anatomic concerns include the following:

- Long lesions requiring more than one stent per lesion
- Small coronary artery reference vessel diameters (<2.5 mm)

- Significant thrombus at the lesion site
- Lesions in saphenous vein grafts, the left main artery, ostial locations, or bifurcated lesions
- Restenotic lesions
- Diffuse disease or poor outflow distal to the identified lesion
- Very tortuous vessels in the region of the obstruction or proximal to the lesion
- Complex CAD with significant impairment of LV function

It should be noted that some patients with contraindications may have no options regarding coronary revascularization, and PCI becomes their only alternative to failed medical therapy.

Complications of PCI

For more information, see Chapter 12. For most elective procedures:

1. Death (0.1%)
2. Myocardial infarction (MI; 1%–3%)
3. Emergency CABG (0.5%–2%)

Of course, any complications that can occur during diagnostic cardiac catheterizations can also occur during PCI, such as femoral access site bleeding, especially with larger sheaths and prolonged anticoagulation (1:250 patients), contrast-medium reactions, cerebral vascular accident, MI, and vascular injury (e.g., pseudoaneurysm of femoral artery, radial artery occlusion).

Restenosis is a biological effect that is not considered a complication but rather a clinical response to angioplasty. Restenosis occurs in 5% to 10% of cases with drug-eluting stents (DES), and 10% to 20% of cases with bare metal stents. Restenosis within the stent or at the edges of the stent occurs in approximately 10% of patients, even with DES, and may lead to recurrence of anginal symptoms. Typically, restenosis occurs most frequently within the initial 12 months after PCI.

Stent thrombosis is the abrupt formation of a blood clot inside the stent and is a potentially catastrophic event that can lead to MI or death. The incidence of stent thrombosis is 1% to 2%. It is more likely to occur if dual antiplatelet therapy (i.e., aspirin and clopidogrel or other P2Y12 platelet inhibitors) is prematurely discontinued or if the stent is suboptimally expanded.

PCI Equipment

Every PCI starts with three basic pieces of equipment: a guiding catheter, a coronary guidewire, and a balloon/stent catheter system

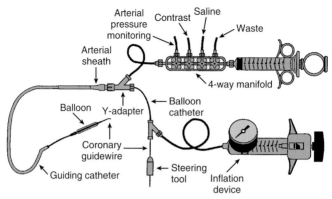

Figure 1.2 Diagram of Components of Percutaneous Coronary Intervention Equipment. The main components include the balloon catheter, which is connected to an inflation device, and a manifold to injection contrast and monitor pressure. The guidewire passes through a Y-connector valve on the guide catheter, permitting continuous pressure readings and access to the guide catheter lumen for contrast media injection. (From Freed M, Grines C, Safian RD. *The New Manual of Interventional Cardiology.* Physicians' Press: 1996.)

(Fig. 1.2). Each piece of PCI equipment is designed to facilitate three major procedural challenges: (1) provide a stable platform (the guide catheter) from which the delivery of the guidewire and balloon/stent catheter can be accomplished; (2) navigate arteries and cross stenoses to deliver the balloon/stent system; (3) expand/implant the stent to the correct vessel size for all plaque types. A large variety of specialized guide catheters, accessories, and lesion modification tools are available to achieve the goal of opening a stenotic vessel. The technique of PCI requires the operator to control all three of the principal movable components (guide catheter, guidewire, and balloon/stent catheter system) simultaneously.

The Guiding Catheter

For more detail, see Chapter 4.

A special large-lumen catheter is used to deliver and help guide the balloon catheter to the stenosis (Fig. 1.3). Compared with a diagnostic catheter, a guiding catheter has a thinner wall and larger lumen, which allows contrast injections with the balloon catheter inside. A large catheter lumen is achieved at the expense of catheter wall thickness and thus may result in decreased catheter wall strength, increased catheter kinking, or less torque control. A guiding catheter is stiffer than a diagnostic catheter to

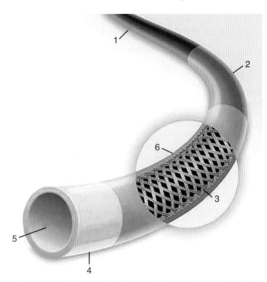

Figure 1.3   Illustration of a Guiding Catheter. 1, Stiffer body; 2, variable softer primary curve; 3, wire braiding; 4, atraumatic tip; 5, large lumen (optional radiopaque marker); 6, lubricous coating. (Courtesy Boston Scientific, Inc.)

provide support for advancing the balloon/stent catheters into the coronary artery. It responds differently to manipulation than a diagnostic catheter. Unlike diagnostic catheters, guiding catheters have relatively shorter, nontapered tips of softer material to decrease catheter-induced trauma.

Use of 6F (or, in some patients, 7F) guide catheters from the radial artery approach is now common practice for most routine PCI. Smaller (<5F) guide catheters may not permit adequate visualization with some stent systems. 7F or 8F guide catheters are used for complex procedures requiring larger PCI devices (e.g., rotoblator) or simultaneous positioning of two stents for treatment of bifurcation lesions. Guiding catheters come in many different shapes for both femoral and radial approaches to meet the need of the numerous anatomic variations encountered in daily practice.

Functions of the Guiding Catheter

The three major functions of a guiding catheter during PCI include balloon/stent catheter delivery, contrast injection, and pressure monitoring:

1. Balloon/stent catheter delivery: The guiding catheter is the delivery device of the coronary guidewire, balloon catheter, or any

other equipment needed for the coronary artery. If the guiding catheter is not seated properly in a coaxial manner, it may not be possible to advance the balloon/stent across the stenotic area. The guiding catheter "sits" in the coronary ostium (a technique called cannulation) and provides backup support or a "platform" to push the balloon/stent catheter across the stenosis. Several important terms are commonly used when referring to guiding catheters:

- Backing out: The guiding catheter moves out of the coronary ostium into the aortic root when pressure is applied to the balloon to cross the lesion. This is caused by an insufficient support position or a vessel or stenosis producing considerable resistance or friction to the balloon or stent movement.

- Deep seating: The guiding catheter moves deeply into the ostium or into the proximal portion of the coronary vessel. This maneuver increases backup support and is typically used as a last resort because of the increased risk for guiding catheter–induced dissection. A guide catheter extension (see later) obviates this maneuver and currently is the preferred approach.

- Coaxial alignment: Good backup support is best achieved when the catheter tip is aligned parallel (i.e., coaxial) to the axis of the ostial part of the left main coronary artery, right coronary artery (RCA), or bypass conduit. Coaxial alignment permits efficient transmission of the force needed to advance the balloon/stent across a stenosis. Alignment may require guide catheter repositioning or occasionally deep seating into the artery. A specialized guide-within-a-guide or guide extension catheter (e.g., guideliner, also called mother-and-child guides; Fig. 1.4) may be required for support in some difficult situations. Although safer than deep guide catheter intubation, use of the guide extension is associated with an increased chance of proximal vessel dissection.

2. Contrast injection: The guiding catheter permits visualization of the target by contrast administration with or without the balloon catheter in place. Reliable visualization of the vessel and stenosis before, during, and after intervention is critical to correct positioning and to success of the balloon/stent systems. Good visualization may be particularly difficult when the lumen is occupied by the PCI devices inside. Large nonballoon PCI devices (e.g., rotoblators, thrombus aspiration catheters) in small guide catheters may not allow adequate contrast delivery

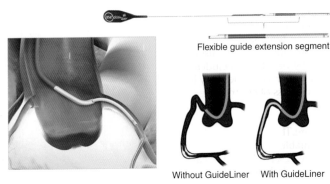

Flexible guide extension segment

Without GuideLiner   With GuideLiner

Figure 1.4   Guide Catheter Extension. Guideliner is inserted through the guide catheter and is soft enough to be deeply positioned in the artery. The guideliner is often advanced with a partially inflated balloon in the tip to prevent vessel dissection. This maneuver is called balloon-assisted tracking. (Courtesy Vascular Solutions, Inc.).

and vessel visualization. This problem has been overcome with larger lumen catheters and contrast media power injectors.

3. Pressure monitoring: The guiding catheter allows the operator to continually assess aortic pressure during the procedure, an essential monitor for patient safety (e.g., avoiding hypotension from vagal episode or ischemia because of guide catheter obstruction). Pressure wave damping may occur if the guide catheter blocks the coronary ostium; if there is noncoaxial seating; or if equipment, clot, or plaque obstructs flow through the coronary ostium. Guide catheter coronary occlusion is noted by the change in the arterial pressure waveform to one of "damping," which shows a flattened diastolic portion or ventricular-like pattern (Fig. 1.5). Guiding catheters with small side holes near

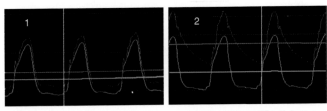

Figure 1.5 Pressure tracings demonstrating guide catheter pressure damping (*left*) and after withdrawal of guide from ostium (*right*). Guide catheter pressure is red, and the pressure wire inside the coronary artery is green.

the tip permit blood to enter the coronary artery when the ostium is blocked by the guide catheter and can reduce damping when the catheter is deeply seated and the tip is obstructing flow. Side holes are used when the guide catheter either partially or totally occludes blood flow into the coronary artery; however, side holes may lead to inadequate artery visualization from loss of contrast media exiting the catheter before entering the artery. Although side holes may provide reliable aortic pressure, coronary flow can still be compromised during the procedure. These catheters should be used with caution and are not suitable for hemodynamic lesion assessment (i.e., fractional flow reserve [FFR]) because of the creation of a pseudostenosis through the side holes (more detail found in Chapter 5).

Balloon Catheter Systems

There are two types of PCI balloon catheters: over-the-wire (OTW; Fig. 1.6) and monorail or rapid-exchange catheters (Fig. 1.7).

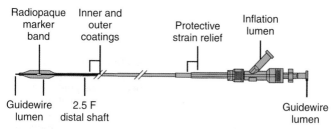

Figure 1.6 Schematic design of a typical over-the-wire (OTW) angioplasty balloon catheter. The guidewire extends the entire length of the catheter.

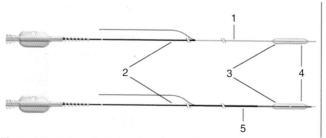

Figure 1.7 Schematic design of a typical rapid-exchange angioplasty balloon catheter. The guidewire extends on "through" the distal part of the catheter allowing for single-operator use. (Image provided courtesy of Boston Scientific. © 2022 Boston Scientific Corporation or its affiliates. All rights reserved.)

OTW Angioplasty Balloon Catheters

An OTW balloon/stent catheter has two lumens: one that runs the length of the catheter, ending in the balloon for inflation/deflation, and a second lumen that runs the entire length of the catheter and serves as the channel for the guidewire. These balloons are approximately 145 to 155 cm long and are designed to be used with guidewires of various dimensions (<0.014 in). The major advantage of OTW catheters is their ability to maintain distal artery access with the balloon beyond the lesion while exchanging one guidewire for another or using the distal lumen to give contrast or administer drugs (e.g., nitrates, thrombolytics, after the guidewire is removed, of course). The OTW system tracks very well because the whole balloon length has a wire in the lumen. Nevertheless, it requires long (300 cm) guidewire exchanges.

To exchange OTW catheters, the balloon is advanced over the wire to a distal position. Although a standard short (145 cm) wire can be used with an OTW balloon/stent, typically an exchange length guidewire (300 cm) is preferred. Guidewire extension devices or magnets can facilitate exchange of OTW balloons/stents if the operator prefers to use a short wire. OTW catheters can accept multiple guidewires, which allows for the exchange of additional devices that may require stronger, stiffer, or specialized guidewires.

The limitations of OTW systems include the slightly larger catheter diameter than the rapid-exchange (monorail) catheters and the need for additional personnel to help with long guidewire catheter exchanges.

Rapid-Exchange (Monorail) Catheters

Rapid-exchange catheters, also called monorail catheters, were developed to permit the exchange of balloon catheters by a single operator. Rapid-exchange catheters have one long lumen to inflate the balloon and a short (30–40 cm) length of the distal catheter shaft, which contains two lumens. The second lumen holds the guidewire over which the catheter travels through the guide and into the vessel. Because only a limited portion of the catheter requires two lumens, rapid-exchange catheters are smaller in diameter than OTW balloon catheters.

Rapid-exchange balloon catheters obviate the need for long exchange wires to change OTW catheters and two operators to participate in the exchange (although one can certainly be used if the operator prefers). The smaller diameter monorail design may also have some advantage.

Limitations of monorail catheters include that it requires more care in manipulation of the guidewire, balloon/stent catheter, and guiding catheter. For example, if the monorail balloon is advanced beyond the distal end of the guidewire, the wire may come out of its short lumen, necessitating catheter withdrawal and reassembly of the balloon and guidewire. This is especially true when with catheters that have relatively short (<2 cm) "rail" segments (e.g., some IVUS catheter systems). Additionally, if the balloon catheter requires substantial force during advancement, a loop of guidewire may form outside the guide catheter in the aorta. This loop is nearly invisible but should be considered if the operator advances the catheter without seeing motion at the balloon tip.

Characteristics of Balloon Catheters

The plastic material of the balloon determines its compliance (defined as the amount of expansion or diameter size for a given amount of pressure), stiffness, and strength. Compliance is the main differentiating feature among balloon catheters. Inflation of a moderately compliant balloon above factory-determined mean inflation pressure (also called nominal pressure to achieve a known balloon size) will lead to approximately a 10% to 20% balloon size over the predicted diameter. NC balloons, on the other hand, remain very close to their rated diameter even when inflated several atmospheres above nominal pressure.

A compliant balloon may result in balloon oversizing, particularly after several high-pressure inflations, and possibly cause a dissection. After stent deployment, high-pressure inflations are routinely performed with NC balloons to assure that the stent struts firmly and completely into the vessel wall and fully expanded.

Operators should understand that there is balloon overinflation at balloon ends beyond the stent. According to Laplace's law, wall stress increases with radius. Artery sites adjacent to the lesion may be traumatized by inflations at high pressures. When inflating a balloon above the rated burst pressure, consider limiting the number and duration of inflations.

Balloon diameters always increase with increasing pressure. Even NC balloons will grow in diameter (usually by <10% over nominal) with high pressure. Compliant balloons may increase by more than 20%. Table 1.4 lists the advantages and limitations of angioplasty balloon catheters.

Selection of Balloon Size (Diameter and Length)

In general, select a balloon size to achieve a less than 1 to 1 size match with the vessel so that some part of the lesion is visible for stent positioning (e.g., use of a 2.5-mm balloon in a 3.0-mm vessel so that a remnant of the lesion will mark the area for stent positioning). Balloon-to-artery ratios of more than 1.2 to 1 are associated with increased complications. Longer balloons (30–40 mm) are

Table 1.4

Advantages and Limitations of Angioplasty Balloon Catheters		
	Advantages	**Limitations**
Over the wire (OTW)	Distal wire position	Needs two people for exchanging balloon catheter/stent
	Accepts multiple wires	
	Distal port for pressure, contrast injection	
Rapid exchange (monorail)	Ease of use, single-operator system	Needs good guide support
	Enhanced visualization	Blood loss at Y valve during exchanges
		Unable to change wire

useful for dilating long and diffuse narrowings. Short (10–15 mm) balloons are used for stent expansion to avoid stretching the vessel wall outside the stent.

The balloon/stent size is determined using the distal arterial reference segment diameter compared with the size of the guiding catheter (conversion of 1 French = 0.33 mm; 6F x 0.33 = 1.98 mm or approximately 2 mm, which is useful as a gauge of artery diameter or distance on the angiogram). Visual estimation of artery diameter is less accurate than quantitative angiographic and intravascular imaging (IVUS or OCT) approaches, but it is the method used by nearly all interventionalists during the procedure. From IVUS studies, most stents selected by visual sizing are 0.5 mm smaller than true vessel dimensions.

Although some consider various technical features of stent systems, including device profile, ease of delivery, and restenosis and acute thrombosis rates, when making a decision, there appears to be only a small difference between different modern balloon and stent systems. Stent profile alone is not the only factor in facilitating a stent to cross a lesion. Resistance to balloon/stent catheter forward motion may also occur because of vessel tortuosity or calcification with the guidewire or friction within the guide catheter.

Balloon/Stent Inflation Strategies

Stenosis resolution occurs when the balloon/stent pressure eliminates the balloon indentation caused by the stenosis (called the *waist*). Unstable or thrombotic lesions are generally soft and are associated with a lower balloon inflation pressure than are chronic, stable, or calcific lesions. Because stenting is now routine, issues regarding optimal balloon inflation strategies (namely, inflation time or pressure) are relatively unimportant. Balloon inflations are generally brief (<60 sec) but should be inflated long enough to permit elastic tissue to relax and stretch and permit some stent metal to expand to its nominal diameter.

PCI Guidewires

PCI guidewires are small-caliber (0.010–0.014 in), steerable wires advanced into the coronary artery branches over which the balloon/stent/device is tracked to address the lesion. The operator imparts a slight bend to the tip, which allows for steering across side branches and through tortuous artery curves.

Guidewires are made with an inner core wire and an outer spring tip. The shorter the distance between the end of the central core and the spring tip, the stiffer and more maneuverable the wire. Differences in core construction affect guidewire handling. Important considerations when selecting a guidewire include diameter, coating, torque control, flexibility, malleability, radio-opacity, and trackability. The most used coronary guidewires are 0.014 in, but a family of specialized guidewires and microcatheters (See Chapters 4 and 8 for further details) are available for crossing and treating CTOs.

Several guidewire characteristics should be considered in their selection. Stiffness of the guidewire determines specific performance. Soft wires may be easier to advance through tortuous artery branches. Stiff wires torque better and are often useful for crossing difficult or total chronic occlusions. Extrastiff guidewires provide better support for difficult stent placement in highly tortuous arteries. "Steerability," "flexibility," and "malleability" are terms used to differentiate various guidewires (Table 1.5).

Radio-Opacity, Marker Bands, and Special Coatings

Visualization of the guidewire is improved by a radio-opaque coating usually applied only to the distal 3 cm of the wire. The limited radio-opaque segment permits lesion visualization without obscuring useful angiographic detail, such as small dissections. Calibrated radio-opaque marker bands on some wires are used to gauge lesion length.

Stent/balloon catheters usually have two markers, one at each end of the balloon. Small balloons (e.g., 1.5 mm in diameter) have one central marker. These markers may be confused for the markers on some marker guidewires.

A variety of different wire coatings increase ease of wire movement within the balloon catheter and artery. Some coated plastic-tipped wires, especially those with hydrophilic tips, have a higher likelihood of dissecting or perforating the arterial wall. With the emergence of the special approaches to CTO, families of

Table 1.5

General Categories of Guidewires			
Category	**Use**	**Features**	**Example**
Workhorse	First-line wire for majority of percutaneous coronary interventions (PCIs)	Safety, 1:1 torque, Good tip shape retention	HT Balance Middleweight Universal
Finesse	Tortuosity	Lubricity, moderate support	HT Pilot 50
Extra-Support	Tortuosity, distal lesions	Soft gentle tip, High-level of support, Does not "spring back"	HT Iron Man
Specialty	Multiple	Depends on need	Sion

specialized guidewires have been developed that increase procedure success (see Chapter 8 on CTO).

An exchange guidewire is like the standard wires previously mentioned except for its length (280–300 cm). This long wire replaces the initial 140-cm wire when an exchange of the OTW balloon catheter is necessary (e.g., upsizing balloon or insertion of stent). Alternatively, a 120- to 145-cm extension wire can be connected to a companion 145-cm guidewire, thus creating a long exchange guidewire to allow balloon catheter exchanges. Some regular-length guidewires can accept an extension wire and thus become an exchange wire.

Accessory Equipment

See Fig. 1.8.

Adjustable Hemostatic Rotating Y-Connector Valves

The Y-connector is attached to the guide catheter to permit introduction of PCI equipment into the guide while allowing contrast injection and pressure measurement through the guide catheter. The end of the Y-connector has a rotating hub and a valve. The valve minimizes back bleeding while the PCI catheter is inserted or removed from the guide catheter.

Balloon Inflation Devices

A disposable syringe device is used to inflate the PCI balloon. A pressure gauge or digital display indicates the precise inflation

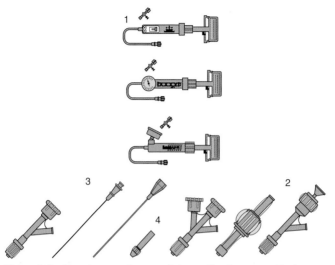

Figure 1.8 **Percutaneous Coronary Intervention Accessory Equipment.** Examples of balloon inflation device and Y connectors, wire introducer needles, and torque tool. (Courtesy Meritt Medical, Inc, Salt Lake City, UT.)

pressure in atmospheres (atm or torr) or pounds/square inch (psi). Typically, the balloon is inflated with sufficient pressure (4–12 atm) to fully expand the stenosis indentation ("dumbbell" or "waist") of the partially inflated balloon. Occasionally, some calcified or highly fibrotic lesions require very high inflation pressures (>18 atm) to expand and eliminate the "dumbbell" appearance of the balloon.

Guidewire Torque (Tool) Device and Guidewire Introducer

A small, cylindrical pin vise clamp slides over the end of a guidewire and permits the operator to perform fine steering manipulations of the guidewire. A guidewire introducer is a very thin, needlelike tube with a tapered conical opening on one end that helps the operator insert the guidewire through a Y-connector valve or into a balloon catheter.

Stents

Stents are used in nearly all PCI procedures. The choice of drug-coated (i.e., DES) or bare metal stents is based on the clinical scenario for a particular individual. Currently, the choice is DES in the majority of, if not all, patients.

There are many different designs for stents (Fig. 1.9). For most coronary arteries, expanded stent diameters range from 2.25 to 5 mm. Stent lengths currently available vary from 8 to 38 mm. For saphenous vein grafts and peripheral vessels, larger stent diameters (>5 mm) are available. Specialized stents are specifically designed for problems. For example, a unique covered stent with a polytetrafluoroethylene (PTFE) coating is designed for coronary perforation or rupture and can be used to cover aneurysms. Dedicated bifurcated stents are in development.

Fig. 1.9C lists stent types, characteristics, and specialized features of material and cell configuration. Figs. 1.10 and 1.11

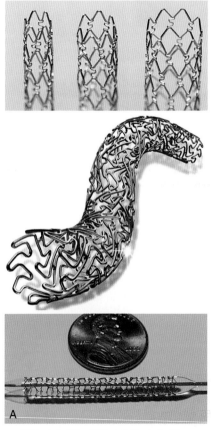

Figure 1.9A Different stent designs.

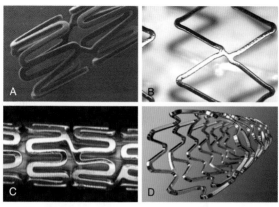

Figure 1.9B (**A, B**) The cobalt chromium Elixir DESyne Novolimus-eluting stent crimped (**A**) and expanded (**B**). (**C, D**) The platinum chromium everolimus-eluting Element stent crimped (**C**) and expanded (**D**). (**A,** Reproduced with permission from Costa JR, Jr, Abizaid A, Costa R, et al. 1-year results of the hydroxyapatite polymer-free sirolimus-eluting stent for the treatment of single de novo coronary lesions: the VESTASYNC I trial. *JACC Cardiovasc Interv.* 2009;2(5):422–427. **C, D,** Courtesy Boston Scientific. From Garg S, Serruys PW. Coronary stents: Looking forward. *J Am Coll Cardiol.* 2010;56:S43–S78.)

Durable polymer-coated stent		Biodegradable polymer-coated stent						Bioresorbable drug-eluting stent
Abbott/ Boston	Medtronic	Biosensors	Terumo	Translumina	Boston	Biotronik		Abbott
Xience/ Promus	Resolute	BioMatrix	Ultimaster	Yukon Choice PC	Synergy	Orsiro		ABSORB
CoCr/PtCr-EES	CoNi-ZES	316L-BES	CoCr-SES	316L-SES	PtCr-EES	CoCr-SES		PLLA-EES

Strut thickness

81 μm	91 μm	120 μm	80 μm	87 μm	74 μm	60 μm	150 μm

Polymer coating

Circumferential	Abluminal	Circumferential

C

Figure 1.9C Overview of principal characteristics of selected current-generation durable polymer and biodegradable polymer drug-eluting stents and fully bioresorbable drug-eluting stents with published large-scale randomized controlled trial data. *BES,* Biolimus-eluting stent; *CoCr,* cobalt chromium; *CoNi,* cobalt nickel; *EES,* everolimus-eluting stent; *PtCr,* platinum chromium; *SES,* sirolimus-eluting stent; *ZES,* zotarolimus-eluting stent. (Byrne RA, Joner M, Kastrati A. Stent thrombosis and restenosis: What have we learned and where are we going? The Andreas Grüntzig Lecture ESC 2014. *Eur Heart J.* 2015;36[47]:3320–3331.)

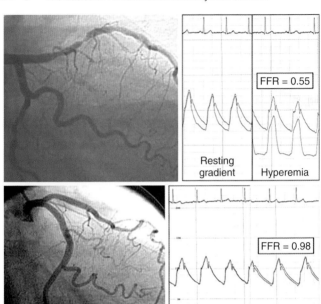

Figure 1.10 **Single-Vessel Stenting.** *Top,* Left anterior descending artery with a 90% narrowing and significant hemodynamic gradient and low fractional flow reserve (FFR) before percutaneous coronary intervention (PCI). *Bottom,* Post PCI result with 0% angiographic residual and normalization of translesional pressure. (Courtesy Drs. Bernard De Bruyne and Nico Pijls.)

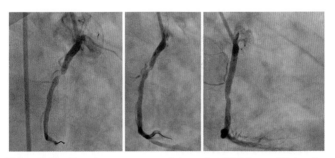

Figure 1.11 Percutaneous coronary intervention (PCI) for non-ST elevation myocardial infarction (STEMI) of right coronary artery (RCA). *Left,* Mid RCA severe stenosis with slow flow to patent ductus arteriosus (PDA). Collaterals from left coronary not shown. *Middle,* After initial balloon inflation. *Right,* After stent implantation. Note PDA fills completely in antegrade fashion.

are examples of stent placement in the left coronary artery and RCA.

Compared with balloon angioplasty, stenting produces a larger minimal luminal diameter, maintains arterial patency, and reduces restenosis with excellent long-term results. Stenting reduces the incidence of acute recoil, abrupt vessel closure, and the need for emergency CABG previously associated with balloon angioplasty alone. DES is favored over a bare metal stent because of the reduced restenosis rates. Stents improve long-term results compared with balloon angioplasty in nearly every angiographic subset examined. Stents prevent abrupt vessel closure from dissections. In reducing recoil and minimizing regrowth of neointima (i.e., hyperplasia) with antiproliferative coatings, drug-coated stents further reduce coronary restenosis compared with uncoated or bare metal stents.

Numerous stent designs are available to overcome patent issues, improve vascular scaffolding mechanisms, provide unique antiproliferative coatings, and, most recently, become resorbable over time. Stents are composed of metal mesh, wire coil, slotted tube, multicellular designs, or unique bioabsorbable materials of custom design. A stent may be made of stainless steel, cobalt-based alloy, tantalum, titanium, or nitinol. DES have drug-impregnated coatings, biodegradable drug carrier coatings, and/or other types of drug delivery systems. Biodegradable and bioabsorbable stents have been developed and studied, but none are currently clinically available.

Stent Deployment Mechanisms

There are two mechanisms of stent expansion: balloon expandable and self-expanding. Most stents are balloon expandable. They are mounted on a balloon catheter, delivered to the lesion, and then the balloon is inflated, deploying the stent.

Self-expanding stents often are used for peripheral vascular disease interventions. They are compressed on a delivery catheter and covered with a sheath to prevent premature deployment. Once the stent system is delivered to the lesion, the cover is withdrawn, permitting the stent to expand on its own. Often nitinol is the memory metal used in these stents.

Considerations for Stent Delivery: Predilation or Direct Stenting?

Delivery of a stent to the lesion is usually performed after initial balloon angioplasty of the lesion (predilation), or it can be performed without predilation (direct stenting). A preliminary balloon dilation informs the operator about the difficulty of negotiating the artery, crossing the lesion, and selecting the correct stent size. After the initial expansion of the stenosis, the increased blood flow produces flow-mediated vasodilation and, on second-look angiography, the vessel diameter is often larger than when seen before dilation, thus altering stent sizing.

Before stent implantation, dilation with a balloon that is slightly undersized relative to the reference vessel diameter is a safe strategy that gives the operator useful information, such as the pressure needed to expand the lesion. Using a slightly undersized balloon also leaves an indication of the lesion so the stent can be optimally positioned. Predilation also allows for the vessel to be repressurized with restored flow, which often produces vasodilation. It is not uncommon to find a vessel enlarged after balloon dilation. This enlargement results in the operator selecting a larger stent than would have been chosen initially with a direct stent strategy.

Stenting without predilation is called "direct" stenting. Although this method saves a small amount of time, the advantage is minimal and poststent vasodilation may lead to suboptimal stent sizing for the vessel with accelerated restenosis.

Standard Guidewire or Extra-Support Guidewire?

Routine stent procedures can be easily performed with regular support guide catheters and guidewires. Extra-support or stiff guidewires (0.014 in) provide a stronger, stiffer "rail" on the stent catheter to cross lesions with extreme angulation, calcification, or tortuosity and for lesions with long dissections. The extra-support guidewire assists both guiding catheter stability and stent delivery. Although often helpful, extra-support guidewires can sometimes create difficulties by straightening the vessel and folding the intima, causing "pseudo" lesions or vessel spasm. Exchanging back to a softer, floppy-tipped wire after stent delivery may prevent these effects. Using two wires, one to straighten the vessel and help the balloon/stent catheter running over the second wire, is called the "buddy" wire technique and is also helpful in tortuous, calcified vessels.

IVUS/OCT for Confirmation of Stent Expansion

See Fig. 1.12. More detail can be found in Chapter 5.

Stent optimization is the expansion of the stent to the maximal safe extent without vessel injury. Optimal stent expansion is determined by the ratio of the stent lumen cross-sectional area (CSA) relative to the vessel CSA at the stent site and relative to the

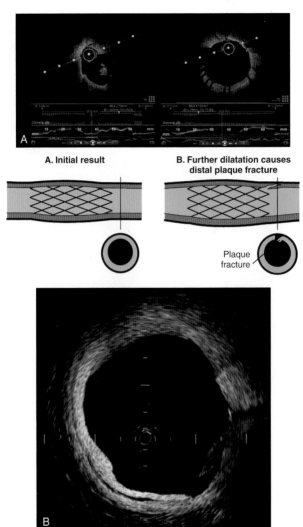

Figure 1.12 Examples of Intravascular Imaging. 12a, Optical coherence tomography (OCT) image of a (*left*) small lumen after balloon expansion with medial fracture and thrombus; poststent (*right*) shows full stent implantation, symmetric expansion, and complete strut apposition. **12b,** OCT frame showing segment distal to stent with dissection at 5 o'clock and separation of the media continuing to 8 o'clock. Small stent edge dissections often can be managed medically.   *Continued*

Incomplete stent expansion

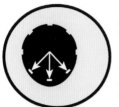

Stent struts are not attached
to the intima

This can occur in the ostial LAD lesion
or in the ectatic vessel (poststenotic
dilation site)

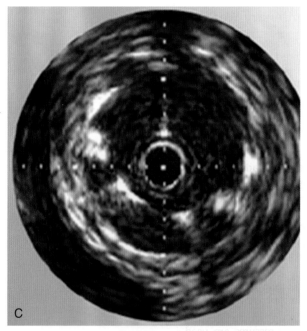

C

Figure 1.12, cont'd 12c, Intravascular ultrasound (IVUS) frame showing
under expansion of the stent with malapposition of struts from 4 o'clock to
9 o'clock. Further inflations with larger balloons are required.

reference lumen CSA. The essential features of the stent optimization technique are:

1. Evaluation of the dimensions of the reference vessel and implanted stent by IVUS/OCT
2. Selection of an appropriately sized, NC balloon based on IVUS/OCT target vessel diameter at the stent site

3. Performance of high-pressure balloon dilatation of the stent (usually >12 atm) or dilation with a larger balloon

Successful stent expansion is achieved when (1) there is no significant difference between the lumen diameters of the stent and the reference site (particularly the distal reference), and (2) there is complete apposition of the stent to the vessel wall. For small vessels (<2.5 mm in diameter), the IVUS criterion of achieving a final stent lumen CSA larger than the distal reference lumen CSA is strongly recommended.

Cautionary Words on Stent Deployment

1. When stenting multiple lesions, stent the distal lesion first, followed by the proximal lesion. Stenting in this order obviates the need to recross the proximal stent with another stent and reduces the chances of stent delivery failure or loss of stent when pulling back an undeployed stent for whatever reason.

2. When recrossing a recently implanted stent, use a large J-wire tip curve or even loop to ensure that the guidewire does not go under the stent or between the stent and the vessel wall, which may result in inadvertent stent damage or dislodgement and failure to advance equipment beyond the stent.

3. If there is stent inflow or outflow obstruction or residual distal vessel narrowing, a freshly prepared balloon catheter can be advanced through the stented area for further dilatations.

4. Eliminate any inflow or outflow narrowing by additional high-pressure balloon inflations or additional stent implantations (especially if the stent margin has a dissection).

5. An acceptable angiographic result is a residual narrowing of less than 10% by visual estimate, but a truly optimal stent result can only be confirmed by IVUS/OCT.

6. Vasospasm may occur during the procedure when high inflation pressures are used for stent optimization. Vasospasm is often self-limiting, nearly always resolves with time or intracoronary nitroglycerin, and has not been associated with any unfavorable clinical events. Extraordinarily high-pressure inflations (>16 atm) are generally unnecessary and have been associated with stent overexpansion, vasospasm, and higher in-stent restenosis rates.

7. Crossing a proximally implanted stent to deliver a stent more distally may be difficult because of the friction of stent-on-stent contact. Excess stent catheter force or deep guide seating may deform the implanted stent. Consider repeated high-pressure

proximal stent expansion, balloon-assisted guide catheter advancement (advance guide over deflated balloon catheter inside the stent), a buddy wire method, or a guideliner to facilitate stent-through-stent advancement.

Stent Expansion Strategies

There are two methods of increasing the stent lumen CSA: (1) high pressure and (2) a larger diameter NC balloon. When an oversized balloon is used, there is an increased likelihood of coronary vessel rupture or dissection. Using high pressure with a balloon that is appropriately sized to the vessel allows for stent expansion to occur within the natural confines of the vessel. To avoid complications, the balloon-to-reference vessel ratio should be approximately 1.0. If a balloon-to-vessel ratio is greater than 1.0, a short, NC balloon with medium pressure (12–16 atm) should be used. Use of a balloon larger than the distal IVUS minimum vessel diameter (MLD, measured media to media) should be avoided.

When there is a large diameter difference between the proximal and distal vessels (e.g., left anterior descending [LAD] artery before and after a diagonal branch), use a lower inflation pressure when treating the distal part of the stent segment and a higher pressure for the proximal. Care should be taken not to overexpand the distal stent edge with an oversized balloon. Occasionally, for significant vessel tapering, two balloons of different diameters are used.

NC balloons are preferable to compliant balloons for final stent inflations for several reasons. NC balloons will expand and dilate uniformly, even in focal areas of resistant lesions, and they are more likely to maintain a uniform diameter even at high pressures, without balloon overexpansion vessel injury in the adjacent unstented segments. Additionally, IVUS has shown that 25% of stents will improve stent expansion with an increase in pressure from 15 to 18 atm or more.

Stent expansion should be symmetric, which is easily accomplished in soft plaques. Hard fibrotic or calcified plaques, seen in approximately 20% to 30% of lesions, are not easily compressed and result in asymmetric stent expansion into the normal arc of the vessel. In lesions with a significant arc ($\geq$270 degrees) of hard fibrocalcific disease, stent expansion has a low symmetry index of less than 0.7 minimum-to-maximum lumen diameter ratio. Further balloon inflation produces focal overstretching or edge dissection, especially if an oversized balloon is used. Using a balloon that is 0.25 to 0.5 mm smaller than the size of the vessel at high pressure may safely improve the symmetry index but will not necessarily increase the CSA of the lumen at the stent site.

Asymmetric overexpansion is associated with a risk of vessel rupture. If the stent lumen CSA is acceptable relative to the distal lumen CSA and the stent is well apposed, avoid efforts to make stent symmetry perfect.

Incomplete Stent Expansion

Full stent expansion is related to the plaque burden and composition. Optimal stent expansion in lesions with 50% to 70% diameter stenosis or lesions with a spiral dissection can be easily accomplished because there is not much atheroma. In lesions with greater than 90% diameter stenosis, full stent expansion is more difficult to achieve with a higher asymmetry. Incomplete stent expansion (i.e., when the stent struts do not contact the intimal surface) can occur, particularly in ectatic vessels (e.g., aneurysm sites) and in the ostial LAD artery near the left main trunk (see Fig. 1.12D). In the latter case, dilation of the ostial lesion with only the shoulder of the balloon does not provide sufficient expansion force to implant the stent fully.

Dissection at the Stent Margin

Stent implantations sometimes cause dissection at the edge of the stent and diseased vessel, and this may require additional stents to stabilize the newly produced injury (see Fig. 1.12B). Misplacement of the postdilation balloon at the edge of the stent, especially if the balloon is clearly oversized, can cause stent margin dissection. Stent margin dissections for elastic or soft lesions may also be seen when the stents are deployed on highly angulated bend points.

Working Through Difficult Stent Delivery and Other Problems

The complex nature of the stent procedure predisposes it to unique complications and technical challenges. Problems of stenting can be broken into six major categories:

A. Delivery Failure: Failure to deliver the stent is most often because of:

1. Suboptimal guide support
2. Failure to cross lesion (e.g., failure to predilate a significant stenosis or calcific segment)
3. Failure to negotiate proximal tortuosity or calcific segment (e.g., unanticipated vessel rigidity or acute angulation)

To manage these problems, predilation rather than direct stenting is recommended and has the advantage of identifying factors associated with delivery failure. A predeployment balloon that tracks easily to the lesion, dilates the lesion simply, and provides evidence of good guide catheter support bodes well for the easy delivery of the stent to the lesion. Difficulties with advancing the balloon, guide catheter instability, and difficulty in dilating through tortuous segments, on the other hand, herald stent delivery problems.

In highly tortuous arteries with multiple bends, guidewire selection is an important factor in stent delivery success. Extra-support guidewires may not be ideal for initially crossing lesions because of vessel straightening, producing intimal folds and pseudostenosis. Conventional softer guidewires may permit stent delivery while avoiding creation of pseudostenosis. Table 1.6 lists several technical manipulations that may help when a stent fails to advance.

B. Underexpanded Stent: The inability to fully expand the stent with persistent narrowing after implantation may be because of calcification or rigid vessels. Images that may be confused for underexpansion of a stent include dissection around the stent originating at stent margins or unsuspected thrombus formation within or adjacent to the stent, which may appear as narrowings related to stent implantation.

Table 1.6

Technical Manipulations When a Stent Fails to Advance

General

- Best technical manipulation: Secure a more stable guide position or, if possible, the guide can be deep-seated safely. A potential late complication is ostial stenosis because of endothelial trauma. The use of a guide extension such as a guideline can obviate dangerous deep seating of the guide catheter.
- Place constant forward pressure on the stent catheter while pulling the wire back to decrease friction inside the stent catheter lumen and to straighten the stent catheter.
- Use additional proximal segment dilation or plaque modification (e.g., rotoblator) to facilitate stent advancement.

Wire Manipulations

- Advance a second stiffer wire to straighten the artery (the buddy wire technique). This stiff wire can cause wire bias and misdirect the stent if not carefully maneuvered.
- Advance the stent on the second, stiffer buddy wire. Occasionally stents may actually advance more easily over a softer wire.
- Shape the wire along the curve of the artery to lessen wire bias so there is less friction or resistance at the outer curve of the vessel and the path of the wire is more coaxial with the path of the vessel.
- Use a "wiggle" wire.

Table 1-6

Technical Manipulations When a Stent Fails to Advance (Continued)

Stent Manipulations

- If the problem is extreme tortuosity of the proximal segment, change to shorter stent.
- Select a stent with better flexibility.
- Gently bend the stent to conform it along the curve of the artery (rarely done).

Guide Manipulations

- Change to a different curve to achieve better backup and more coaxial to allow less friction at the ostium.
- Use a larger or smaller guide to achieve better backup.
- Use guideliner extension.

Techniques Facilitating Recrossing of a Stented Area by a Balloon or Another Stent

GENERAL

- Best technical manipulation: Steer the wire into a different direction or to a different branch to lessen wire bias and increase wire centering.
- Rotate the balloon catheter while advancing it and let the catheter enter the stent by itself through its rotational energy (like torquing the Judkins Right catheter).

GUIDEWIRE MANIPULATIONS

- Bend the wire and place the bent segment near the ostium of the stent to be crossed to position the wire more at the center of the entrance of the stented segment and to decrease wire bias.
- Insert a second, stiffer wire to straighten the vessel.
- Change the current wire to a stiffer one.

BALLOON/STENT MANIPULATIONS

- Use a shorter balloon or stent.
- Use a more flexible balloon or stent.
- Use partial tip inflation to deflect the nose of stent away from struts.
- If only the balloon needs to enter the stented segment, inflate the balloon with 1 to 2 atm so the balloon centers the wire in the lumen and facilitates the crossing of the wire and balloon.

(Modified from Nguyen T, Douglas JS, Jr, Hieu NL, Grines CL. Basic stenting. *J Interventional Cardiol.* 2002;15:237–241.)

During the balloon inflation, if an indentation persists, higher balloon inflation pressures or a larger, short balloon should be used. Failure of full stent expansion is usually the result of an inadequate predilation approach. In cases where stent deployment appears suboptimal, intravascular imaging (IVUS/OCT) will confirm the mechanism of persistent narrowing caused by tissue prolapse, incomplete apposition, heavy calcification, or, in some cases, thrombus. Failure to adequately expand the stent is associated with increased restenosis rates and/or acute thrombosis. Caution is needed when extracting the balloon from the underexpanded stent so that the guide catheter is not drawn into the vessel and causes proximal vessel dissection.

C. Loss of Access to the Stent

1. Loss of guidewire access may prevent successful recrossing for postdilation balloon inflations. Failure to recross through the central stent lumen and not under a strut may result in stent deformation. Recrossing a recently deployed stent is facilitated by using a soft guidewire with an exaggerated tip loop to prolapse through the stent. All efforts should be made to prevent the guidewire from entering between the strut and the arterial wall.

2. Recrossing stents with balloons may be difficult when the proximal border of the stent is on a tortuous vessel segment, thus forcing the balloon tip into the vessel wall where it is blocked by the stent struts. Stent-on-stent friction also makes distal stent positioning difficult. Several approaches can be used to overcome this problem:

   a. The guide catheter can be repositioned in a more coaxial manner.

   b. A stiffer guidewire or buddy wire can be advanced to reshape the curve of the artery. Several operators have recommended putting a curve into a stiff part of the guidewire and using it to advance across a tortuous segment proximal to a stent and placing a curve on the balloon by using a technique similar to that of putting a gentle curve on a guidewire.

D. Embolized Stent: Several techniques for recovery of embolized stents have been proposed and include loop snares, basket retrieval devices, biliary forceps, biopsy forceps, and other specifically designed retrieval systems.

E. Artery Perforation: First, reposition a balloon catheter to tamponade the perforation then quickly consider your options, which include using a covered stent (see Chapter 10, Complications of Percutaneous Coronary Interventions) or emergency CABG.

F. Stent-Related Dissection, Thrombosis, and Ischemia: The following factors are associated with an increased risk for stent thrombosis and ischemia:

1. Inadequate stent expansion (e.g., highly calcified lesion that did not undergo rotoblator)

2. Dissection, not covered by the stent

3. Poor distal runoff or infarct in related vessel
4. Presence of thrombus or no reflow
5. Subtherapeutic anticoagulation
6. Vessels less than 2.5 mm in diameter
7. Subacute thrombotic occlusion is rare within the first week after implantation but may happen during the week after discharge if dual antiplatelet therapy is not maintained. Risk factors for subacute occlusion were noted earlier. The risk of subacute thrombosis is increased when multiple overlapping stents are used. Subacute occlusion is treated with repeat balloon dilatations, confirmation of adequate implantation by IVUS/OCT, and continuation antiplatelet agents.
8. Ruptured inflation balloon: Although uncommon, loss of inflation pressure during expansion of the stent can indicate balloon rupture or perforation. The ruptured balloon must be exchanged for a new one. If balloon rupture occurs after the ends of the stent are flared and anchored in the artery wall, the balloon can be deflated, rotated two or three times inside the stent, and gently pulled back inside the sheath and removed.

The Pre-PCI Workup

Noninvasive testing for ischemia provides an objective basis and support to proceed with PCI in stable patients. The most common ischemic tests are: (1) exercise stress with/without perfusion imaging or echo LV wall motion, as indicated; (2) pharmacologic stress study (e.g., dipyridamole); and (3) two-dimensional echocardiogram (as indicated for assessment of LV function or valvular heart disease) or computed tomography angiography (CTA) with an FFR.

In the absence of objective evidence of noninvasive ischemia testing, invasive assessment of the ischemic potential of a stenosis can be obtained during coronary angiography measuring translesional pressure–derived FFR or nonhyperemic pressure ratios (Fig. 1.13).

Pre-PCI Preparation: Holding Area

- Patient preparation (intravenous [IV] access, meds, review of relevant precatheterization testing, and consent)
- Patient and family teaching (procedure, results, complications)
- Cardiothoracic surgeon consultation, particularly for high-risk, multivessel disease or decreased LV function
- Appropriate laboratory data (type and crossmatch, complete blood cell and platelet counts, prothrombin time [PT], partial

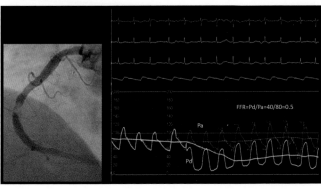

Figure 1.13   Measurement of fractional flow reserve (FFR) across severe right coronary artery (RCA) stenosis (*left panel*) shows initial matching of the aortic guide catheter pressure (Pa, red) and pressure sensor guidewire (Pd, white). Immediately after the sensor passes the stenosis, the distal pressure drops, demonstrating a large gradient at rest without much more change during hyperemia. FFR = Pd/Pa = 40/80mm Hg = 0.5.

thromboplastin time [PTT], electrolytes, blood urea nitrogen [BUN], creatinine)

Patient Preparation in Catheterization Suite

- Electrocardiogram (ECG; inferior and anterior wall leads): 12-lead (radiolucent) ECG
- 1 or 2 IV lines
- Sterile preparation for vascular access (right radial artery for most cases, left radial for CABG or short patients [<5 ft 5 in]); femoral to be considered in dialysis patients or those who may require larger than 7F equipment
- For high-risk PCI (e.g., acute MI, new left bundle branch block) or RCA rotoblator or mechanical thrombus aspiration, venous access for temporary pacemaker may be needed.
- Aspirin (325 mg PO): Failure to administer aspirin before PCI is associated with a two to three times higher acute complication rate.
- P2Y12 oral antagonist agent (e.g., clopidogrel, ticagrelor orally or cangrelor IV if indicated). Best outcomes are associated with antiplatelet preloading.
- Continue routine medications, particularly the antihypertensive agent(s).

- Heparin, 70 u/kg IV bolus. Target activated clotting time (ACT) greater than 250 sec. Heparin is critical for PCI despite controversies regarding dosing and unpredictable therapeutic responses. Higher levels of anticoagulation are roughly correlated with reduced complications during PCI, albeit at the expense of increased bleeding complications at higher heparin doses. Weight-adjusted heparin provides a clinically superior anticoagulation method over fixed heparin dosing. Bivalirudin may be substituted for heparin in some patients (see Chapter 3, Interventional Pharmacology).
- Premedication is the same as for diagnostic angiography (e.g., fentanyl 25–50 mg IV and midazolam [Versed] 1 to 2 mg IV).

Concluding the Procedure

- Final angiography should be made with the guidewire removed (the guidewire hides dissection flaps) and after intracoronary nitroglycerin (relieves vasospasm).
- For patients with femoral access, femoral artery angiography is needed before vascular closure device insertion. Perform a right anterior oblique (RAO) view for right femoral artery (FA) and left anterior oblique (LAO) for left FA. If the artery is not suitable for closure device, secure arterial and venous sheaths in place for transfer to a holding area. Remove sheath with manual compression hemostasis when the ACT is less than 150 to 200 seconds.
- For the radial approach, apply radial artery compression band for hemostasis after final coronary angiography.
- Do not give routine postprocedure heparin unless there are clinical indications beyond the stent procedure (e.g., deep vein thrombosis [DVT], pulmonary embolism [PE]).

Postprocedure Care: Recovery Area

Nurses should begin patient teaching on hospital course, potential bleeding problems, late complications, and restenosis. After the PCI, the cath lab team notifies the referring physician, the family, the recovery area, the intensive care unit (ICU) if needed, and any standby surgical team. Postprocedure labs and ECG are obtained.

Postprocedure Care: Step-Down Area

After PCI, chest pain may occur in about less than 10% of patients. ECG evidence of ischemia identifies those at significant risk for acute vessel closure. When angina pectoris with ischemic ECG changes occurs within the first 24 hours, a return to the cath lab for diagnosis and possible thrombolysis and/or restenting is often needed. The decision to proceed with further interventional procedures, CABG surgery, or medical therapy must be individualized based on factors such as hemodynamic stability, amount of myocardium at risk, and the likelihood that the treatment will be successful. After PCI, the hospital care team should monitor the patient for recurrent myocardial ischemia, puncture site complications, and contrast-induced renal failure.

Post-PCI Care: Medications

- Aspirin (81 mg/day PO)
- P2Y12 oral platelet inhibitor agents (clopidogrel 300-mg or 600-mg loading dose and 75 mg/day, prasugrel 60-mg loading with 10 mg/day, or ticagrelor 180 mg PO with 90 mg PO b.i.d.)
- Initiate statin drugs, if not already prescribed.
- Restart or initiate antihypertensive or antianginal medications depending on the patient's clinical needs.
- Resume prior medications for other conditions (e.g., gastroesophageal reflux disease [GERD]).

Appropriate secondary atherosclerosis prevention programs should be started involving adherence to recommended medical therapies and behavior modifications to reduce morbidity and mortality from coronary heart disease.

Patients with renal dysfunction and diabetes should be monitored for contrast-induced nephropathy. In addition, those patients receiving higher contrast loads (>5 mL/kg) or a second contrast load within 72 hours should have their renal function assessed over several days. Whenever possible, nephrotoxic drugs (certain antibiotics, nonsteroidal antiinflammatory agents [NSAIDs], and cyclosporin) and metformin (especially in those with preexisting renal dysfunction) should be withheld for 24 to 48 hours after PCI.

After discharge, the patient then returns to activities of daily living within 1 to 2 days. Factors preventing rapid return to work include access site complications and persistent symptoms. A functional (ischemic test) evaluation for patients with multivessel coronary angioplasty or incomplete revascularization after angioplasty will identify cardiac limitations, if any, on return to work status.

CAD Risk-Factor Modification

All patients should be instructed about risk-factor modification and medical therapies for secondary atherosclerosis prevention before leaving the hospital. The interventional cardiologist should emphasize these measures directly to the patient and family. Failure to do so suggests that secondary prevention therapies are not important. The interventional cardiologist should contact the primary care physician regarding the secondary prevention therapies initiated and those to be maintained, including aspirin therapy, hypertensive control, diabetic management, aggressive control of serum lipids with a high-intensity statin, abstinence from tobacco use, weight control, regular exercise, and angiotensin-converting enzyme (ACE) inhibitor therapy as recommended in the AHA/ACC consensus statement on secondary prevention.

Follow-Up Planning

- Access site check on first office visit, 2 to 4 weeks
- Routine stress testing is not performed after PCI. Annual stress testing is not recommended by guidelines unless symptoms appear. There is no indication for annual exercise testing in asymptomatic patients. The AHA/ACC practice guidelines recommend selective evaluation in patients considered to be at particularly high risk (e.g., patients with decreased LV function, multivessel CAD, proximal LAD disease, previous sudden death, diabetes mellitus, hazardous occupations, and suboptimal PCI results). For many reasons, stress imaging is preferred to evaluate symptomatic patients after PCI. If the patient's exertional capacity is significantly limited, coronary angiography may be more expeditious to evaluate symptoms of typical angina. Exercise testing after discharge is helpful for activity counseling and/or exercise training as part of cardiac rehabilitation. Neither exercise testing nor radionuclide imaging is indicated for the routine, periodic monitoring of asymptomatic patients after PCI without specific indications.
- If symptoms or signs of ischemia are present early after PCI, coronary angiography is repeated.

PCI Programs Without Surgical Backup

PCI is performed in laboratories without on-site surgical backup. Criteria for the performance of PCI at hospitals without on-site cardiac surgery have been summarized as follows:

1. The operators must be experienced interventionalists who regularly perform elective intervention at a surgical center

(75 cases/year). The institution must perform a minimum of 36 primary PCI procedures per year.

2. The nursing and technical catheterization laboratory staff must be experienced in handling acutely ill patients and comfortable with interventional equipment. They must have acquired experience in dedicated interventional laboratories at a surgical center. They participate in a 24-hour, 365-day call schedule.

3. The catheterization laboratory itself must be well equipped, with optimal imaging systems, resuscitative equipment, and LV support devices (e.g., intra-aortic balloon pump [IABP], Impella, Tandem Heart) and must be well stocked with a broad array of interventional equipment to handle any emergency.

4. The cardiac care unit nurses must be adept in hemodynamic monitoring and LV support device management.

5. The hospital administration must fully support the program and enable the fulfillment of the preceding institutional requirements.

6. There must be formalized written protocols in place for immediate (within 1 hour) and efficient transfer of patients to the nearest cardiac surgical facility that are reviewed/tested on a regular (quarterly) basis.

7. Primary intervention must be performed routinely as the treatment of choice around the clock for a large proportion of patients with acute MI to ensure streamlined care paths and increased case volumes.

8. Case selection for the performance of primary angioplasty must be rigorous. Criteria for the types of lesion appropriate for primary angioplasty and for the selection for transfer for emergency aortocoronary bypass surgery are shown in Table 1.7.

9. There must be an ongoing program of outcomes analysis and formalized periodic case review.

10. Institutions should participate in a 3- to 6-month period of implementation, during which time the development of a formalized primary PCI program is instituted that includes establishing standards, training staff, detailed logistic development, and creation of a quality assessment and error management system. (Levine G, et al. *Circulation.* 2011;124: e574–e576)

Training for Coronary Angioplasty

Advances in interventional procedures have maintained high and durable success rates despite increasingly complex procedures.

Table 1.7

Patient Selection for Percutaneous Coronary Intervention (PCI) at Hospitals Without On-Site Cardiac Surgery

Avoid intervention in hemodynamically stable patients with:

1. Significant unprotected left main coronary artery narrowing upstream from an acute occlusion in the left coronary system that might be disrupted by the angioplasty catheter
2. Extremely long or angulated infarct-related lesions with thrombolysis in myocardial infarction (TIMI) grade 3 flow
3. Infarct-related lesions with TIMI grade 3 flow in stable patients with three-vessel disease
4. Infarct-related lesions of small or secondary vessels
5. Lesions in other places besides the infarct artery
6. Patients with high-grade residual left main or multivessel coronary disease and clinical or hemodynamic instability should be transferred to a coronary artery bypass graft-capable center by prearrangement ambulance agreement.

(Adapted from Wharton TJ, Jr, McNamara NS, Fedele FA, et al. Primary angioplasty for the treatment of acute myocardial infarction: Experience at two community hospitals without cardiac surgery. *J Am Coll Cardiol.* 1999;33:1257–1265.)

The need for appropriate training and guidelines for the procedure is obvious. Recent guidelines for the assessment and proficiencies of coronary interventional procedures have been summarized in a report from a joint task force from the AHA/ACC. American Board of Internal Medicine (ABIM) board certification in interventional cardiology requires documentation of training in an accredited fellowship program during which a minimum of 125 coronary angioplasty procedures must have been performed, including 75 performed with the trainee as primary operator (Table 1.8).

Angiography for PCI

Angiography for PCI expands on the fundamentals of diagnostic angiography and requires establishing details regarding the best method of stent delivery and deployment. Before PCI, the angiographer should acquire the following additional angiographic detail:

1. Establish the relationship of coronary ostium to aorta for guide catheter selection.
2. Verify target vessel, pathway, and angle of entry.
3. Confirm lesion length and morphology using additional angulated views to eliminate vessel overlap.

Table 1.8

American Heart Association (AHA) Proficiencies

Considerations for the Assessment and Maintenance of Proficiency in Coronary Interventional Procedures

Institutions

- Quality assessment monitoring of privileges and risk-stratified outcomes
- Provide support for a quality assurance staff person (e.g., nurse) to monitor complications
- Minimal institutional performance activity of 200 interventions per year with the ideal minimum of 400 interventions per year
- Interventional program director who has a career experience of more than 500 percutaneous coronary intervention (PCI) procedures and is board certified by the American Board of Internal Medicine (ABIM) in interventional cardiology
- Facility and equipment requirements to provide high-resolution fluoroscopy and digital video processing
- Experienced support staff to respond to emergencies
- Establishment of a mentoring program for operators who perform fewer than 75 procedures per year by individuals who perform 150 procedures per year

Physicians

- Procedural volume of 75 per year
- Continuation of privileges based on outcome benchmark rates with consideration of not granting privileges to operators who exceed adjusted case-mix benchmark complication rates for a 2-year-period
- Ongoing quality assessment comparing results with current benchmarks, with risk stratification of complication rates
- Board certification by ABIM in interventional cardiology

(From Hirshfeld JW, Ellis SG, Faxon DP, et al. Recommendations for the assessment and maintenance of proficiency in coronary interventional procedures. *J Am Coll Cardiol* 1998;31:722–743. See Naidu SS, Aronow HD, Box LC, et al. SCAI Expert Consensus Statement: 2016 Best Practices in the Cardiac Catheterization Laboratory: Endorsed by the Cardiological Society of India, and Sociedad Latino Americana de Cardiologia Intervencionista; Affirmation of Value by the Canadian Association of Interventional Cardiology–Association Canadienne de Cardiologie d'intervention.)

4. Separate associated side branches and degree of ostial atherosclerosis.

5. Visualize distribution of collateral supply.

6. Determine the true (maximally vasodilated) diameter of the coronary artery at the target site.

7. An optimal definition of the ostial and proximal coronary segments is critical to plan the procedure and select an appropriate PCI guide catheter.

8. Assessment of calcium from angiography is less reliable than IVUS but is still useful in assessing the need for rotational atherectomy and its associated risks.

Visualization of vessel bifurcations, origin of side branches, the portion of the vessel proximal to a significant lesion, and previously "unimportant" lesion characteristics (length, eccentricity, calcium, and the like) will assist in device selection and identifying potential procedural risk. For total chronic vessel occlusions, the distal vessel should be visualized as clearly as possible by injecting the coronary arteries that supply collaterals and imaging long enough with panning to visualize late collateral vessel filling and the length of the occluded segment.

Optimal radiographic imaging technique is also critical to a successful intervention by enhancing accurate interpretation of procedure results. Modification of panning technique to reduce motion artifact, optimal use of beam restrictors (collimation) to reduce scatter, and improved contrast media delivery all can enhance clinical results. A working knowledge of the principles of radiographic imaging permits the interventionalist to improve their imaging outcomes.

Radiation exposure is higher in PCI than in diagnostic procedures. Continued awareness of the inverse square law of radiation propagation will reduce the exposure to patient, operators, and the cath lab team. Obtaining quality images should not necessitate increasing the ordinary procedural radiation exposure to either the patient or catheterization personnel.

Common Angiographic Views for Angioplasty

The routine coronary angiographic views described here should include those that best visualize the origin and course of the major vessels and their branches in at least two different (preferably orthogonal) projections.

Anteroposterior Imaging

The image intensifier positioned is directly over the patient, with the beam perpendicular to the patient lying flat on the x-ray table (Figs. 1.14 and 1.15). The anteroposterior (AP) view or shallow RAO displays the left main coronary artery in its entire perpendicular length. In this view, the branches of the LAD and left circumflex coronary arteries branches overlap. Slight RAO or LAO angulation may be necessary to clear the density of the vertebrae and the

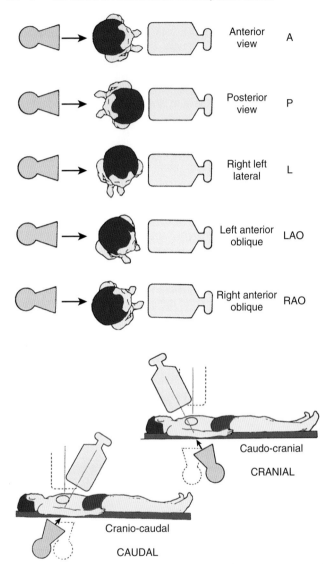

Figure 1.14 Nomenclature for angiographic views. (Modified from Paulin S. Terminology for radiographic projections in cardiac angiography. *Cathet Cardiovasc Diagn*. 1981;7:341.)

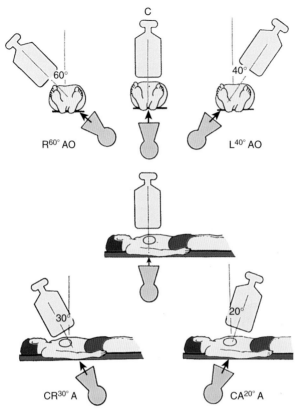

Figure 1.15 Nomenclature for Angiographic Views. (Modified from Paulin S. Terminology for radiographic projections in cardiac angiography. *Cathet Cardiovasc Diagn*. 1981;7:341.)

catheter shaft in the thoracic descending aorta. In patients with acute coronary syndromes, AP caudal or cranial is useful to identify left main stenosis. The AP cranial view is excellent for visualizing the LAD with septal perforating arteries moving to the left (on screen) and diagonal branches to the right, thus helping direct wire placement.

Right Anterior Oblique Imaging

The image intensifier is to the right side of the patient. The RAO caudal view shows the left main coronary artery bifurcation with the origin and course of the circumflex/obtuse marginals, intermediate or ramus branch, and proximal LAD segment well seen. The RAO, caudal view is one of the best two views for visualization of the circumflex artery. The LAD beyond the proximal segment is often obscured by overlapped diagonals.

The RAO or AP cranial view is used to open the diagonals along the mid and distal LAD. Diagonal branch bifurcations are well visualized. The diagonal branches are projected upward. The proximal LAD and circumflex usually are overlapped. Marginals may overlap, and the circumflex is foreshortened.

For the RCA, the RAO view shows the mid RCA and the length of the posterior descending artery and posterolateral branches. Septal perforators supplying an occluded LAD via collaterals may be clearly identified. The posterolateral branches overlap and may need the addition of the cranial view.

Left Anterior Oblique Imaging

In the LAO position, the image intensifier is to the left side of the patient. The LAO/cranial view also shows the left main coronary artery (slightly foreshortened), LAD, and diagonal branches. Septal and diagonal branches are separated clearly. The circumflex and marginals are foreshortened and overlapped. Deep inspiration will move the density of the diaphragm out of the field. The LAO angle should be set so that the course of the LAD is parallel to the spine and stays in the "lucent wedge" bordered by the spine and the curve of the diaphragm. Cranial angulation tilts the left main coronary artery down and permits a view of the LAD/circumflex bifurcation (Fig. 1.16). Too steep a LAO/cranial angulation or shallow inspiration produces considerable overlapping with the diaphragm and liver, thus degrading the image.

For the RCA, the LAO/cranial view shows the origin of the artery, its entire length, and the posterior descending artery bifurcation (crux). Cranial angulation tilts the posterior descending artery down to show vessel contour and reduces foreshortening. Deep inspiration clears the diaphragm. The posterior descending artery and posterolateral branches are foreshortened.

The LAO/caudal view ("spider" view) shows a foreshortened left main coronary artery and the bifurcation of the circumflex and LAD. Proximal and midportions of the circumflex and the origins of obtuse marginal branches are usually seen excellently. Poor image quality may be because of overlapping of diaphragm and spine. The LAD is considerably foreshortened in this view.

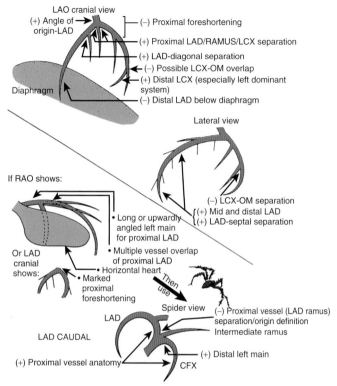

Figure 1.16 Diagrammatic view of left coronary artery demonstrating special positioning to best observe branch segments. (From Boucher RA, Myler RK, Clark DA, Stertzer SH. Coronary angiography and angioplasty. *Cathet Cardiovasc Diagn.* 1988;14:269–285.)

Angulations for Saphenous Bypass Grafts

Coronary artery saphenous vein grafts are visualized in at least two views (LAO and RAO). It is important to show the aortic anastomosis, the body of the graft, and the distal anastomosis. The distal runoff and continued flow or collateral channels are also critical. The graft vessel anastomosis is best seen in the view that depicts the native vessel best. A general strategy for graft angiography is to perform the standard views while assessing the vessel key views for specific coronary artery segments (Table 1.9) to determine the need for contingency views or an

Table 1.9

Recommended "Key" Angiographic View for Specific Coronary Artery Segments

Coronary Segment	Origin/Bifurcation	Course/Body
Left main	AP	AP
	LAO cranial	LAO cranial
	LAO caudal[a]	
Proximal LAD	LAO cranial	LAO cranial
	RAO caudal	RAO caudal
Mid LAD	LAD cranial	
	RAO cranial	
	Lateral	
Distal LAD	AP	
	RAO cranial	
	Lateral	
Diagonal	LAO cranial	RAO cranial, caudal, or straight
	RAO cranial	
Proximal circumflex	RAO caudal	LAO caudal
	LAO caudal	
Intermediate	RAO caudal	RAO caudal
	LAO caudal	Lateral
Obtuse marginal	RAO caudal	RAO caudal
	LAO caudal	
	RAO cranial	(distal marginals)
Proximal RCA	LAO	
	Lateral	
Mid RCA	LAO	LAO
	Lateral	Lateral
	RAO	RAO
Distal RCA	LAO cranial	LAO cranial
	Lateral	Lateral
PDA	LAO cranial	RAO
Posterolateral	LAO cranial	RAO cranial
	RAO cranial	RAO cranial

[a]Horizontal hearts
AP, Anteroposterior; *LAD,* left anterior descending artery; *LAO,* left anterior oblique; *PDA,* posterior descending artery (from RCA); *RAO,* right anterior oblique; *RCA,* right coronary artery.
(From Kern MJ, ed. *The Cardiac Catheterization Handbook.* Mosby, 1995:286.)

alteration/addition of special views. Therefore the graft views can be summarized as follows:

1. RCA graft: LAO cranial/RAO and lateral

2. LAD graft (or internal mammary artery): Lateral, RAO cranial, LAO cranial, and AP (the lateral view is especially useful to visualize the anastomosis to the LAD)

3. Circumflex (and obtuse marginals) grafts: LAO and RAO caudal

Angiographic Classification of Blood Flow: The TIMI Grade, Frame Count, and Blush Score

Thrombolysis in myocardial infarction (TIMI) flow grading has been used to qualitatively assess the degree of restored perfusion achieved after thrombolysis or angioplasty in patients with acute MI. Table 1.10 provides descriptions used to assign TIMI flow grades. The distal angiographic contrast runoff is classified into four stages (also known as *TIMI grade*):

- Normal distal runoff (TIMI 3)
- Good distal runoff (TIMI 2)
- Poor distal runoff (TIMI 1)
- Absence of distal runoff (TIMI 0)

TIMI flow grades 0 to 3 have become a standard description of coronary blood flow in clinical trials. TIMI grade 3 flows have been associated with improved clinical outcomes.

Table 1.10

Thrombolysis in Myocardial Infarction (TIMI) Flow	
TIMI Flow Grade	**Description**
Grade 3 (complete reperfusion)	Anterograde flow into the terminal coronary artery segment through a stenosis is as prompt as anterograde flow into a comparable segment proximal to the stenosis. Contrast material clears as rapidly from the distal segment as from an uninvolved, more proximal segment.
Grade 2 (partial reperfusion)	Contrast material flows through the stenosis to opacify the terminal artery segment, but contrast enters the terminal segment perceptibly more slowly than more proximal segments. Alternatively, contrast material clears from a segment distal to a stenosis noticeably more slowly than from a comparable segment not preceded by a significant stenosis.
Grade 1 (penetration/with minimal perfusion)	A small amount of contrast flows through the stenosis but fails to fully opacify the artery beyond.
Grade 0 (no perfusion)	There is no contrast flow through the stenosis.

Modified from Sheehan F, Braunwald E, Canner P, et al. The effect of intravenous thrombolytic therapy on left ventricular function: a report on tissue-type plasminogen activator and streptokinase from the Thrombolysis in Myocardial Infarction (TIMI) Phase I Trial. *Circulation.* 1987;72:817–829.

TIMI Frame Count

Myocardial blood flow can be quantitated by using cine frame counts from the first frame of the filled catheter tip to the frame where contrast is last seen filling a predetermined distal arterial end point; the rate is called the TIMI frame count.

Typically, a normal frame count reflecting normal flow is corrected for the length of the LAD, called the *corrected TFC (CTFC)*. The CTFC accounts for the distance the dye travels in the LAD relative to the other arteries. The CTFC divides the absolute frame count in the LAD by 1.7 to standardize the distance of dye travel in all three arteries. The LAD CTFC 21 ± 2; for the circumflex artery, TFC is 22 ± 4; for the RCA, TFC is 20 ± 3. High TFC may be associated with microvascular dysfunction despite an open artery. A CTFC of less than 20 frames was associated with low risk for adverse events in patients after MI. A contrast injection rate increase of more than 1 mL/sec by hand injection can decrease the TFC by two frames. TIMI flow grades do not correspond well to measured Doppler flow velocity or CTFC.

TIMI Myocardial Blush Grades

Washout of contrast from the microvasculature in the acute infarction patient is coupled to prognosis. Better blush scores indicate better myocardial salvage. Myocardial blush grade (MBG) scoring is shown in Table 1.11.

Angiographic Classification of Collateral Flow

Collateral flow can be seen and classified angiographically. The late opacification of a totally or subtotally (99%) occluded vessel

Table 1.11

Myocardial Blush Grade
Myocardial Blush Grade
0 No myocardial blush or contrast density; or myocardial blush persisted ("staining")
1 Minimal myocardial blush or contrast density
2 Moderate myocardial blush or contrast density but less than that obtained during angiography of a contralateral or ipsilateral noninfarct-related coronary artery
3 Normal myocardial blush or contrast density, comparable with that obtained during angiography of a contralateral or ipsilateral noninfarct-related coronary artery

through antegrade or retrograde channels will assist in correct guidewire placement, lesion localization, and a successful procedure. The collateral circulation is graded angiographically as follows:

- Grade 0: No collateral branches seen
- Grade 1: Very weak (ghostlike) opacification
- Grade 2: Opacified segment is less dense than the source vessel and filling slowly
- Grade 3: Opacified segment is as dense as the source vessel and filling rapidly

Collateral visualization will help establish the size of the recipient vessel for the purposes of selecting an appropriately sized balloon. Determining whether the collateral circulation is ipsilateral (e.g., proximal RCA to distal RCA collateral supply) or contralateral (e.g., circumflex to distal RCA collateral supply) and exactly which region will be affected should collateral supply be disrupted is important to gauge procedural risk. The evaluation of collaterals must be included when making decisions on which vessels should be addressed by CTO techniques.

Assessment of Coronary Stenoses

The degree of an angiographic narrowing (stenosis) is reported as the estimated percentage lumen reduction of the most severely narrowed segment compared with the adjacent angiographically normal vessel segment, seen in the single worst x-ray projection Table 1.12. Because the operator uses visual estimations, an exact evaluation is impossible. There is a plus or minus 20% variation between readings of two or more experienced angiographers. Stenosis severity alone should not always be assumed to be associated with abnormal physiology (flow) and ischemia. Moreover, CAD is a diffuse process and thus minimal luminal irregularities on angiography may represent significant, albeit nonobstructive, CAD at the time of angiography. The stenotic segment lumen is compared with a nearby lumen that does not appear to be obstructed but may have diffuse atherosclerotic disease. This explains why postmortem examinations and IVUS describe much more plaque than is seen on angiography. The percent diameter is estimated from the angiographically normal adjacent proximal segment. Because coronary arteries normally taper as they travel to the apex, proximal segments are always larger than distal segments, often explaining the large disparity between several observers' estimates of stenosis severity. *Area stenosis* is always greater than *diameter stenosis* and assumes the lumen is circular, whereas most of the time the lumen is eccentric. In general, four categories of lesion severity can be assigned:

1. Minimal or mild CAD; narrowings less than 50%
2. Moderate; stenosis between 50% and 75%
3. Severe; stenosis between 75% and 95%
4. Total occlusion

Technical note: Stenosis anatomy should not be confused with abnormal physiology (flow) and ischemia, especially for lesions 40% to 70% narrowed. For nonquantitative reports, the length of a stenosis is simply mentioned (e.g., LAD proximal segment stenosis diameter 25%, long or short). Other features of the coronary lesion may not be appreciated by angiography and may require IVUS imaging. Anatomic factors producing resistance to coronary flow across a coronary stenosis include entrance angle, length of disease, length of stenosis, minimal lumen diameter, minimal lumen area, eccentricity of lumen, area of reference vessel segment, and viscosity (Fig. 1.17).

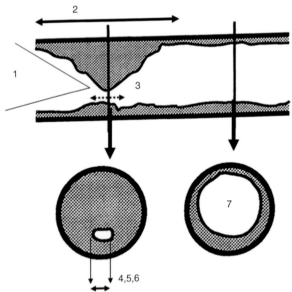

Figure 1.17 Factors of Stenosis Resistance. 1, Entrance angle; 2, disease length; 3, stenosis length; 4, 5, 6, shape and size of lumen; 7, area of normal reference vessel. These factors determine the hemodynamic significance of a lesion and explain the visual function mismatch between angiography and ischemic testing.

New Importance of Quantitative Coronary Angiography

In clinical practice, coronary stenosis severity is reported from a visual estimation of the angiographic percentage of diameter narrowing relative to the normal appearing proximal segment diameter. Although universally employed, visual estimate is crude with a plus or minus 20% variation among trained observers. The interobserver variability is highest for intermediate stenoses ranging from 40% to 80% diameter stenosis. Quantitative angiography uses an automated edge detection system and can reconstruct a vessel in three dimensions (3D) from two orthogonal views. Applying computational fluid dynamics to the 3D artery reconstruction will yield a virtual FFR to accompany a more precise stenosis quantitation. Quantitative coronary angiography (QCA) is frequently used for research studies that require a high level of reproducibility.

Terminology for Coronary Lesion Characterization and Vessel Morphology

Various and distinct characteristics of coronary lesions and vessels are associated with different clinical outcomes (Table 1.12). These characteristics help assess risk for adverse cardiac events during PCI. General characteristics of the artery proximal to the lesion dilated are as follows:

1. Tortuosity: None/mild, straight proximal segment or only one bend of at least 60 degrees; Moderate, two bends of at least 60 degrees proximal to the lesion; Severe, three or more bends of at least 60 degrees proximal to the lesion

2. Arterial calcification: Light, proximal artery wall calcification (not necessarily the lesion) seen as thin line(s); heavy, easily seen calcification.

    Angiographic characteristics of the PCI target lesion are as follows:

1. Arrangement of the lesion(s)

    a. Tandem: Two lesions located within one balloon length (i.e., both lesions can be covered during a single balloon inflation)

    b. Sequential: Two lesions located at a distance longer than the balloon

2. Length

    a. Discrete: 5 mm or more in length

    b. Tubular: 5 to 10 mm in length

    c. Diffuse: more than 10 mm in length

Table 1.12

Classifications of Lesion Severity

ACC/AHA Lesion-Specific Characteristics

Type A Low Risk	Type B Medium Risk	Type C High Risk
Discrete (<10 mm length)	Tubular (10–20 mm length)	Diffuse (length >2 cm)
Concentric	Eccentric	Excessive tortuosity of proximal segment
Readily accessible	Moderate tortuosity of proximal segment	Extremely angulated segments >90 degrees
Nonangulated segment <45 degrees	Moderately angulated segment, 45–90 degrees	Total occlusions >3 mos. old ± bridging collaterals
Smooth contour	Irregular contour	Inability to protect major side branches
Little or no calcification	Moderate to heavy calcification	Degenerated vein grafts with friable lesions
Less than totally occlusive	Ostial in location	
Not ostial in location	Bifurcation lesions requiring double guidewires	
No major branch involvement	Some thrombus present	
Absence of thrombus	Total occlusion less than 3 months old	
Procedure success rate: 92%	Procedure success rate: 76%	Procedure success rate: 61%
Complication rate: 2%	Complication rate: 10%	Complication rate: 21%

Note: If more than two medium risk factors are present, lesion is classified as Type B2 and is considered complex.
National Cardiovascular Disease Registry, Cath PCI Registry v4.3.1 Coder's Data Dictionary, 2008.

SCAI Lesion-Specific Characteristics

Type I	Type II	Type III	Type IV
Patent and does not meet criteria for ACC/AHA type C lesion	Patent and meets any criteria for type C lesion	Occluded and does not meet any criteria for type C lesion	Occluded and meets any criteria for type C lesion
Procedure success rate 98%	Procedure success rate 94%	Procedure success rate 91%	Procedure success rate 80%
Complication rate 2.4%	Complication rate 5.1%	Complication rate 9.8%	Complication rate 10.1%

Note: Major complications were the composite of in-hospital death, acute myocardial infarction, emergency angioplasty, or emergency coronary artery bypass surgery. Lesion success was defined as a more than 20% decrease in stenosis with a residual stenosis of less than 50%.
From Krone RJ, Shaw RE, Klein LW, et al. Evaluation of the American College of Cardiology/American Heart Association and the Society for Coronary Angiography and Interventions lesion classification system in the current stent era of coronary interventions (from the ACC-National Cardiovascular Data Registry). *Am J Cardiol.* 2003;92:389–394.

Table 1.12

Classifications of Lesion Severity (Continued)

Ellis Lesion-Specific Classification

Class I Low Risk	Class II Moderate Risk	Class III High Risk	Class IV Highest Risk
No risk factors	1 to 2 moderate correlates and the absence of strong correlates	3 or more moderate correlates and the absence of strong correlates	Either of the strongest correlates
Complication rate: 2.1%	Complication rate: 3.4%	Complication rate: 8.2%	Complication rate: 12.7%

Moderately strong correlates:
Length at least 10 mm
Lumen irregularity
Large filling defect
Calcium + angle at least 45 degrees
Eccentric
Severe calcification
SVG age at least 10 years old

Strongest correlates:
Nonchronic total occlusion
Degenerated SVG

Note: Complication defined as death, myocardial infarction, or emergent coronary artery bypass grafting.
ACC, American College of Cardiologists; *AHA*, American Heart association; *SCAI*, Society for Cardiac Angiography and Interventions; *SVG*, saphenous vein graft.
(From Ellis SG, Guetta S, Miller D, et al. Relation between lesion characteristics and risk with percutaneous intervention in the stent and glycoprotein IIb/IIIa era - an analysis of results from 10 907 lesions and proposal for new classification scheme. *Circulation.* 1999;100:1971–1976.)

3. Eccentricity: A concentric, central lumen axis is located along the long axis of the artery or on either side of it but by no more than 25% of the normal arterial diameter.

4. Ostial: Lesion is located at the aorto-ostial or bifurcation origin

5. Side branch: minor branch greater than 1.5 mm diameter

6. Contour: Smooth, irregular, or ulcerated

7. Thrombus:

   a. Definite is defined as an intraluminal, filling defect, visible in two views, a lucency surrounded on three sides by contrast media and/or documentation of embolization of this material.

   b. There are other possible filling defects not associated with calcification, lesion haziness, irregularity with ill-defined borders, or intraluminal staining at the total occlusion site.

8. Stenosis calcification: Calcification at the actual lesion site

9. Angulation:

   a. None/mild: Lesion located on a straight segment or a bend of less than 45 degrees.

   b. Moderate: 45- to 90-degree bend.

   c. Severe: Bend of greater than 90 degrees; angulation should be evaluated in end-diastolic frames.

Use of the SYNTAX Score to Select PCI or CABG

In 2009 the SYNTAX trial compared multivessel PCI (including patients with left main narrowings) cases with CABG cases. The angiograms of the patients were analyzed and given SYNTAX scores. The SYNTAX score is an angiographic grading tool to determine the complexity of CAD. The results of this randomized study demonstrated that patients who had high SYNTAX scores (>34) did better with CABG compared with PCI than did those with lower SYNTAX scores, in whom PCI had similar major adverse cardiac events with lower stroke rates.

The SYNTAX score is the sum of the points assigned to each individual lesion identified in the coronary tree with greater than 50% diameter narrowing in vessels of more than 1.5 mm diameter. The coronary tree is divided into 16 segments according to the AHA classification (Fig. 1.18). Each segment is given a score of 1 or 2 based on the presence of disease, and this score is then weighted, based on a chart, with values ranging from 3.5 for the proximal LAD to 5.0 for left main and 0.5 for smaller branches. Branches of less than 1.5 mm in diameter, despite having severe lesions, are not included in the SYNTAX score. The percent diameter stenosis is not a consideration in the SYNTAX score, only the presence of a stenosis of 50% to 99% diameter, less than 50% diameter narrowing, or total occlusion. A multiplication factor of 2 is used for nonocclusive lesions, and 5 is used for occlusive lesions, reflecting the difficulty of PCI.

Further characterization of the lesions adds points. For example, a total occlusion duration of more than 3 months, a blunt stump, a bridging collateral image, the first segment visible beyond the total occlusion, and a side branch of greater than 1.5 diameter all receive one point. For bifurcation lesions, one point is given for simple types; two points are given for complex types; and one point is given for an angulation of greater than 70 degrees. For trifurcations, one diseased segment gets three points, two diseased segments get four points, three diseased segments get five points, and four disease segments get six points.

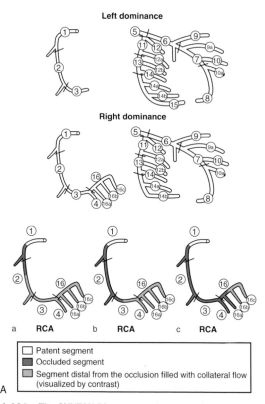

Figure 1.18A   The SYNTAX Diagram. Definition of the coronary tree segments: 1, Right coronary artery (RCA) proximal: From the ostium to one-half the distance to the acute margin of the heart. 2, RCA mid: From the end of first segment to acute margin of heart. 3, RCA distal: From the acute margin of the heart to the origin of the posterior descending artery. 4, Posterior descending artery: Running in the posterior interventricular groove. 16, Posterolateral branch from RCA: Posterolateral branch originating from the distal coronary artery distal to the crux. 16a, Posterolateral branch from RCA: First posterolateral branch from segment 16. 16b, Posterolateral branch from RCA: Second posterolateral branch from segment 16. 16c, Posterolateral branch from RCA: Third posterolateral branch from segment 16. 5, Left main: From the ostium of the left coronary artery (LCA) through bifurcation into the left anterior descending (LAD) and left circumflex (LCX) branches. 6, LAD proximal: Proximal to and including first major septal branch. 7, LAD mid: LAD immediately distal to origin of first septal branch and extending to the point where LAD forms an angle (right anterior oblique [RAO] view). If this angle is not identifiable, this segment ends at one-half the distance from the
Continued

first septal to the apex of the heart. 8, LAD apical: Terminal portion of LAD, beginning at the end of the previous segment and extending to or beyond the apex. 9, First diagonal: The first diagonal originating from segment 6 or 7. 9a, First diagonal a: Additional first diagonal originating from segment 6 or 7, before segment 8;.10, Second diagonal: Originating from segment 8 or the transition between segment 7 and 8. 10a, Second diagonal a: Additional second diagonal originating from segment 8. 11, Proximal circumflex artery: Main stem of circumflex from its origin of left main and including origin of first obtuse marginal branch. 12, Intermediate/anterolateral artery: Branch from trifurcating left main other than proximal LAD or LCX. It belongs to the circumflex territory. 12a, Obtuse marginal a: First side branch of circumflex running in general to the area of obtuse margin of the heart. 12b, Obtuse marginal b: Second additional branch of circumflex running in the same direction as 12; 13, Distal circumflex artery: The stem of the circumflex distal to the origin of the most distal obtuse marginal branch, and running along the posterior left atrioventricular groove. Caliber may be small or artery absent; 14, Left posterolateral: Running to the posterolateral surface of the left ventricle. May be absent or a division of obtuse marginal branch; 14a, Left posterolateral a: Distal from 14 and running in the same direction; 14b, Left posterolateral b: Distal from 14 and 14a and running in the same direction; 15, Posterior descending: Most distal part of dominant left circumflex when present. It gives origin to septal branches. When this artery is present, segment 4 is usually absent. (From Sianos G, Morel M, Kappetein Ap, et al. The SYNTAX Score: An angiographic tool grading the complexity of CAD. *Eurointerv.* 2005;1:219–227.)

Additionally, an aorto-ostial lesion is worth one point, severe tortuosity of vessel is worth two points, lesion length greater than 20 mm is worth one point, heavy calcification is worth two points, thrombus is worth one point, and diffuse disease or small-vessel disease is worth one point per segment involvement. Multiple lesions that are less than three reference vessel diameters apart are scored as a single lesion, but tandem lesions at a distance of more than three vessel diameters are considered separate lesions. Segments in which bifurcations are evaluated are those involving the proximal LAD and left main, the mid LAD, the proximal circumflex, the midcircumflex, and the crux of the RCA. The SYNTAX score algorithm then sums each of these features for a total SYNTAX score. Table 1.13 summarizes the SYNTAX grade categories. A computer algorithm is then queried, and a summed value is produced.

Low SYNTAX scores are less than 22, intermediate SYNTAX scores range from 23 to 32, and high SYNTAX scores are greater than 33. High scores are associated with increasing cardiac mortality, major adverse cardiac events, and a specific, predefined combination

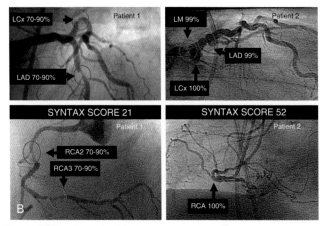

Figure 1.18B Example of SYNTAX score and specific angiographic anatomy.

Table 1.13

The SYNTAX Score Algorithm

1. Dominance
2. Number of lesions
3. Segments involved per lesion, with lesion characteristics
4. Total occlusions with subtotal occlusions:
   a. Number of segments
   b. Age of total occlusions
   c. Blunt stumps
   d. Bridging collaterals
   e. First segment beyond occlusion visible by antegrade or retrograde filling
   f. Side branch involvement
5. Trifurcation, number of segments diseased
6. Bifurcation type and angulation
7. Aorto-ostial lesion
8. Severe tortuosity
9. Lesion length
10. Heavy calcification
11. Thrombus
12. Diffuse disease, with number of segments

of end points. When comparing all clinical and angiographic factors, it was evident that the SYNTAX score, in addition to age, gender, smoking, diabetes, and acute coronary syndromes, is one of the highest predictors of cardiac mortality and major adverse cardiac events in patients undergoing multivessel and, specifically, unprotected left main PCI. A SYNTAX score greater than 34 also identifies a subgroup with a particularly high risk for cardiac death independent of age, gender, acute coronary syndrome, ejection fraction, Euro score, and degree of revascularization.

Examples of the types of SYNTAX scores are provided in figures from the original paper (Fig. 1.19). The SYNTAX scores can be

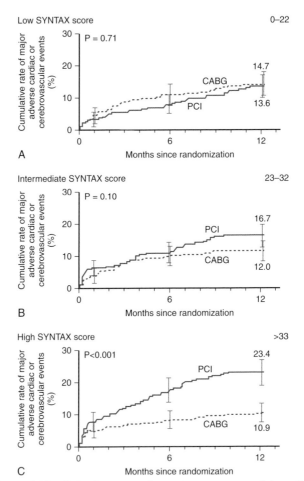

Figure 1.19 **(A–C)**, Outcomes of percutaneous coronary intervention (PCI) versus coronary artery bypass graft (CABG) by SYNTAX scores. (Data from Serruys PW, Morice M-C, Kappetein AP, et al. Percutaneous coronary intervention versus coronary artery bypass grafting for severe coronary artery disease. The SYNTAX Trial. *N Engl J Med*. 2009:360[10]:961–972.)

divided into three tertiles. The high scores indicate complex conditions and represent the greatest risks to patients undergoing PCI. High scores have the worst prognosis for revascularization with PCI compared with CABG. Equivalent or superior outcomes for percutaneous intervention were noted in comparison to CABG surgery for patients in the lowest two tertiles.

A discussion of the most challenging angiographic scenarios, including aorto-ostial lesions, bifurcations, and anomalous coronary arteries is provided in Chapter 3 of *Kern's Cardiac Catheterization Handbook*, 7e. PCI for lesions in these arteries can be performed in a routine fashion once difficulty of achieving a stable guide catheter position is overcome.

Radiographic Contrast Media for PCI

The most common contrast media for PCI involves nonionic or low-osmolar contrast agents because of safety, patient tolerance, and cost. Selection of a nonionic or low-osmolar contrast agent for the interventional procedure is, to a large extent, a matter of personal preference.

Radiation Exposure During PCI

Because more time is involved in positioning intravascular equipment and assessing the result of the intervention, x-ray exposure is higher than diagnostic studies. Operator exposure for PCI is nearly double what it is for routine diagnostic coronary angiography. This increase is largely because of longer fluoroscopy times without correspondingly longer cineradiography time. Device-specific procedure times may be longer than routine stent placement (Table 1.14).

Working in an angled projection for PCI also increases x-ray exposure (Fig. 1.20). LAO views produce 2.6 to 6.1 times the dose of radiation for the operator of equivalently angled RAO views (Table 1.15). Steeper LAO views also increased operator dose. An LAO of 90 degrees produces eight times the dose of an LAO of 60 degrees and three times the dose of an LAO of 30 degrees. Fluoroscopy produced more radiation than cine during angioplasty, by a factor of 6 to 1. Reducing the steepness of angulation reduces operator radiation dosage.

Pacemakers During PCI

The routine use of pacemakers for PCI is not required. Cardiac pacemakers may be used prophylactically during PCI to reduce

Table 1.14

Estimated Radiation Entrance Exposure of Patients Using Phantom Model Data

Procedure	Fluoroscopy (R)	Cine (R)
Isolated balloon angioplasty	43	25
Isolated directional coronary atherectomy	32	23
Directional coronary atherectomy + balloon angioplasty	66	29
Isolated laser coronary angioplasty	45	18
Laser coronary angioplasty + balloon angioplasty	57	27
Elective stenting	52	27
Emergency stenting	96	41

(From Federman J, Bell MR, Wondrow MA, et al. Does the use of new intracoronary interventional devices prolong radiation exposure in the cardiac catheterization laboratory? *J Am Coll Cardiol.* 1994;23:347–357.)

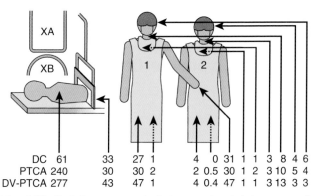

DC	61	33	27	1	4	0	31	1	1	3	8	4	6
PTCA	240	30	30	2	2	0.5	30	1	2	3	10	5	4
DV-PTCA	277	43	47	1	4	0.4	47	1	1	3	13	3	3

Figure 1.20   Radiation exposure rates for two operators during coronary angioplasty. *DC,* Diagnostic catheterization; *DV-PTCA,* double-vessel percutaneous transluminal coronary angioplasty; *XA,* x-ray amplifier in plane A; *XB,* x-ray amplifier in plane B. (Modified from Finci L, Meier B, Steffenino G, et al. Radiation exposure during diagnostic catheterization and single- and double-vessel percutaneous transluminal coronary angioplasty. *Am J Cardiol.* 1987;60:1401–1403.)

the hemodynamic compromise of heart block and are needed to rescue patients after the development of conduction abnormalities associated with hypotension. External pacing patches are useful for emergency pacing when a temporary pacing wire cannot be immediately positioned. When using pacing patches, the patient must be sedated because each electrical stimulation causes contraction of chest muscles and the heart muscle and may be painful.

Table 1.15

Radiation Dose and Angulation	
View	**Dose (Relative Increase)**
Image intensifier position	
RAO 30–60 degrees	1
LAO 30–60 degrees	2.6–6.1
Increasing angulation	
LAO 30 degrees	1
LAO 60 degrees	3
LAO 90 degrees	9

LAO, Left anterior oblique; *RAO,* right anterior oblique.

Indications for Pacemaker During PCI

1. Previously demonstrated high-degree conduction block
2. Symptomatic bradycardia (after contrast or angiography of RCA)
3. Acute MI with trifascicular block
4. Prophylactic use for rotational atherectomy and thrombectomy procedures, especially involving the RCA
5. Transluminal alcohol septal artery ablation in hypertrophic obstructive cardiomyopathy (HOCM) patients.

Atropine may be used to prevent bradycardia, but a pacemaker should always be on standby in the lab.

Venous access for a temporary transvenous pacemaker can use the internal jugular, subclavian, brachial, or femoral vein. The easiest access is usually the vein close to the arterial entry site. A 5F balloon-tipped pacing catheter is preferred because there is a reduced chance of perforation of the thin free wall or apex of the right ventricle when the balloon is inflated.

Cutaneous patch pacemakers are also effective until secured venous pacing routes can be established. Muscle contractions induced by the cutaneous pacing patches are uncomfortable, so the patient should be well sedated.

Competency Requirements for Interventional Cardiologists

Interventional cardiology, a subspecialty of adult cardiology, requires a minimum 1-year interventional cardiology fellowship in addition to the specialized training required for cardiology. Interventional cardiology requires multiple skills including the cognitive and procedural competencies enumerated in detail in the ACCF/ AHA/SCAI 2013 Clinical Competence Statement (see Suggested Readings). This document should be required reading for every cardiac interventionalist.

Key References

Lofti A, Davies JE, Fearon WF, et al. Focused update of expert consensus statement: use of invasive assessments of coronary physiology and structure: a position statement of the society of cardiac angiography and interventions. *Catheter Cardiovasc Interv*. 2018;92:336-347. https://doi.org/10.1002/ccd.27672.

Naidu SS, Abbott JD, Bahai J, et al. SCAI expert consensus update on best practices in the cardiac catheterization laboratory. *Catheter Cardiovasc Interv*. 2021;98: 255-276. https://doi.org/10.1002/ccd.29744.

Neumann FJ, Sousa-Uva M, Ahlsson A, et al. 2018 ESC/EACTS Guidelines on myocardial revascularization. *Eur Heart J*. January 07, 2019;40(2):87-165. https://doi.org/10.1093/eurheartj/ehy394.

Patel MR, Calhoon JH, Dehmer GJ, et al. ACC/AATS/AHA/ASE/ASNC/SCAI/SCCT/STS 2017 appropriate use criteria for coronary revascularization in patients with stable ischemic heart disease: a report of the American College of Cardiology Appropriate Use Criteria Task Force, American Association for Thoracic Surgery, American Heart Association, American Society of Echocardiography, American Society of Nuclear Cardiology, Society for Cardiovascular Angiography and Interventions, Society of Cardiovascular Computed Tomography, and Society of Thoracic Surgeons. *J Am Coll Cardiol*. 2017;69:2212-2241.

Shroff AR, Gulati R, Drachman DE, et al. SCAI expert consensus statement update on best practices for transradial angiography and intervention. *Catheter Cardiovasc Interv*. 2020;95:245-252. https://doi.org/10.1002/ccd.28672.

References

Al-Hijji MA, Lennon RJ, Gulati R, et al. Safety and risk of major complications with diagnostic cardiac catheterization. *Circ Cardiovasc Interv*. 2019;12:e007791.

Blankenship JC, Gigliotti OS, Feldman DN, et al. Ad hoc percutaneous coronary intervention: a consensus statement from the Society for Cardiovascular Angiography and Interventions. *Catheter Cardiovasc Interv*. 2013;81:748-758.

Byrne RA, Joner M, Kastrati A. Stent thrombosis and restenosis: what have we learned and where are we going? The Andreas Grüntzig Lecture ESC 2014. *Eur Heart J*. 2015;36(47):3320-3331. doi:10.1093/eurheartj/ehv511.

Dehmer GJ, Blankenship JC, Cilingiroglu M, et al. SCAI/ACC/AHA expert consensus document: 2014 update on percutaneous coronary intervention without on-site surgical backup. *J Am Coll Cardiol*. 2014;63:2624-2641.

Harold JG, Bass TA, Bashore TM, et al. ACCF/AHA/SCAI 2013 Update of the Clinical Competence Statement on Coronary Artery Interventional Procedures: a Report of the American College of Cardiology Foundation/American Heart Association/ American College of Physicians Task Force on Clinical Competence and Training (Writing Committee to Revise the 2007 Clinical Competence Statement on Cardiac Interventional Procedures). *J Am Coll Cardiol*. 2013;62:357-396.

Layland J, Oldroyd KG, Curzen N, et al. Fractional flow reserve vs. angiography in guiding management to optimize outcomes in non-ST-segment elevation myocardial infarction: the British Heart Foundation FAMOUS-NSTEMI randomized trial. *Eur Heart J*. 2015;36:100-111.

Moscucci M. *Baim's Cardiac Catheterization*, Angiography, and Intervention. 9th ed. Philadelphia: Wolters/Kluwer/Lippincott Williams; 2021.

Nishimura RA, Otto CM, Bonow RO, et al. 2014 AHA/ACC guideline for the management of patients with valvular heart disease: a report of the American College of Cardiology/American Heart Association Task Force on Practice Guidelines. *J Thorac Cardiovasc Surg*. 2014;148:e1-e132.

Rao SV, Tremmel JA, Gilchrist IC, et al. Best practices for transradial angiography and intervention: a consensus statement from the Society for Cardiovascular Angiography and Intervention's Transradial Working Group. *Catheter Cardiovasc Interv*. 2014;83:228-236.

Sorajja P, Lim MJ, Kern MJ, eds. *Kern's Cardiac Catheterization Handbook*. 7th ed. Philedelphia: Elsevier; 2019.

Van Nunen LX, Zimmermann FM, Tonino PA, et al. Fractional flow reserve versus angiography for guidance of PCI in patients with multivessel coronary artery disease (FAME): 5-year follow-up of a randomised controlled trial. *Lancet*. 2015;386: 1853-1860.

Vascular Access

MICHAEL J. LIM

KEY POINTS

- A significant source of complications from catheterization procedures continues to arise from the site of access.

- Ultrasound-guided access is the preferred method regardless of access site.

- There are several options for the best site of access, including the distal radial, radial, and femoral artery.

- Operators should adopt a consistent approach to vascular access to gain efficiency and minimize complications.

Vascular access techniques for interventional procedures are the same as those used for diagnostic catheterization but require greater precision because of the increased risk for bleeding with most interventions and their associated anticoagulation regimens. For both diagnostic and interventional procedures, vascular access is the most frequent cause of procedural morbidity. The site and size of the access and sheath are determined by the anatomic and clinicopathologic conditions (e.g., peripheral vascular disease) and the anticipated interventional techniques required.

To avoid known pitfalls and complications, operators should review previous procedure notes and any difficulties encountered during prior procedures. At the minimum, assessment of all arterial pulses before and after the procedure is mandatory. The use of ultrasound to guide all access is now routine and all cath lab personnel should be very familiar with ultrasound imaging of the vasculature. For procedures requiring "large-bore" access (≥10 F), additional imaging from preprocedure computed tomography (CT) scans has also become essential in the planning phase.

Percutaneous Radial and Femoral Artery Access

Although the femoral artery approach had been standard for decades, the radial approach has become the new standard for both the diagnostic and interventional coronary procedures in many labs. This is largely attributable to the fact that compared to the femoral approach, the radial approach has significantly fewer access-related complications and, in most comparative studies, better late outcomes, including bleeding and mortality. Conditions in which radial artery access should be favored are listed in Table 2.1.

Radial Artery Access for Percutaneous Coronary Intervention

In 1996, to reduce bleeding complications associated with early stent procedures, Kiemeneij of the Netherlands pioneered the radial approach for coronary interventions, increasing the success rate, improving patient comfort, and providing a method for excellent hemostasis in fully anticoagulated patient. Rates of major bleeding are significantly lower for transradial procedures, even in populations at high risk for arterial access complications, such as women and the elderly. Data from patients of all ages suggest that reduced bleeding may translate into reduced rates of death and ischemic events. In addition, patient comfort and satisfaction are enhanced by the transradial procedure because patients can sit up immediately and ambulate as soon as their sedation has worn off.

Table 2.1

Conditions in Which Radial Artery Access Should Be Favored
1. Claudication
2. Absent leg pulses
3. Femoral bruits
4. Prior femoral artery graft surgery
5. Extensive inguinal scarring from previous procedures
6. Surgery or radiation treatment near inguinal area
7. Excessively tortuous iliac system and lower abdominal aorta
8. Abdominal aortic aneurysm
9. Severe back pain or inability to lie flat
10. Downward origin of renal arteries (for renal artery stenting)
11. Patient request

Patient Selection for Transradial Intervention

Transradial intervention (TRI) presents an important first-line option for many patients undergoing coronary intervention. Proper patient selection remains central to achieving optimal outcomes. In general, TRI is *avoided* in patients in whom:

1. The radial artery is being considered for use in coronary artery bypass graft (CABG) surgery or in whom hemodialysis via arteriovenous fistula (AVF) may be necessary and in patients with an existing AVF.

2. There is known upper extremity vascular disease (severe atherosclerosis, active carotid disease, extreme tortuosity), vascular anomalies, or vasospastic disorders (Raynaud disease, Buerger disease, or systemic sclerosis).

3. The procedure will likely require guide catheters of 7F or larger (unless a sheathless guide is to be used).

Prior CABG is not a contraindication to the radial approach because right or left internal mammary artery graft conduits may be approached from the ipsilateral or even contralateral wrist. Although one small randomized study suggested that CABG patients require more time and guide catheters from the radial approach, most TRI for CABG patients can be successfully performed from the left radial artery with sufficient experience.

Transradial catheterization for ST-elevation acute myocardial infarction (STEMI) can be performed without significant delays in door-to-balloon time and without increasing procedure duration, radiation exposure, or contrast if used in experienced labs by experienced operators. STEMI patients have demonstrated a reduction in mortality with transradial access, likely because of an ability to apply the maximal antithrombotic regimen necessary with less concern for bleeding.

TRI is an especially good option for patients on systemic anticoagulation with elevated international normalized ratio (INR), especially those with mechanical heart valves. The ability to perform angiography without interrupting or bridging anticoagulation is a major logistical advantage. For patients with suspicion of descending aortic dissection or peripheral vascular disease (which preferentially affects the lower extremities), TRI overcomes these potential barriers. In all cases, TRI patient selection should balance the risks and benefits of radial versus femoral access.

Radial Access Technique

Operators should familiarize themselves with the relevant anatomy of the arm and wrist (Fig. 2.1) to avoid cannulation of the radial

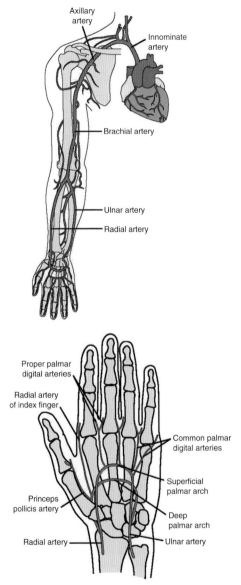

Figure 2.1 Vascular Anatomy of the Arm. *Top:* Brachial, radial, and ulnar arteries and their connections. *Bottom:* Radial and ulnar arteries as they join the palmar arch. Note that the thumb has its own arterial supply.

artery too distally and appreciate anatomic variants that may make moving through the radial artery to ascending aorta challenging.

Use of the Allen Test

Although demonstration of contralateral flow through the ulnopalmar arch was commonly recommended before performing radial catheterization, more recent data have demonstrated the lack of utility in this assessment. The RADAR study showed that in the 30% of patients with an abnormal Allen test there were no clinical or subclinical signs of hand ischemia after the procedure. If testing of the palmar arch patency is to be performed, it can be done by the Allen test (Fig. 2.2) or by the Barbeau test (Fig. 2.3).

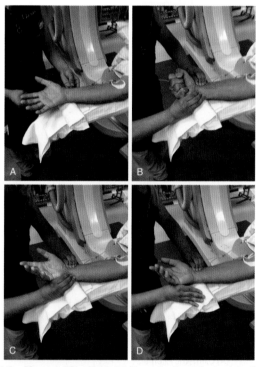

Figure 2.2 **Manual Allen Test.** (A) Normally, the palm is pink. (B) A fist is made and the radial and ulnar arteries are compressed. (C) The hand is opened and blanches after compression of both ulnar and radial artery. (D) The palm is pink after release of ulnar artery with radial artery occluded.

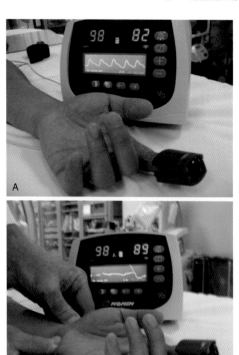

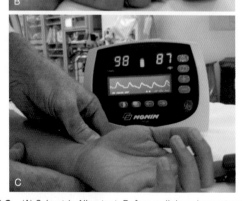

Figure 2.3 (A) Oximetric Allen test. Before radial or ulnar artery compression, pulse oximeter waveform is normal. (B) Waveform is flat when both radial and ulnar arteries are compressed. (C) Pulse waveform is normal when only ulnar is released. Radial artery is still compressed. This is a type A response. Type B is blunted waveform, and type C is a flattened wave.

Room and Patient Setup

Transradial coronary angiography can be performed from either the right or left arm. In general, the right arm is more convenient because most catheterization labs are set up with the operator on the right side of the patient and the video screens on the left. Use of the right arm obviates the need to reach over the patient. Recent comparisons have suggested that left radial access and catheter manipulation more closely approximates that of femoral angiography and may take less time and use less contrast than the right radial approach. During catheterization via the left radial artery, the left arm should be comfortably adducted over the patient's belly toward the operator (standing on the right side) after access has been obtained.

For either the right or left radial approach, correct positioning and preparation of the patient's arm are important steps for successful arterial access (Fig. 2.4). Preparation and placement of the arm and hand are the same as for the diagnostic procedure. Some operators may employ additional radiation-protective drapes. An optional short (elbow to hand) cushioned arm board typically used for arterial pressure lines can also help secure the wrist in an optimal position. An innovative way to keep the patient's hand both sterile and free of blood during the procedure is to place a sterile glove on the patient's hand before the top drape (Fig. 2.5).

Whether the groin should also be prepped for a transradial case depends on the comfort and experience of the operator and lab and the type of intervention needed. Access-site crossover rates range from 5% to 10% in most studies. For elective cases, converting to the contralateral radial site is preferable to femoral access.

Ultrasound Imaging for Radial Artery Access

Ultrasound-guided access has been shown to improve the first-pass success rate, decreasing the total number of attempts and reducing time to access. Ultrasound can also help rescue a failed access by manual palpation, reducing the need for crossover to another access site. Nevertheless, clinical events such as spasm and bleeding are not changed with ultrasound.

Some operators would prefer to use ultrasound guidance up front, whereas others may only turn to it when initial palpation attempts have failed. Absent any benefit in clinical outcomes, either approach is reasonable, although not necessarily as efficient. Nevertheless, the transradial operator should become comfortable with the technique because failure of palpation guidance can be avoided.

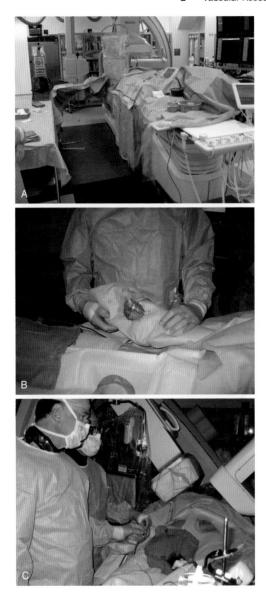

Figure 2.4 (A) Right arm is positioned extended on arm board. (B) After radial sheath insertion, the arm is moved to the patient's hip for introduction of catheters and (C) performance of angiography and intervention.

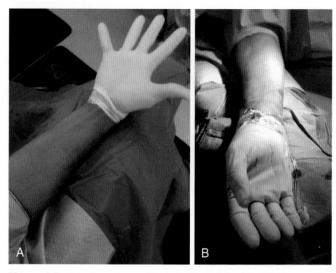

Figure 2.5 An alternative method for draping the hand is to cover the hand with a sterile glove. (A) Arm is prepared with betadine and put through a drape with elastic hole. The glove is then put on the hand. (B) Radial access with sheath in artery and Tegaderm dressing securing the sheath to the skin and part of the glove.

The following characteristics should lead the operator to consider up front or very early use of ultrasound guidance:

1. Significant hypotension (e.g., shock)
2. Weak pulses (hypotension, peripheral vascular disease [PVD], or obesity)
3. Prior transradial catheterization to rule out radial occlusion
4. Patients at risk for spasm or transradial failure (women, PVD, prior coronary bypass patients)
5. STEMI

The size of the radial artery can be assessed with ultrasound before the procedure, which may affect the likelihood of spasm or radial artery occlusion. A very small artery might suggest that smaller sheath sizes, sheathless approaches, or alternative access sites (i.e., ulnar) may be helpful. Preprocedure ultrasound screening may also detect calcified radial arteries (Fig. 2.6), dual radial artery systems (Fig. 2.7), and radial artery loops (Fig. 2.8) in up to 10% of patients, which can make the transradial procedure difficult or unfeasible.

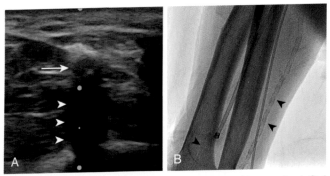

Figure 2.6 Calcified Radial Artery. (A) Ultrasound image of calcified ulnar artery. Note the prominent posterior shadowing (*white arrowheads*) below the artery (*arrow*). (B) Fluoroscopy demonstrating extensive calcification of ulnar artery (*black arrowheads*) and, to a lesser extent, the radial artery. Ultrasound located a segment of radial artery that was less calcified and successfully cannulated.

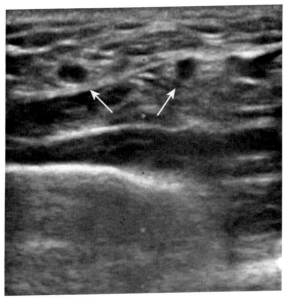

Figure 2.7 Dual radial systems or high radial bifurcations (*arrows*) are evident on ultrasound, where one branch may be small or have a radial loop that can make navigation difficult.

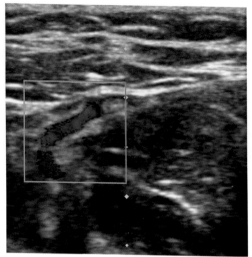

Figure 2.8 **Radial Artery Loop.** Preprocedure Doppler ultrasound in axial plane.

Duplex ultrasonography is the gold standard for detection of radial artery occlusion and may be useful for confirming patent hemostasis. Other complications such as dissections and pseudoaneurysms (Fig. 2.9) are easily detected with ultrasound.

Stepwise Approach to Ultrasound-Guided Radial Access

Table 2.2 lists tips for successful radial access. There are 2 methods of artery entry: 1) anterior wall punction only and 2) through and through both walls (see below); Both techniques begin with the following steps.

Step 1: Prepare the ultrasound probe with a sterile cover. Place sterile gel inside and on the front of the covered probe. The image display settings should be set at a minimum of depth penetration (i.e., 2 cm) and high gain. Turn on the centerline guide markers (see ultrasound setup for femoral access).

Step 2: Image the radial artery in the axial plane by holding the ultrasound probe perpendicular to the course of the artery (Fig. 2.10). The artery will be an echolucent circle that pulsates on gentle compression.

Step 3: Align the artery with the centerline guide on the display by moving the probe. This ensures that the artery is directly beneath the center of the probe.

Step 4: Inject lidocaine above the radial artery with a small (25-gauge) needle.

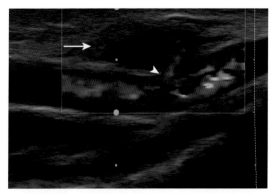

Figure 2.9 Radial pseudoaneurysm (*arrow*) after transradial catheterization. Color Doppler shows the pseudoaneurysm neck with active flow (*arrowhead*).

Table 2.2

Key Points for Radial Access

1. The ideal puncture site is greater than 2 cm proximal to the radial styloid, the bony prominence of the distal radius (Fig. 2.11).
2. Mid-forearm punctures are more difficult to compress and can result in hematoma formation but may be necessary if the distal vessel is too small or obstructed.
3. The double-wall technique is very effective with the two-component needle (Fig. 2.12). Be sure to advance needle and its cannula beyond the back wall before removing the needle.
4. There should be no resistance to wire advancement. If resistance is encountered, fluoroscopy should be used to immediately visualize the wire. Fig. 2.13 shows the steps for radial sheath insertion.
5. Use only the included metal guidewires with metal needles because hydrophilic wires can be shredded if they are pulled back against the bevel.
6. A small skin incision facilitates sheath introduction.
7. Hydrophilic-coated sheaths can reduce radial artery spasm and pain upon sheath withdrawal.
8. A large Tegaderm with a slit cut into it can be placed over the sheath to secure the system without the need for sutures and to provide ready access for catheters and guidewires.
9. A radial arterial loop does not necessarily preclude a transradial approach because passage of a 0.014-inch hydrophilic coronary wire can sometimes straighten out tortuous loops, allowing for smooth advancement of catheters.
10. If 7F or larger guide catheters are needed, consider using the slender guides or sheathless guide insertions. Most coronary interventions are possible through 6F guide catheters, including 1.5-mm Rotablator burrs and bifurcation stenting techniques using rapid exchange systems.

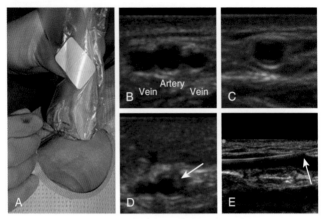

Figure 2.10 Technique of Ultrasound-Guided Radial Access. (A) Ultrasound transducer, sterilely wrapped and placed over the radial artery for needle puncture guidance. (B) Visualization of radial artery and veins. (C) Compression causes closure of radial veins and reveals the pulsatility of the artery. (D) Visualization of the needle tip (*arrow*) compressing and puncturing the artery. (E) Confirmation of wire position (*arrow*) in the radial artery in longitudinal plane.

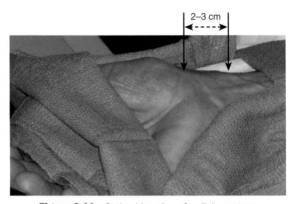

Figure 2.11 Optimal location of radial puncture.

Step 5: Insert the access needle into the skin directly underneath the center marking of the probe at about a 45-degree angle. Keep or move the probe close to the needle after skin puncture.

Step 6: Use short "strokes" (short in-and-out movements of the needle) to track the approximate course of the needle.

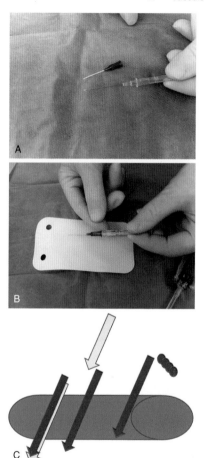

Figure 2.12 (A,B) Radial two-component needle. (C) "Through-and-through" technique for radial puncture. (Reprinted from Nguyen TN, Hu D, Chen SL, et al. *Practical Handbook of Advanced Interventional Cardiology*. 3rd ed. Blackwell; 2008.)

Adjust the probe position or angulation if the tip of the needle is not seen. Adjust the needle angle or puncture location if needed to have the needle move toward the artery. Eventually, you should see the needle compress and puncture the artery wall.

Step 7: The ultrasound can be used to follow the guidewire up the arm to confirm appropriate intravascular placement.

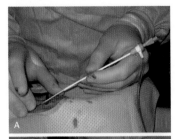

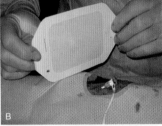

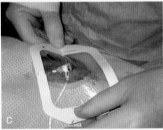

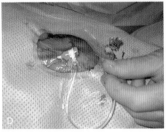

Figure 2.13 Radial Artery Access and Sheath Introduction. Once draped, the radial pulse is palpated. The point of puncture should be 1 to 2 cm cranial to the bony prominence of the distal radius. Administer a small amount of lidocaine into the skin. Use the micropuncture needle at 30- to 45-degree angulation; slowly advance until blood pulsates out of needle. It will not be a strong pulsation because of the small bore of the needle. Fix needle position and carefully introduce 0.018-inch guidewire with twirling motion. There should be little or no resistance to wire introduction. Remove needle. Make a small incision over the wire to prepare for introducing the sheath. Advance sheath over wire into artery (A). If sheath moves easily, advance to hub. If resistance is felt with sheath halfway in artery, remove wire, and administer vasodilator cocktail. Reinsert wire and continue to advance sheath. Secure sheath with clear plastic dressing or suture (B,C). After sheath is positioned and flushed (D), the arm can now be moved to patient's side for catheter introduction.

Through-and-Through Technique

Some operators choose to use an angiocath (or short micropuncture needle) and advance into the anterior wall (blood will fill the proximal hub) and then further advance to puncture the posterior wall. At this point, the needle is removed from the angiocath and the catheter is then slowly withdrawn until pulsatile blood flow is seen. A 0.021-inch guidewire can then be advanced, the angiocath can be removed, and the access sheath can be advanced over the guidewire.

The through-and-through technique is has a similar incidence of hematoma and 30-day radial artery patency compared with the anterior wall approach but with faster access times with a lower number of attempts to gain successful access.

Hemostasis After Sheath Removal

Hemostasis after radial artery catheterization is achieved easily given that the radius bone lies just beneath the artery and provides a firm surface for compression. Manual compression can certainly be used, but, more commonly, dedicated radial bands have been developed by multiple manufactures to provide hemostatic compression of the site. Using a dedicated band, the following steps are followed to achieve hemostasis and prevent future radial artery occlusion:

1. Apply the band on the wrist centered on the access site.
2. Increase pressure in the band while removing the sheath from the artery; increase the pressure in the band to achieve complete hemostasis.
3. Gradually decrease the pressure in the band until a small amount of blood is seen at the access site and then increase the pressure just enough to eliminate this bleeding.
4. Assess the presence of antegrade flow from the radial artery by artery or using a "reverse Barbeau" procedure. If antegrade flow cannot be detected, attempts should be made to decrease the pressure in the band over the first 10 to 15 minutes to allow hemostasis with objective antegrade flow. (i.e. patent hemostasis, see below).

Radial Artery Hemostasis and Postprocedure Care

Radial hemostasis is achieved by applying radial artery compression devices (multiple varieties commercially available). The inflatable Terumo TR Band is popular for its ease of use and the ability to directly visualize the puncture site. Regardless of the device chosen, there are several important steps to promote radial artery patency after hemostasis.

Given the superficial position and easy compressibility of the radial artery, checking an activated clotting time is not necessary before sheath removal. Another dose of antispasmotic agent may minimize radial artery spasm and patient discomfort. After applying the compression band, the sheath should be removed slowly and smoothly while slowly tightening the band. Tightening the band too aggressively before the sheath is completely removed increases patient discomfort and may strip any clot in the sheath into the artery.

When using a band, the sheath should be pulled out several centimeters (Fig. 2.14) so that the band does not cover the valve

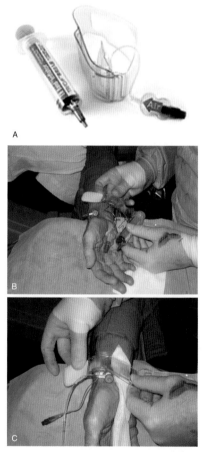

Figure 2.14 (A) Terumo band with inflatable compression pad. (B) Band applied around wrist with green dot over puncture. (C) A thin gauze wick is placed beneath band to absorb blood when pressure is released to assess proper compression pressure in pad.

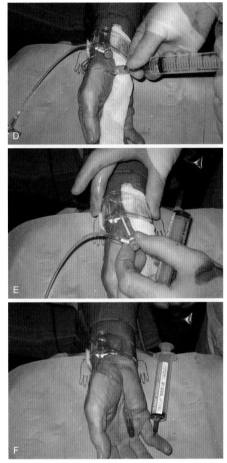

Figure 2.14, cont'd   (D) Compression pad inflated. (E) Sheath removed.
(F) Final result.

portion of the sheath. After applying the band, inflate with 15 to
17 mL of air and pull the sheath out at the same time. Next, the
band is slowly deflated until bleeding occurs, at which point 1 to
2 mL of air should be reinserted into the band. This technique,
known as "patent hemostasis," reduces the incidence of radial artery occlusion. In the recovery area, the band is left undisturbed for
1 to 2 hours (for diagnostic procedures) or 2 to 4 hours (for interventional procedures) after achievement of hemostasis. Once the

band is deflated and removed, a sterile dressing is applied. After discharge, activity restrictions include not using the affected wrist for 24 hours. Patients are instructed to elevate the arm and hold pressure in the event of small hematoma formation and to report large hematomas or significant forearm or hand pain.

Radial Artery Spasm

Radial spasm causes resistance against catheter movement and arm pain to the patient. It arises frequently often as a consequence of catheter manipulation and can preclude completion of a procedure. Risk factors for radial artery spasm include female gender, younger age, small radial artery diameter, large sheaths, diabetes, anxiety, unsuccessful access at first attempt, and prolonged catheter manipulation. Use of sedation, analgesia, and spasmolytic agents is important for both prevention and treatment of spasm. The use of smaller sheaths (including slender systems) or guide catheters can prevent and relieve spasm.

Overcoming severe spasm during sheath removal requires gentle but steady withdrawal of the sheath to minimize patient discomfort. Excessive force should never be applied because this may result in avulsion or rupture of the radial artery. Antispasmodics, sedation, nerve blocks, and anesthesia may be used in escalating fashion for spasm that prevents easy sheath removal.

Radial Complications

Arm Hematoma

Most hematomas develop after transradial sheath removal, but a hematoma can develop during the procedure. Patients complaining of pain or paresthesia (numbness) warrant a close evaluation. During the procedure, checking under the drapes for enlarging hematoma formation is recommended.

A developing forearm hematoma can be managed with compression with a careful arm-wrapping technique. Elastic tape, compression (Ace wrap) bandage, or a manual blood pressure cuff can provide compression to the forearm. Recheck your hemostasis device and reposition if needed. After a few minutes, remove the tape and recheck the forearm; if it is not softer, rewrap with higher tension and check for hemostasis.

The most serious complication of forearm bleeding and hematoma is a compartment syndrome with resultant hand ischemia. This extremely rare but dangerous problem requires surgical fasciotomy when it occurs. A less dangerous but debilitating complication is chronic regional pain syndrome, or reflex sympathetic dystrophy. This complication, thought to be related to prolonged

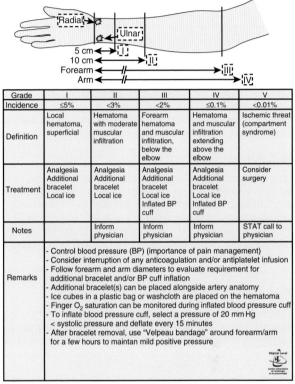

EASY HEMATOMA CLASSIFICATION
AFTER TRANSRADIAL/ULNAR PCI

Grade	I	II	III	IV	V
Incidence	≤5%	<3%	<2%	≤0.1%	<0.01%
Definition	Local hematoma, superficial	Hematoma with moderate muscular infiltration	Forearm hematoma and muscular infiltration, below the elbow	Hematoma and muscular infiltration extending above the elbow	Ischemic threat (compartment syndrome)
Treatment	Analgesia Additional bracelet Local ice	Analgesia Additional bracelet Local ice	Analgesia Additional bracelet Local ice Inflated BP cuff	Analgesia Additional bracelet Local ice Inflated BP cuff	Consider surgery
Notes		Inform physician	Inform physician	Inform physician	STAT call to physician
Remarks	- Control blood pressure (BP) (importance of pain management) - Consider interruption of any anticoagulation and/or antiplatelet infusion - Follow forearm and arm diameters to evaluate requirement for additional bracelet and/or BP cuff inflation - Additional bracelet(s) can be placed alongside artery anatomy - Ice cubes in a plastic bag or washcloth are placed on the hematoma - Finger O_2 saturation can be monitored during inflated blood pressure cuff - To inflate blood pressure cuff, select a pressure of 20 mm Hg < systolic pressure and deflate every 15 minutes - After bracelet removal, use "Velpeau bandage" around forearm/arm for a few hours to maintan mild positive pressure				

Bertrand et al. Circulation 2006;114(24):2646-53 ©Hôpital Laval 2002 213-08

Figure 2.15 Diagram of forearm hematoma classification and its management. (From Bertrand OF, De Larochellière R, Rodés-Cabau J, et al. A randomized study comparing same-day home discharge and abciximab bolus only to overnight hospitalization and abciximab bolus and infusion after transradial coronary stent implantation. *Circulation*. 2006;114[24]:2646–2653.)

access site compression, is also very rare and requires only conservative management. Fig. 2.15 provides a guide to radial artery hematoma complications and the management of these problems.

Radial Artery Occlusion

Aside from bleeding, which is typically minor, the most frequent complication of transradial coronary intervention (TRI) is radial artery occlusion, which affects 3% to 5% of patients. It is typically asymptomatic, and 50% of such occlusions undergo spontaneous recanalization at 30 days. Risk factors for radial artery occlusion include duration of catheterization time, longer sheaths, high sheath-to-artery diameter ratio, insufficient anticoagulation, and prolonged compression time. Systemic heparin is often given after radial access or after positioning of the catheter in the aortic root to help minimize radial occlusion postprocedure. Patent hemostasis, confirmed with oximetry or a reverse Allen test, is the most effective technique to avoid radial artery occlusion. Treatment of asymptomatic radial artery occlusion is typically unnecessary, although studies have described using ulnar occlusion and catheter-directed techniques to encourage recanalization.

Rare Complications

Pseudoaneurysm is an uncommon complication that can be diagnosed by ultrasound and treated with compression or thrombin injection. Radial artery dissections and perforations are also rare events that will both seal internally with guide catheter placement. The use of hydrophilic sheaths has been infrequently associated with the formation of sterile abscesses or granulomas. These typically develop 2 to 3 weeks postprocedure and rarely require drainage.

Distal Radial Access

One method to reduce the risk of subsequent radial artery occlusion and potential compartment syndrome is to access the radial artery between the thumb and forefinger. With further exploration, this technique also has been advocated to be more comfortable to the patient given that there is no "forced" supination of the forearm during setup and there is an increased freedom of movement after the procedure.

Stepwise Technique

See Fig. 2.16.

1. The patient is positioned with the arm in a neutral position with the snuffbox facing upwards. Some have advocated having the patient hold a roll of 4x4 gauze or a small towel to keep the dorsal area of the hand open for access. The snuffbox area is then prepped in the usual sterile technique.
2. Ultrasound guidance is preferred because the artery is very superficial.
3. Subcutaneous lidocaine is used for local anesthesia (same as standard radial technique).

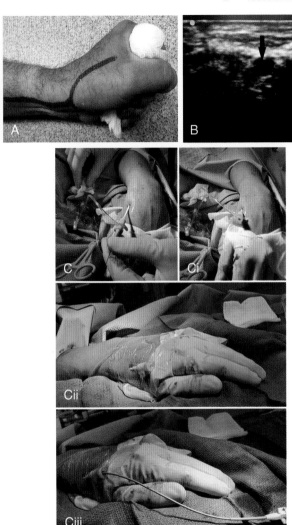

Figure 2.16 Stepwise Approach to Distal Radial Arterial Access.
(A) Showing the hand gripping sterile gauze. Note the red lines drawn on the hand to demonstrate the course of the artery. (B) Ultrasound image of the artery (*black arrow*). (C) Typical placement of the sheath after which the arm can be mobilized and placed in the best position for the operator to manipulate catheters and wires. (From Davies RE, Gilchrist IC. Back hand approach to radial access: The snuff box approach. *Cardiovasc Revasc Medicine.* 2018;19(3 Pt B):324–326.)

4. A 21-gauge open needle is used for access. With a 30- to 45-degree angle, the needle is directed to the point of the strongest pulse. The needle entry point is preferred to be at the dorsum of the hand where the artery is more superficial as opposed to the middle of the snuffbox. A "through-and-through" puncture is not recommended.

5. After successful anterior wall puncture, a flexible, soft j-tipped wire is then advanced.

6. A small skin-nick can be made to facilitate passing the sheath without damaging the tip of the dilator.

The remainder of the procedure takes place with the same steps as a standard radial artery catheterization, including vasodilators and anticoagulation with heparin. After the procedure, some operators have removed the sheath and placed radial bands for hemostasis, whereas others have fashioned "custom" gauze compression dressings. Dedicated distal radial compression devices have also been developed for use because the traditional radial bands rely on the immobility of the wrist to provide pressure on the artery, which is more difficult in the distal snuff-box location.

Ulnar Artery Access

Although not used as a "preferred" access site routinely over the radial or distal radial technique, the ulnar artery has been used for access when the radial artery otherwise is not available for access or cannot be accessed successfully. In general, ulnar access has been shown to be noninferior to that of radial access from a standpoint of safety and efficacy, making it perhaps safer than moving to femoral access when the radial artery cannot be cannulated. From an anatomic standpoint (see Fig. 2.7), the ulnar artery courses along the medial aspect of the ulna bone in the forearm with less tortuosity and loops than are encountered with the radial artery.

The technique of ulnar artery access is almost identical to that of accessing the radial artery with the following differentiating points:

1. The ulnar nerve is located just lateral to the artery, and one should bias the needle path away from this location to avoid contact with the nerve itself.

2. The point of access should be slightly more distal in the ulnar artery than the radial artery.

3. Hemostasis after the procedure may be slightly more difficult than for the radial as the ulnar artery is deeper in the forearm. Use of radial bands placed "backward" to apply pressure over

the ulnar site can be used, but operators should emphasize hemostasis over the more common "patent hemostasis" technique for the radial artery.

Medications for Radial Catheterization

Radial artery spasm is a concern for TRI, particularly for female or small patients and when using 6F or larger sheaths. Common antispasmodic medications include verapamil (2.5 to 5 mg IA) and nitroglycerin (100–200 mcg IA). Anxiety and high sympathetic tone are also significant contributors to vasospasm, making the use of adequate local anesthesia, sedation, and analgesia important factors for a smooth procedure.

Heparin is mandatory to reduce the risk of radial artery occlusion but should be given intravenously after the sheath is inserted to reduce pain in the hand. Use heparin 2000 to 5000 U for diagnostic procedures to maintain postprocedure radial artery patency. A higher dose of heparin (70–100 U/kg) is used to prevent clotting during the percutaneous coronary intervention (PCI) procedure.

Table 2.3 provides a sample regimen of drugs and doses used in our lab.

Femoral Artery Puncture Technique

1. The basic access techniques for both the femoral and radial arteries are presented in detail in the *Cardiac Catheterization*

Table 2.3

Medical Regimen for Radial Catheterization

Before the procedure: Topical anesthetic cream over the radial artery (optional)

1. Sedation: 0.5-1.0 mg versed and 50 mcg fentanyl
   a. Typically given together but one or the other may be used in the elderly or in patients with respiratory compromise.
2. Local anesthetic: 1% lidocaine
   a. Use no more than 0.5-1 mL of lidocaine
3. After the sheath is inserted (before catheter insertion), give intraarterial spasmolytic (one of the following):
   a. Nitroglycerin 100 to 200 mcg for most patients
   b. Verapamil 2.5 mg diluted into 10 mL of blood or saline
6. Intravenous unfractionated heparin 40 U/kg bolus up to a maximum of 5000 U
7. After the procedure and before sheath removal: Verapamil 1 to 2.5 mg (optional) intra-arterial (IA).

Handbook, 6th ed., in chapter 2. This section will highlight issues and advanced techniques pertinent to vascular access for the interventional procedures. It is strongly advised that a "standard" technique be adopted for accessing the femoral artery regardless of sheath size or procedure (diagnostic catheterization or known PCI) to maximize the efficiency and reproducibility of good patient outcomes. With an emphasis on the safety of the PCI procedure, operators must emphasize a careful and meticulous approach to femoral access, because multiple studies have shown that femoral access site complications remain the most frequent complications of patients undergoing these procedures. The following technique now has become the standard for minimizing the occurrence of access complications.

2. Anatomic landmarks now are used to provide a general initial guidance for preparation of the area rather than providing knowledge of the location of the common femoral artery. The proper entry site for femoral artery puncture is the common femoral artery (CFA), defined as the segment above the femoral artery bifurcation and below the inferior epigastric artery (Figs. 2.17–2.18). This "target zone" is located by visualizing the head of the femur with a metal marker (e.g., hemostat), indicating the planned path of the needle by fluoroscopy.

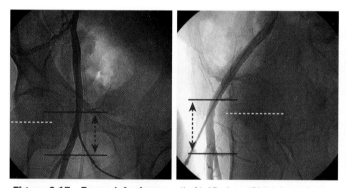

Figure 2.17 Femoral Angiogram. (*Left*) AP view. (*Right*) Lateral view. The common femoral artery (CFA) has the inferior epigastric artery and bifurcation of the superficial and profunda femoral arteries as the top and bottom markers. The *yellow dotted line* is the middle of the femoral head. *Lower red line* is bifurcation of superficial and profunda femoral arteries, and *top red line* is lower border of inferior epigastic artery. The *arrow* shows the target zone for proper puncture in the CFA over the femoral head, with the center third of the femoral head being the optimal location.

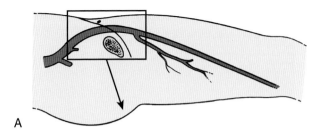

A

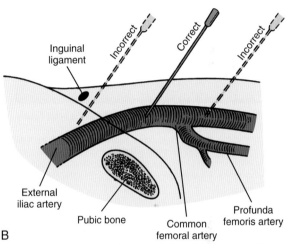

B

Figure 2.18 Technique of Single-wall Arterial Puncture. Parasagittal cross-sectional diagram of inguinal region at level of femoral artery. Correct needle entry position is below inguinal ligament and above femoral artery bifurcation. Correct access is particularly critical for procedures. (From Kern MJ, ed. *The Interventional Cardiac Catheterization Handbook.* 3rd ed. Elsevier; 2012. Originally from Kulick DL, Rahimtoola SH, eds. *Techniques and Applications in Interventional Cardiology.* Mosby, 1991:3.)

3. Ultrasound is then used to confirm the exact location of the common femoral artery and identify the exact area of needle entry into the vessel. Ultrasound imaging can identify the CFA bifurcation consistently and ensure the access is above it. In the longitudinal view, ultrasound can also identify the femoral head, the posterior course of the external iliac artery, and the soft-tissue inguinal ligament (which appears as an echodense

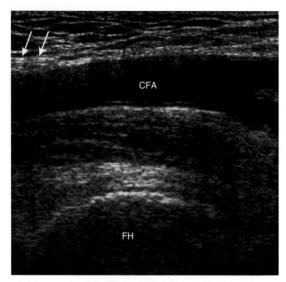

Figure 2.19   Longitudinal Ultrasound of Common Femoral Artery. Ultrasound image shows the inguinal ligament (*arrows*) and femoral head (FH) along the longitudinal plane and common femoral artery (CFA) with its bifurcation. (From Yun SJ, Nam DH, Ryu JK. Femoral artery access using the US-determined inguinal ligament and femoral head as reliable landmarks: Prospective study of usefulness and safety. *J Vasc Interv Radiol.* 2015;26[4]:552–559.)

triangle; Fig. 2.19). Table 2.4 lists several tips for success ultrasound-guided access.

a. Prepare the ultrasound probe by placing transducer gel in the base of the probe cover. Cover the probe with the sterile sheath cover and place gel on the front. The image display settings should be set at a minimum of depth penetration needed (i.e., 3–4 cm) and high gain. Turn on the centerline guide markers.

b. Image the vessel in the axial plane by holding the ultrasound probe perpendicular to the course of the vessel. Gently compress the vessels by applying downward pressure on the probe. An artery will be an echolucent circle that pulsates on gentle compression. A vein will often be larger, easily compressible or collapsing with respiration, and without visible pulsation. Ultrasound is able to image the CFA bifurcation (Fig. 2.20) and guard against an overly low or inferior cannulation.

c. Align the target vessel with the centerline guide on the display by moving the probe. This ensures that the target vessel is directly beneath the center of the probe.

Table 2.4

Tips for Ultrasound Femoral Arterial Access

1. Attempting to cannulate just above the bifurcation will generally avoid a high stick and can be performed consistently with some practice.
2. Combining axial ultrasound with manual palpation of landmarks, fluoroscopic guidance, or longitudinal views of the femoral head can help avoid arteriotomies that are superior to the desired location.
3. Avoid puncturing locations that are heavily calcified on ultrasound to ensure successful access and closure.
4. If a single artery and vein are not well separated laterally and the vein is often located posterior to the artery, it likely represents the superficial femoral artery. Puncture here should be avoided.
5. A needle guide is of particular utility in the femoral artery because it helps control the superior course of the needle.
6. Tilting the probe and needle guide together is a good way of inserting the needle at a flatter/shallower angle (reduced risk of wire/sheath kinking). Nevertheless, doing so will make the point of insertion more superior. Any time that you tilt the transducer, you change the cranial–caudal site of cannulation.
7. The most common cause of a high stick is *tilting the probe cranially* after successfully imaging the CFA bifurcation in a perpendicular angle. Instead, one should image the needle insertion and bifurcation at the same angle and translocate the probe at the fixed desired angle rather than tilting the probe.

  d. Inject lidocaine subcutaneously under the center of the probe.
  e. Insert the needle into the skin underneath the center marking of the probe at about a 45- to 60-degree angle (Fig. 2.21). For a deep vessel, the needle can be inserted some distance (a) from the probe to match the depth (b) of the vessel, so that a 45-degree angled needle intersects the ultrasound plane at the depth of the vessel.
  f. Use short strokes (short in-and-out movements of the needle) to see the approximate course of the needle. Adjust the probe position distance from the needle or angulation (f) (fanning) if the tip of the needle is not seen. Adjust the needle angle or puncture location to move the needle toward the vessel. Eventually, you should see the needle tip compress and puncture the vessel wall. (With a needle guide, the needle is preloaded into a guide attached to the transducer, and the needle angle is fixed to intersect the ultrasound plane at a specified depth. This provides superior control, such that the needle is guaranteed to insert at the specified depth.)
  g. When appropriate blood flashback is seen, the guidewire is inserted through the needle and into the vessel. The ultrasound image can be used to confirm appropriate intravascular placement of the guidewire and that the arteriotomy does not involve the CFA bifurcation.

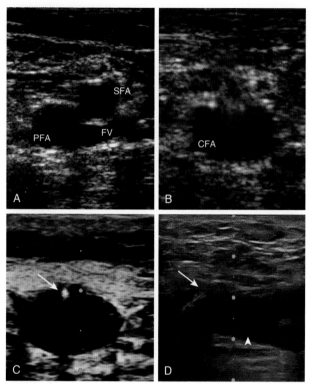

Figure 2.20 Axial Ultrasound of Common Femoral Artery. (A) The right common femoral bifurcation is imaged in the axial plane, demonstrating the profunda femoral artery and superficial femoral artery. Compression is used to differentiate arteries from the femoral vein. (B) The probe is moved or angled superiorly to the common femoral artery (CFA). During needle advancement, the anterior wall of the vessel is indented by the needle tip. (C) The guidewire insertion point (*arrow*) can be imaged in the axial plane after cannulation to confirm that the insertion is above the CFA bifurcation. (D) Longitudinal view shows the guidewire entry (*arrow*) is superior to the CFA bifurcation (*arrowhead*).

Micropuncture Technique

See Fig. 2.22.

Micropuncture access has the potential to improve the safety and accuracy of femoral access, which is particularly useful for large bore sheath placement. There are several available "kits" now, generally consisting of a low-profile needle or needle (21- vs. 18-gauge),

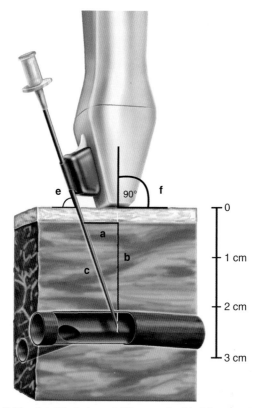

Figure 2.21 Axial Technique of Ultrasound-guided Access. The probe is aligned perpendicular (f) to the vessel, creating a circular image of the vessel. Without a needle guide, the needle is inserted at an angle (e) and at a distance (a) from beneath the center of the probe. The needle is not visible until it crosses the imaging plane of the probe at a depth (b). Changes of needle angle (c), to (a), (b), (e), and (f) are interrelated, such that the success of this technique depends on experience, repeated jabbing motions of the needle, and adjustment to probe angle (f) to visualize the course of the needle. With a needle guide selected based on the depth (b) of the vessel, the needle angle (e) is fixed to intersect the ultrasound plane at the set distance below the ultrasound plane, guaranteeing needle puncture at the location imaged. The probe angle (f) can and should be adjusted to allow for a more shallow entry of the needle. (Modified from Seto AH, Abu-Fadel MS, Sparling JM, et al. Real-time ultrasound guidance facilitates femoral arterial access and reduces vascular complications: FAUST (Femoral Arterial Access With Ultrasound Trial). *JACC Cardiovasc Interv.* 2010;3:751–758.)

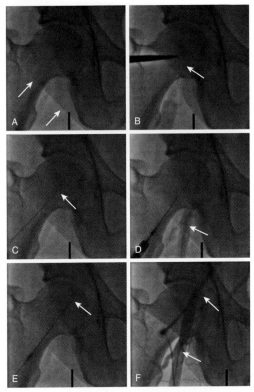

Figure 2.22 **Micropuncture Arterial Access Technique.** (A) Using fluoroscopy, the midfemoral head is identified. The arrows show the femoral skin crease. (B) A hemostat marks the midfemoral head, and the local anesthesia needle is just below the skin surface (*arrow*). This provides some idea of where the micropuncture needle should be introduced into the skin. (C) Repeat fluoroscopy once the needle is deep in the subcutaneous tissue, but not yet into the femoral artery, is required to achieve an ideal location of femoral puncture at the level of the midfemoral head. The arrow shows the tip of the micropuncture needle. (D) Contrast injection through the micropuncture needle shows the level of needle entry in the common femoral artery (CFA; *arrow* shows the level of CFA bifurcation). (E) A 0.018-inch guidewire is advanced into the femoral artery. The arrow shows the guidewire exit point from the needle tip, which is the site of needle entry into the CFA lumen. (F) Angiography via a 6F sheath confirms the arterial entry site. The arrows show the takeoff of the inferior epigastric artery and the CFA. The sheath entry is above the midfemoral head but clearly inferior to the inferior sweep of the inferior epigastric artery (*upper arrow*) and above the bifurcation (*lower arrow*). (From Cilingiroglu M, Feldman T, Salinger MH, Levisay J, Turi ZG. Fluoroscopically-guided micropuncture femoral artery access for large-caliber sheath insertion. *J Invasive Cardiol.* 2011;23[4]:157–161.)

a 0.018-inch nitinol or hydrophilic guidewire, and a 4F or 5F tapered micropuncture sheath with an inner dilator. When access is achieved and the inner dilator and wire are removed, a standard 0.035- or 0.038-inch guidewire can be inserted to facilitate final sheath placement.

Advantages of the micropuncture access technique include a smaller initial puncture with less arterial trauma (which is particularly important if multiple attempts are needed to access the vessel) and contrast angiography through the 4F or 5F micropuncture catheter or inner dilator to confirm an optimal location of the arteriotomy before large sheath placement. If the operator is not satisfied with the position of entry, the small catheter can be removed and access reattempted after 5 minutes of manual compression. The micropuncture needle also has a lower crossing profile, which can be helpful in highly resistant (calcified) arteries. Most operators now will access the femoral artery with the micropuncture technique during ultrasound-guided access (as previously described).

Percutaneous Femoral Vein Puncture

Indications for femoral venous sheath placement in patients undergoing PCI include the need for transseptal access, intracardiac imaging, temporary pacemaker, or pulmonary artery pressure monitoring. Avoid unnecessary or "routine" venous access because bleeding complications are more frequent in combined arterial–venous procedures. Safety indicates avoiding an inadvertent arterial puncture. Common practice accesses the vein first then the artery. If the artery is accidentally punctured, check the location and, if acceptable, place the arterial sheath. Then, with an angle slightly more medial, try another puncture. Ultrasound guidance is particularly helpful for cannulation of decompressed veins.

The most common cause of failed transradial catheterization is unsuccessful arterial access. Note that the first radial attempt has the highest chance of success. An injured artery may spasm, making subsequent attempts more difficult. Operators should thus proceed slowly and carefully, especially when first learning to obtain radial artery access. Key to reducing local vasospasm is general conscious sedation and adequate but limited local anesthesia. Ultrasound-guided access has high success rates for first-pass entry and increases the likelihood of a successful and quicker procedure.

Percutaneous Brachial Artery Access

In general, percutaneous brachial artery puncture should be abandoned. The rate of bleeding complications is highest in the brachial artery, followed by femoral and radial arteries. The brachial approach may be advantageous in some lower extremity or renal procedures when equipment of sufficient length is unavailable but has larger been supplanted by radial, distal radial, and ulnar access.

Additional Arterial and Venous Access for High-Risk Interventions

For patients at high risk for complications who may require urgent placement of a temporary pacemaker or mechanical circulatory support (MCS), an additional arterial or venous access is helpful. As a standby procedure, a small 4 to 5F sheath introducer can be placed in the opposite femoral artery or vein at the beginning of the procedure, permitting immediate vascular access if urgent hemodynamic or pacing support is required. Before MCS or other large device insertion, abdominal and iliac angiography should be performed to identify any significant peripheral vascular disease.

Arterial Access Management for Large-Bore Devices

The increase in percutaneous management of structural heart disease and the increased use of mechanical support devices have brought increased vascular complications because of larger size (bore) catheters. The first step in successful management of the vascular access is proper location of the arteriotomy. Ultrasound-guided access is strongly recommended to avoid the bifurcation and to ensure anterior wall puncture. Some centers will obtain contralateral access using landmarks from angiography. Initial access is often obtained with a smaller 6F sheath followed by "preclosure" preparation with a suture-mediated closure device. Currently, the Perclose ProGlide and ProStar XL devices are the only ones used. In both systems, the needles are deployed and the sutures set aside for closure after the procedure. Upsizing of the sheath can commence after the preclosure has been performed. At the conclusion of the procedure, completion of the vascular closure with the predelivered sutures can be performed.

Crossover Technique for Transfemoral Access and Closure

See Fig. 2.23.

An additional helpful technique to control bleeding is crossover balloon hemostasis. This method uses a peripheral balloon to occlude the iliac artery after introduction from the contralateral

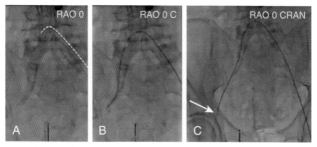

Figure 2.23 Crossover Angiographic Technique. Basic crossover wire technique. (A) The dotted line outlines the path of a left internal mammary 5F diagnostic catheter used to engage the iliac bifurcation. (B) A standard 0.035-inch J-wire has been passed across the bifurcation. (C) The left mammary catheter has been tracked over the wire to just above the contralateral femoral head, as noted by the white arrow. (From Perlowski AA, Levisay JP, Salinger MH, Feldman TE. Access and closure for TAVR. *Cardiac Interventions Today.* 2014.)

side. It is inflated while closure is being performed. Once completed, hemostasis is confirmed with an angiogram from the contralateral catheter. For complications including incomplete closure or vessel rupture, the peripheral balloon is used for stabilization of the arteriotomy prior to placement of a covered stent.

Technique

1. Contralateral angiography (e.g., left femoral artery access is performed with a 5F angiographic catheter positioned over the iliac bifurcation) is used to identify the desired location in the target artery (e.g., right common femoral artery). The iliac crossover is generally straightforward, using an internal mammary artery or Omniflush catheter and a standard 0.035-inch hydrophilic wire.

2. Closure of arterial access sites used for large-bore catheters uses percutaneous vascular suture devices like the Prostar XL (Abbott Vascular, Santa Clara, CA) or ProGlide (Abbott Vascular), which are placed at the beginning of access. At the conclusion of the procedure, the large-bore sheath is withdrawn over a 0.035-inch wire to the pelvic brim.

3. To reduce bleeding and have better control of the access site, a crossover balloon is advanced over the iliac bifurcation and inflated. Low-pressure balloon occlusion with a modestly oversized balloon provides proximal hemostasis, thus permitting rapid and easy deployment of the closure sutures. The retrograde 0.035-inch wire is removed, provided adequate hemostasis has been achieved.

Overcoming Difficult Vascular Access Problems

Excessive Vessel Tortuosity

The most frequently encountered difficulty in advancing guide catheters is tortuosity of the iliac or subclavian vessels, a condition often found in elderly patients. A steerable 0.038-inch flexible guidewire (e.g., Wholey, Benson) is excellent for negotiating tortuous vessels. Its flexible, atraumatic, gently curved tip is steerable, thus increasing safety. In cases of extreme tortuosity, a JR diagnostic catheter may be used to help direct the guidewire tip and control the advancement of the guidewire. Angiograms will delineate the arterial course and any other obstructive lesions. Once the guidewire is beyond the tortuous or narrowed segments, further catheter exchanges should use a long exchange-length guidewire. A longer (>30 cm) or braided vascular sheath can be positioned and is often effective in straightening tortuous segments.

Commonly selected equipment for tortuous vessels includes:

1. Wholey 0.035-inch steerable guidewires (crossing)
2. Angled hydrophilic wire (crossing)
3. Angled hydrophilic glide catheter
4. Long 300-cm regular exchange guidewires
5. Long 300-cm extrastiff exchange guidewires
6. Long arterial sheaths of 23 to 90 cm

Peripheral Vascular Disease

PVD complicates access and guide catheter manipulation. Weak femoral pulses often indicate atherosclerotic obstruction at the level of the femoral, common iliac, or aortoiliac bifurcation. Inability to advance the guidewire to the central aortic position requires angiography to determine further maneuvers needed to negotiate the femoral approach. In such patients, abdominal aortography and peripheral angiography are necessary to evaluate the extent of obstructive disease with focal iliac stenosis. Should a coronary intervention be required, some operators advocate iliac stent placement before proceeding with PCI. PVD may require the use of the radial approach. In patients with PVD of the lower extremities, coexistent subclavian atherosclerosis may also complicate arm access.

Access Through Inguinal Scarring, Previous Vascular Closure Device, or Synthetic Vascular Graft

Inguinal scarring may be present in patients having multiple prior interventional procedures, aortofemoral bypass surgery, femoral bypass cannula access, intra-aortic balloon pump (IABP) repair, or radiation therapy. In some of these patients, a synthetic arterial conduit graft may be present but is often calcified. If possible, select an alternative access site. Otherwise, access of a severely fibrotic or scarred groin or through a femoral bypass graft may require successive dilations with 5, 6, 7, and 8F dilators before inserting a vascular sheath one size smaller than the largest dilator. Perclose and Starclose closure devices have difficulty penetrating calcified or fibrotic arteries and should be used with caution only if the tract is well dilated. Entrapment of a StarClose clip during placement in a scarred groin has been reported.

Most vascular closure device manufacturers indicate that re-access through a site with a recently placed closure device can be performed without a problem if the device has no internal artery fixation component. Caution should be used when reaccessing all sites but especially those closed with Angio-Seal, although there are no reports of Angio-Seal anchor dislodgement during reaccess. Access of sites closed with such devices after 2 to 4 weeks is thought to be safe. Nevertheless, the contralateral femoral artery should be considered in most cases for patient comfort.

Hemostasis After Femoral PCI

Complications related to vascular access management are the most significant cause of morbidity and prolonged hospitalization. Timely and safe removal of the arterial sheath with minimal patient discomfort is the goal of a successful intervention. Improved outcomes have been associated with using smaller sheaths, discontinuing post-PCI heparin infusions, and removing the sheath early. Although results are improving, resources (both staff and equipment) necessary for appropriate sheath care and hemostasis are critically important to good outcomes.

Immediate Sheath Removal

The femoral arterial and venous sheaths are not routinely left in place after PCI. The presence of a vascular sheath in a heavily anticoagulated patient predisposes to hemorrhage and retroperitoneal hematoma. Most laboratories remove sheaths within a few hours after the procedure or immediately remove the sheath in the laboratory after hemostasis with a vascular closure device.

Femoral PCI Sheath Removal

Sheath removal after PCI may occur in the lab, holding area, or at patient's bedside. Manual sheath removal proceeds as described for diagnostic procedures. Several points should be kept in mind for manual sheath removal:

1. Adjust bed height or use a footstool to exert maximal pressure downward for puncture site compression with minimal fatigue.

2. Ensure good intravenous (IV) access.

3. Give local anesthetic (10–20 mL of 1% lidocaine) to the skin around the sheath and IV analgesics before sheath removal.

4. Have atropine and pain medication available.

5. Before removing the sheath, check that the heparin is stopped, the activated clotting time (ACT) is less than 150 seconds, vital signs are stable, no chest pain is present, and there are no plans for recatheterization.

6. If both arterial and venous sheaths were used, remove the arterial sheath first, preserving good venous access in case the peripheral IV stops working. Avoid prolonged pressure on the femoral vein. Prolonged venous occlusion, especially with pressure devices, may cause venous thrombosis. Check the leg and foot for cyanosis.

7. The duration of pressure holding, usually 15 to 20 minutes, depends on the sheath size, ACT, and ease of bleeding control.

8. When longer pressure application is needed after removal of a large sheath, IABP catheter, or cardiopulmonary support cannula, the FemoStop (St. Jude Medical, St. Paul, MN) or a similar compression device is one of the preferred methods of mechanical arterial compression (see later). Compression devices provide a constant stable pressure, relative patient comfort, and easy adjustment of the degree of pressure applied. Compression devices are not intended for unsupervised use. The duration of pressure application should be kept to a minimum to decrease complications such as skin necrosis, nerve compression, or venous thrombosis.

Femoral Compression Systems

The FemoStop system (St. Jude Medical, St. Paul, MN; Fig. 2.24) is an air-filled, clear plastic compression bubble that molds to the skin contours. It is held in place by straps passing around the hips. The amount of pressure applied is controlled with an insufflator connected to a sphygmomanometer gauge. The clear plastic dome permits visualization of the puncture site. The FemoStop is mostly used for patients in whom prolonged compression is anticipated or if bleeding persists despite prolonged manual compression. The duration of FemoStop compression and time to removal of the

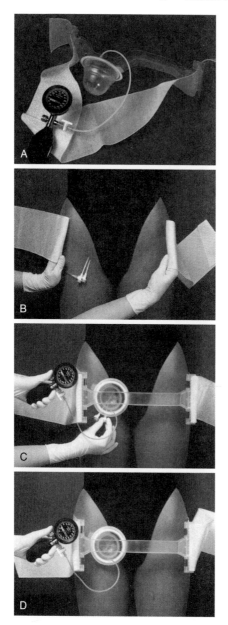

Continued

Figure 2.24 Use of the FemoStop. (A) Before proceeding, examine the puncture site carefully; note and mark edges of any hematoma; record current blood pressure. (B) Position belt. The belt should be aligned with the puncture site equally across both hips. Center the dome and adjust the belt. (C) The dome should be centered over the arterial puncture site above and slightly toward the midline of the skin incision. The sheath valve should be below the rim of the pressure dome. Attach belt to ensure a snug fit. The center arch bar should be perpendicular to the body. (D) Connect dome pressure pump. Right side, for the arterial sheath, pressurize dome to 60 to 80 mm Hg and remove sheath and increase pressure in dome to 10 to 20 mm above systolic arterial pressure. Maintain full compression for 3 minutes. Reduce pressure in dome by 10 to 20 mm Hg every few minutes until 0 mm Hg. Check arterial pulse. Observe for bleeding. After hemostasis is obtained, remove FemoStop and dress wound. (From Kern MJ. *The Cardiac Catheterization Handbook*, 4th ed. Mosby, 2003:67–69.)

device varies depending on the patient and staff protocols. In some hospitals, the time from application to removal may be less than 30 minutes. In other patients in whom hemostasis is required, the device may be left at a lower pressure for longer. Mechanical C-clamp systems are rarely used. Femoral compression systems should not be used in patients with lower extremity bypass grafts (fem-pop) at the access site because of the risk of graft thrombosis.

Vascular Closure Devices and In-Lab Hemostasis

Immediate hemostasis can be achieved in the catheterization suite using one of several vascular closure devices. Before selecting the device, femoral angiography from an oblique projection will indicate the suitability of the device insertion. Note that the ipsilateral oblique view (e.g., the right anterior oblique [RAO] for right femoral artery) best displays the bifurcation of the profunda and superficial femoral branches.

Vascular closure devices (VCDs) were developed both to obtain quick, safe hemostasis and to improve patient comfort by decreasing the time patients lie flat after the procedure. The safety of VCDs has been demonstrated in diagnostic catheterization and interventions. Most catheterization laboratories report high success rates for various closure devices used directly after PCI in fully anticoagulated patients receiving antithrombins, heparin, or glycoprotein receptor blockers. Commonly used VCDs are shown in Table 2.5.

Table 2.5

Vascular Closure Devices

Device	On the Market	Mechanism	Advantages	Disadvantages	Sheath Sizes	Ipsilateral Access <90 Days
AngioSeal (St. Jude Medical, St. Paul, MN) 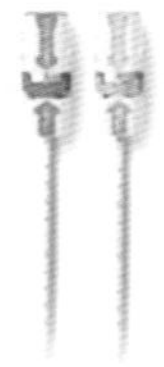	1997 to present	Collagen and suture mediated	Secure closure, long track record	Intra-arterial component, possible thromboembolic complications, infection related to suture serving as a wick	6 and 8F	1 cm higher
Perclose (Abbott Vascular, Redwood City, CA) 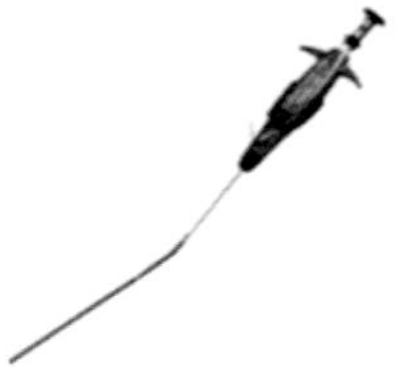	1997 to present	Suture mediated	Secure closure	Intra-arterial component, steep learning curve, device failure may require surgical repair	5–8F	No restrictions

Continued on following page

Table 2.5

Vascular Closure Devices (Continued)

Device	On the Market	Mechanism	Advantages	Disadvantages	Sheath Sizes	Ipsilateral Access <90 Days
StarClose (Abbott Vascular, Redwood City, CA)	2005 to present	Nitinol clip	No intraarterial component	Adequate skin tract needed to prevent device failure	5–6F	Not fully established
Mynx (Access Closure, Mountain View, CA)	2007 to present	PEG hydrogel plug	No intra-arterial component, potential use in peripheral vascular disease (PVD)	Possible intra-arterial injection of sealant, failure rate	5–7F	No restrictions

For repeat procedures, restick in the same vessel should be directed 1 to 2 cm above or below the site of the previous device placement site.

Key Points in Postprocedure Sheath Care and Hemostasis

1. "Do it right the first time." The best results stem from a meticulous arterial puncture, correct sheath placement, and careful removal and hemostasis.
2. For transport to the holding area, if the sheath is left in place, placing an appropriately sized obturator in the sheath may prevent sheath kinking (and bleeding) before sheath removal.
3. Use a clear transparent dressing over the puncture site for easy visualization of bleeding. Do not use a wad of gauze under the dressing because the combination of blood and gauze is an excellent culture media for bacteria.
4. Inspect and palpate the puncture site and distal pulses at each postprocedure check.
5. A downward trend in blood pressure and upward trend in heart rate are early warning signs of bleeding, especially occult bleeding such as a retroperitoneal hematoma (RPH). Hypotension after PCI should be assumed to be because of bleeding until the operator has identified an alternate cause (e.g., vagal reaction, ischemia, tamponade, overmedicated). If in doubt about whether there is an RPH and the patient is stable, a CT scan may be helpful.

Complications of Femoral Arterial Access

Hemorrhage

The most common complication from femoral cardiac catheterization is hemorrhage and local hematoma formation, increasing in frequency with the increasing size of the sheath, the amount of anticoagulation, and the degree of obesity of the patient.

Other common complications (in order of decreasing frequency) include RPH, pseudoaneurysm, AVF formation, arterial thrombosis secondary to intimal dissection, stroke, sepsis with or without abscess formation, and cholesterol or air embolization. The frequency of these complications is increased in high-risk procedures; critically ill elderly patients with extensive atheromatous disease; patients receiving anticoagulation, antiplatelet, and fibrinolytic therapies; and patients receiving concomitant interventional procedures. Compared with the femoral approach, the brachial (but not radial) approach carries a slightly higher risk of vascular complications.

Infections and Other Rare Events

Infections are more frequent in patients undergoing repeat ipsilateral (same site) femoral punctures or prolonged femoral sheath maintenance (within 1–5 days). Cholesterol embolism, manifesting with abdominal pain or headache (from mesenteric or central nervous system ischemia), skin mottling ("blue toes"), renal insufficiency, or lung hemorrhage, may be a clinical finding in up to 30% of high-risk patients.

Retroperitoneal Hematomas and Pseudoaneurysms

An RPH should be suspected in patients with hypotension, tachycardia, pallor, a rapidly falling hematocrit postcatheterization, lower abdominal or back pain, or neurologic changes in the leg with the puncture. An RPH may also manifest with back pain and symptoms similar to a vagal reaction, with bradycardia and hypotension not responsive to medications. This complication is associated with *high femoral arterial puncture* and full anticoagulation. Consider a return to the cath lab to identify and control femoral bleeding. Access the contralateral artery for angiography of the suspected site and possible treatment in patients with a high clinical risk of RPH.

Pseudoaneurysm is a complication associated with *low femoral arterial puncture* (usually below the head of the femur). In the past, to avoid further neurovascular complication or rupture, the vascular surgeon routinely repaired all femoral pseudoaneurysms. With ultrasound imaging techniques, these false channels can be easily identified, and nonsurgical closure can be selected. Manual compression of the expansile growing mass, guided by Doppler ultrasound with or without thrombin or collagen injection, is an acceptable therapy for femoral pseudoaneurysm.

Fig. 2.25 shows a femoral artery dissection induced by access difficulties. Fig. 2.26 shows a femoral AVF. Note simultaneous contrast filling of both artery and vein. These complications are not applicable to radial artery PCI.

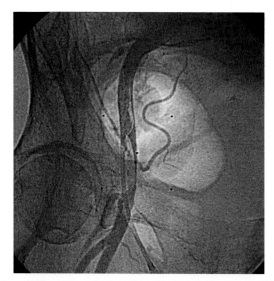

Figure 2.25 A femoral artery dissection induced by access difficulties.

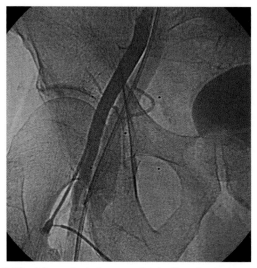

Figure 2.26 A femoral arteriovenous fistula. Note simultaneous contrast filling of both artery and vein. These complications are not applicable to radial artery percutaneous coronary intervention (PCI).

Key References

Davies RE, Gilchrist IC. Back hand approach to radial access: the snuff box approach. *Cardiovasc Revasc Med*. 2018;19:324-326.

Mason PJ, Shah B, Tamis-Holland JE, et al. An update on radial artery access and best practices for transradial coronary angiography and intervention in acute coronary syndrome: a scientific statement from the American Heart Association. *Circ Cardiovasc Interv*. 2018;11:e000035.

Naidu SS, Abbott JD, Bahai J, et al. SCAI expert consensus update on best practices in the cardiac catheterization laboratory. *Catheter Cardiovasc Interv*. 2021;98: 255-276.

Shroff AR, Gulati R, Drachman DE, et al. SCAI expert consensus statement update on best practices for transradial angiography and intervention. *Catheter Cardiovasc Interv*. 2020;95:245-252.

Yun SJ, Nam DH, Ryu JK. Femoral artery access using the US-determined inguinal ligament and femoral head as reliable landmarks: prospective study of usefulness and safety. *J Vasc Interv Radiol*. 2015;26(4):552-559.

References

Ferrante G, Rao SV, Jüni P, et al. Radial versus femoral access for coronary interventions across the entire spectrum of patients with coronary artery disease: a meta-analysis of randomized trials. *JACC Cardiovasc Interv*. 2016;9:1419-1434.

Gokhroo R, Kishor K, Ranwa B, et al. Ulnar artery interventions non-inferior to radial approach: AJmer Ulnar ARtery (AJULAR) intervention working group study results. *J Invasive Cardiol*. 2016;28:1-8.

Kwok CS, Khan MA, Rao SV, et al. Access and non–access site bleeding after percutaneous coronary intervention and risk of subsequent mortality and major adverse cardiovascular events: systematic review and meta-analysis. *Circ Cardiovasc Interv*. 2015;8:e001645.

Moussa Pacha H, Alahdab F, Al-Khadra Y, et al. Ultrasound-guided versus palpation-guided radial artery catheterization in adult population: a systematic review and meta-analysis of randomized controlled trials. *Am Heart J*. 2018;204:1-8.

Pancholy S, Coppola J, Patel T, Roke-Thomas M. Prevention of radial artery occlusion-patent hemostasis evaluation trial (PROPHET study): a randomized comparison of traditional versus patency documented hemostasis after transradial catheterization. *Catheter Cardiovasc Interv*. 2008;72:335-340.

Pancholy SB, Bernat I, Bertrand OF, Patel TM. Prevention of radial artery occlusion after Transradial catheterization: the PROPHET-II randomized trial. *JACC Cardiovasc Interv*. 2016;9:1992-1999.

Seto AH, Roberts JS, Abu-Fadel MS, et al. Real-time ultrasound guidance facilitates transradial access: RAUST (radial artery access with ultrasound trial). *JACC Cardiovasc Interv*. 2015;8:283-291.

Shah RM, Patel D, Abbate A, Cowley MJ, Jovin IS. Comparison of transradial coronary procedures via right radial versus left radial artery approach: a meta-analysis. *Catheter Cardiovasc Interv*. 2016;88:1027-1033.

Van Leeuwen MAH, Hollander MR, van der Heijden DJ, et al. The ACRA anatomy study (assessment of disability after coronary procedures using radial access): a comprehensive anatomic and functional assessment of the vasculature of the hand and relation to outcome after transradial catheterization. *Circ Cardiovasc Interv*. 2017;10:e005753.

Interventional Pharmacology

ARNOLD H. SETO • MICHAEL J. LIM • MORTON J. KERN

KEY POINTS

- Anticoagulant and antiplatelet medications are required for the safe percutaneous coronary intervention (PCI).

- Recent studies have demonstrated that shorter durations of dual antiplatelet therapy (DAPT) are safe.

- Vasodilators and vasopressors may often be necessary in some complicated or critical in-lab scenarios.

This chapter will describe common medications used in the cardiac catheterization laboratory for interventional procedures. It is not intended to be all inclusive, and the reader is referred elsewhere for a comprehensive review of the doses, indications, contraindications, and side effect of these important drugs. A list of the medications commonly used in the cath lab is provided in Table 3.1.

Anticoagulation and Antiplatelet Agents

Antithrombotic and antiplatelet agents for percutaneous coronary intervention (PCI) are summarized in Table 3.2. Fig. 3.1 depicts the mechanism of action of these agents. Recommendations from the American College of Cardiology (ACC)/American Heart Association (AHA) for pharmacology during acute coronary syndromes (ACS) are summarized in Table 3.3. Fig. 3.2 diagrams the mechanism of action of available anticoagulant drugs.

Unfractionated Heparin

Unfractionated heparin (UFH), the most common anticoagulation for PCI, accelerates the activity of antithrombin III (AT III), a

Table 3.1

Medications Commonly Used in the Cardiac Catheterization Laboratory[a]

Inotropic Agents

Digoxin 0.125–0.25 mg IV >4 hr apart
Dobutamine 2–10 μg/kg/min IV drip
Dopamine 2–10 μg/kg/min IV drip
Epinephrine 1:10,000 IV

Antiarrhythmic Agents, Anticholinergic Agents, β-Blockers, Calcium Blockers

Adenosine 5–12 mg IV bolus
Amiodarone 150 mg IV × 10 min (15 mg/min)
Atropine 0.6–1.2 mg IV
Diltiazem 10 mg IV
Esmolol 4–24 mg/kg IV drip
Lidocaine 50–100 mg IV bolus; 2–4 mg/min IV drip
Propranolol 1 mg bolus; 0.1 mg/kg in three divided doses
Verapamil 2–5 mg IV, may repeat dose to 10 mg

Analgesic Agents, Sedatives

Diazepam 2–5 mg IV
Diphenhydramine 25–50 mg IV
Meperidine 12.5–50 mg IV
Morphine sulfate 2.5 mg IV
Naloxone 0.5 mg IV

Anticoagulants

Heparin 2000–5000 U IV; 1000 U/hr IV drip; 40–70 U/kg for PCI
Low-molecular-weight heparin (LMWH; See Table 3.6)
Bivalirudin, bolus: 0.75 mg/kg with infusion of 1.75 mg/kg/h

Antiplatelet Agents

ORAL AGENTS
Clopidogrel – 600 mg loading with 75 mg daily PO
Prasugrel - 60-mg loading dose with 10 mg daily PO
Ticagrelor - Loading dose 180 mg with 90 mg q12hr PO

INTRAVENOUS AGENTS
IV abciximab – A 0.25 mg/kg IV bolus given 10–60 minutes before PCI with a continuous infusion of 0.125 μg/kg/min (to a maximum of 10 μg/min) for 12 hours
IV eptifibatide – **180 mcg/kg intravenous bolus** administered immediately before the initiation of PCI followed by a continuous infusion of 2 mcg/kg/min and a second 180 mcg/kg bolus 10 minutes after the first bolus. Patients >120 kg, given maximum bolus of 22.6 mg with infusion of 15 mg/h.
Patients with renal impairment (CrCl <50 mL/min) should receive the standard 180 mcg/kg loading dose followed by infusion at 1 mcg/kg/min.

Table 3.1

Medications Commonly Used in the Cardiac Catheterization Laboratory (Continued)

IV tirofiban – A high-dose bolus 25 mcg/kg over 3 minutes with 0.15 mcg/kg/min for up to 18 hours. In patients with creatinine clearance ≤60 mL/min, give 25 mcg/kg over 3 minutes and then 0.075 mcg/kg/min.

IV cangrelor – In patients who have not been treated with a P2Y12 platelet inhibitor and are not being given a glycoprotein IIb/IIIa inhibitor
- 30 mcg/kg IV bolus infused over 1 minute before PCI, immediately follow bolus injection with 4 mcg/kg/min IV infusion; continue for at least 2 hr or duration of PCI, whichever is longer

Vasodilators

Nitroglycerin 0.4 mg sublingual; intracoronary 100–300 μg
Nitroprusside 5–50 μg/kg/min IV

Vasoconstrictors

Metaraminol 10 mg in 100 mL saline, 1 mL IV
Epinephrine, for weight >50 kg; 0.5 mg (0.5 mL of epinephrine 1 mg/mL)
Phenylephrine 0.1–0.5 mg bolus, 100–180 μg/min IV drip
Norepinephrine 1:10,000 IV, 1-mL doses IV

IC, Intracoronary; *IV*, intravenous; *PCI*, percutaneous coronary intervention; *PO*, per os.
[a]The list is not meant to be all-inclusive or to exclude emergency life support techniques or standards.

Table 3.2

Antithrombotic, Antiplatelet, and Anticoagulant Drugs

Antithrombotic Therapy

- Heparin (unfractionated)
- Low-molecular-weight heparin (enoxaparin [Lovenox], dalteparin [Fragmin], tinzaparin [Innohep])
- Direct thrombin inhibitor— Polypeptide inhibitor (bivalirudin [Angiomax])
- Low-molecular-weight inhibitor (argatroban [Acova])

Antiplatelet Therapy

- Cyclooxygenase inhibitors (aspirin)
- Adenosine diphosphate (ADP) receptor inhibitors (clopidogrel [Plavix], prasugrel [Effient], ticlopidine [Ticlid], ticagrelor [Brilinta], cangrelor [Kengreal])
- Phosphodiesterase inhibitors (cilostazol [Pletal])
- Glycoprotein IIb/IIIa receptor inhibitors (abciximab [ReoPro], eptifibatide [Integrilin], tirofiban [Aggrastat])
- Adenosine reuptake inhibitors (dipyridamole [Persantine])
- Platelet activating receptor (PAR-1) antagonist [vorapaxar (Zontivity)]

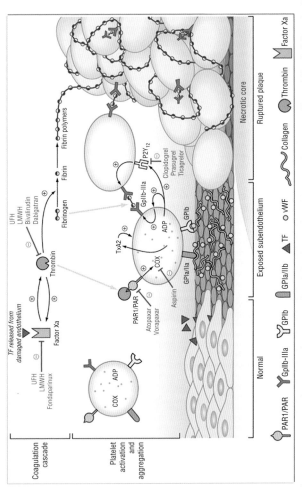

Figure 3.1 Acute coronary syndromes and targets of antiplatelet and antithrombotic agents. From Lilly, S Wilensky RL. Emerging therapies for acute coronary syndromes. *Front Pharmacol.* 2011:2:61.

Table 3.3

ACC/AHA Recommendations for Pharmacologic Management of Patients Undergoing PCI for Acute Coronary Syndromes

Drug	Unstable Angina/NSTEMI	STEMI	Comments
Aspirin	I (LOE A)	I (LOE B)	162–325 mcg loading, 81 mg maintenance
Clopidogrel	I (LOE B)	I (LOE B)	Loading dose of 600 mg recommended as early as possible
Prasugrel	I (LOE B)	I (LOE B)	Contraindicated in patients with prior stroke or TIA. Not recommended before PCI.
Ticagrelor	I (LOE B)	I (LOE B)	IIa recommendation to use in preference to clopidogrel in PCI patients.
Unfractionated heparin	I (LOE B)	I (LOE C)	
Low-molecular-weight heparin	I (LOE A)	I (LOE A) only for postlytic patient	Not recommended for primary PCI.
Bivalirudin	I (LOE B)	I (LOE B)	Especially for patients at high risk for bleeding.
Fondaparinux	I (LOE B)	III (LOE B) for use as sole anticoagulant	Requires an additional antithrombin during PCI. Preferred for conservative strategy.
Glycoprotein IIb/IIIa inhibitors	I (LOE A) in patients not pretreated with P2Y12 inhibitor, IIa (LOE B) when pretreated	IIa (LOE A-B) IIb for intracoronary or prehospital use	

ACC, American College of Cardiology; *AHA,* American Heart Association; *NSTEMI,* non-ST-segment elevation myocardial infarction; *PCI,* percutaneous coronary intervention; *STEMI,* ST-segment elevation myocardial infarction.
From O'Gara et al, J Am Coll Cardiol. 2013 Jan 29;61(4):485-510, and Amsterdam et al, J Am Coll Cardiol. 2014 Dec 23;64(24):e139-228.

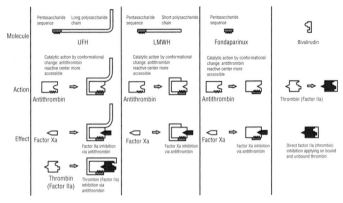

Figure 3.2 Mechanism of action of unfractionated heparin (UFH), low-molecular-weight heparin (LMWH), fondaparinux, and bivaliruden. From Clinical practice/controversy: Selection of initial anticoagulant therapy. *Thoracic Key. https://thoracickey.com/clinical-practicecontroversy-selection-of-initial-anticoagulant-therapy/.*

molecule that breaks down the procoagulant factor IIa (thrombin) and factor Xa by forming a complex with AT III and thrombin. Because heparin has a variable effect, it requires monitoring of its activity during a procedure with a goal of an activated partial thromboplastin time (aPTT) of 50 to 75 seconds for most non-PCI applications, or 1.5 to 2.5 times the upper limit of normal. For PCI, anticoagulation is measured using the whole blood activated clotting time (ACT), with a goal of 250 to 350 seconds, or 200 to 250 seconds if using a GP IIb/IIIa inhibitor.

Typically, bolus intravenous (IV) UFH doses in the catheterization laboratory are 70 to 100 units (U)/kg. ACT values measured using the Hemochron tend to run higher than with the I-Stat ACT (Abbott). Repeated ACT measurements should be made approximately every 20 to 30 minutes. Contamination of the blood sample with heparin or contrast from within the guide catheter may artefactually prolong ACT measurements. Continuing heparinization after a successful PCI procedure increases the risk for bleeding without ischemic benefit and is not recommended.

The half-life of IV UFH is 1.5 hours, resulting in normalization of the clotting cascade a few hours after UFH discontinuation. If there is a need to reverse the anticoagulant effect of UFH, protamine sulfate can be given because it binds to the negatively charged heparin molecule, neutralizing it. Protamine dosage for UFH reversal is 1 mg IV per 100 units of remaining active UFH (max 50 mg/dose at 5 mg/min). The routine use of protamine after elective PCI or catheter ablation is not required from the radial approach but may be useful (and safe) to facilitate early femoral sheath removal. Protamine is unnecessary with femoral vascular closure devices.

Protamine allergic reactions include hypotension and bronchoconstriction caused by the histamine released. Reactions can be mitigated with a slow IV infusion. Although most of the protamine sulfate used today is recombinant, caution should be taken in patients with fish allergies because some proportion may still be derived from fish sperm. Patients taking protamine-containing insulin preparations (e.g., NPH insulin) are at increased risk for severe protamine reactions.

Heparin-Induced Thrombocytopenia

Heparin can cause an immune-mediated thrombocytopenia that can lead to thrombosis, stroke, loss of limb, or other ischemic events (e.g., heparin-induced thrombocytopenia with thrombosis [HITT]). Although relatively rare after brief heparin exposures, heparin-induced thrombocytopenia (HIT) should be of concern if platelets fall below 100,000 or by more than 50%.

There are two types of HIT (Table 3.4). Type I HIT (HIT-1) is caused by direct (non–immune-mediated) platelet activation, with mild thrombocytopenia and a benign clinical course. Type II HIT

Table 3.4

Heparin-Induced Thrombocytopenia		
	Type I Heparin-Induced Thrombocytopenia	**Type II Heparin-Induced Thrombocytopenia**
Incidence	10%	Rare (0.2%)
Mechanism	Direct platelet aggregating effect of heparin	Autoantibody (IgG) directed against platelet factor IV–heparin complex
Onset	Early (within 2 days)	Later (4–10 days)
Platelet count	50,000–150,000/mm³	<50,000/mm³
Duration	Transient; often improves even if heparin is continued	Requires discontinuation of all heparin; gradual recovery in platelet count in most patients
Clinical	Benign	Recalcitrant venous and arterial course thromboses and thromboembolism; may be fatal
Heparin	Unfractionated or low-molecular-weight heparin may be continued	Argatroban for longer treatment. Bivalirudin for PCI or short-term treatment Danaparoid and lipirudin not available in USA.

IgG, Immunoglobulin G; *IV*, intravenous; *PCI*, percutaneous coronary intervention

(HIT-2) is caused by immune-mediated platelet activation, with moderate or severe thrombocytopenia and serious thromboembolic complications.

Anticoagulation to prevent thrombosis is the main treatment of HIT-2 patients; typical drugs are the direct-acting thrombin antagonists argatroban or bivalirudin. Patients presenting to the catheterization laboratory with a history of potential HIT should have procedures with heparin-free saline and bivalirudin for anticoagulation.

Low-Molecular-Weight Heparin

Low-molecular-weight heparins (LMWHs; enoxaparin, tinzaparin, dalteparin) are fractionated heparins with molecular weights between 3000 and 7000 daltons (UFH is 3000–30,000 daltons). Like UFH, LMWH binds to antithrombin, causing inhibition of factor Xa and thrombin. Because of improved subcutaneous absorption, LMWH can be administered either subcutaneously (SQ) or IV. LMWHs have features distinct from UFH, including:

1. More predictable anticoagulation effect
2. Lack of inhibition by platelet factor 4
3. Lack of need for monitoring
4. Lower risk for HIT
5. SQ or IV bolus administration

Table 3.5 compares features of LMWHs with UFH.

Absorption and Clearance

Peak plasma anti-Xa levels are achieved 3 to 4 hours after subcutaneous dosing and are detectable for up to 12 hours. LMWH is eliminated via the kidneys and should be used with caution in patients with creatinine clearance of less than 30 mL/min. LMWH has a half-life of 2 to 4 hours longer than UFH.

Monitoring

The ACT assay does not reliably measure the LMWH effect. LMWH activity is measured using blood anti-Xa levels. Routine monitoring is not readily available in many catheterization laboratories and not necessary in most cases. LMWHs have very predictable antithrombotic effects; monitoring and dose adjustment is necessary only in obese patients (body mass index [BMI] > 40) or patients with renal insufficiency.

Clinical Use

Enoxaparin, the best studied among the LMWH, is used mainly for precatheterization treatment of ACS. The therapeutic dose is 1 mg/kg SQ every 12 hours or 0.75 to 1 mg/kg IV for elective PCI

Table 3.5

Comparison of Low-Molecular-Weight and Unfractionated Heparin

Characteristic	Unfractionated Heparin	Low-Molecular-Weight Heparin
Composition	Heterogeneous mix of polysaccharides; molecular weight 3000–30,000	Homogeneous glycosaminoglycans; molecular weight 4000–6000
Mechanisms	Activates antithrombin III*[a]; equivalent activity against factor Xa and thrombin; releases TFPI from endothelium; unable to inactivate clot-bound thrombin or FDP; inactivates fluid phase thrombin	Less activation of antithrombin III; greater activity against factor Xa than thrombin; releases TFPI for endothelium; unable to inactivate clot-bound thrombin or FDP; weaker inactivation of fluid-phase thrombin
Pharmacokinetics	Variable binding to plasma proteins, endothelial cells, and macrophages leads to unpredictable anticoagulant effects (less available to interact with antithrombin III); short half-life	Minimal binding to plasma proteins, endothelial cells, and macrophages leads to predictable anticoagulation; longer half-life
Laboratory monitoring	Unpredictable anticoagulant effects; use aPTT or ACT	Unable to use aPTT or ACT except in renal failure to body weight <50 kg or >80 kg; use antifactor-Xa levels
Clinical uses	Venous thrombosis; unstable angina, acute myocardial infarction, ischemic stroke, PCI	Venous thrombosis in surgery and trauma patients, unstable angina, ischemic stroke. No advantage during PCI
Reversal	Protamine neutralizes antithrombin activity	Protamine neutralizes antithrombin activity but only partially reverses antifactor-Xa activity
History of HIT-2	Should not be used in patients with a history of HIT-2	Should not be used in patients with a history of HIT-2
Cost	Inexpensive	10–20 times more expensive than unfractionated heparin

ACT, Activated clotting time; *aPTT,* activated partial thromboplastin time; *FDP,* fibrin degradation product; *HIT,* heparin-induced thrombocytopenia; *PCI,* percutaneous coronary intervention; *TFPI,* tissue factor pathway inhibitor.
[a]Antithrombin III is now commonly referred to as antithrombin.
Modified from Safian R, Grines C, Freed M. *The new manual of interventional cardiology.* Physicians' Press, 1999.

Table 3.6

Dosing of Enoxaparin Before Percutaneous Coronary Intervention	
Preprocedural Enoxaparin	**IV Bolus Enoxaparin Dose at Time of PCI**
No prior enoxaparin	0.75 mg/kg IV
Prophylactic doses of enoxaparin only	0.5 mg/kg IV
1–2 1 mg/kg SQ doses, last <8 hrs before	0.3 mg/kg IV
1–2 SQ doses, last 8–12 hrs before	0.3–0.5 mg/kg IV
Adequate (>3) SQ doses, last <8 hrs before	No additional enoxaparin
Adequate (>3) SQ doses, last 8–12 hrs before	0.3 mg/kg IV
Any doses, >12 hours	Can use alternative antithrombin

IV, Intravenous; *PCI,* percutaneous coronary intervention; *SQ,* subcutaneous.

where no other anticoagulant has been given. To optimize anti-Xa activity for PCI, an additional IV booster dose of 0.3 mg/kg is given if PCI is performed 8 to 12 hours after the prior SQ dose, particularly if fewer than three previous SQ doses have been received by the patient. Table 3.6 provides dosing of enoxaparin for PCI.

Switching from one anticoagulant strategy to another (i.e., LMWH to UFH) is associated with increased bleeding risk and is discouraged.

Overall, LMWH is considered equivalent to UFH for ACS and PCI. Its advantages include a predictable dosing, ease of administration, and lower risk for HIT. LMWH has primarily been used in ACS in Europe and Canada, whereas it is only occasionally used in the US.

Fondaparinux

The heparinoid fondaparinux is a synthetic pentasaccharide that is derived from the binding regions of UFH and LWH. It inhibits factor Xa with antithrombin at high potency, with a SQ dose of 2.5 mg daily. Unexpected episodes of catheter thrombosis were noted with fondaparinux (0.9% vs. 0.4%), and therefore, this agent should not be used for anticoagulation during PCI. Operators should routinely use a standard bolus of UFH at the time of PCI for patients pretreated with fondaparinux.

Direct Thrombin Inhibitors

Direct thrombin inhibitors are polypeptide or low-molecular-weight inhibitors of thrombin that do not require antithrombin for

Table 3.7

Direct Thrombin Inhibitors

Polypeptide Inhibitors

Hirudin (lepirudin[b], desirudin[b])
Bivalirudin

Low-Molecular-Weight Inhibitors

Argatroban[a]
Dabigatran

[a]Approved for use in patients with heparin-induced thrombocytopenia (HIT).
[b]Discontinued in the US.

anticoagulant effect (Table 3.7). Low-molecular-weight inhibitors inactivate circulating thrombin at the active binding site but do not inactivate clot-bound thrombin.

Bivalirudin is a 20-amino acid polypeptide with a chemical structure like hirudin that is frequently used in PCI. It binds bivalently (at both the active site and exosite-1) and reversibly to both circulating and clot-bound thrombin with prompt recovery of thrombin function after drug discontinuation. This specific pharmacology potentially leads to reductions in bleeding complications and increased efficacy against thrombus.

Bivalirudin is given as an IV bolus of 0.75 mg/kg, with an infusion of 1.75 mg/kg/hr. It has a rapid onset of action of 5 minutes. Bivalirudin is excreted by the kidney and has a short half-life of 25 minutes in patients with normal renal function. The infusion should be dose-adjusted in renal insufficiency, but PCI procedures may be so brief that dose adjustment may be unnecessary unless the infusion is continued post-PCI.

Clinical Use

Compared with UFH with glycoprotein inhibitors, bivalirudin demonstrates equal efficacy with a reduced risk for bleeding in patients with unstable angina/non–ST-segment elevation myocardial infarction (UA/NSTEMI; see the REPLACE-2, ACUITY, MATRIX trials) and in ST-segment elevation myocardial infarction (STEMI; the HORIZONS-AMI trial). In the absence of glycoprotein IIb/IIIa receptor inhibitors (GPI) and particularly with radial access, bleeding is not necessarily reduced (VALIDATE-SWEDEHEART trial).

Bivalirudin is associated with an increased risk for acute stent thrombosis because the drug's short duration of action may not sufficiently protect against thrombosis while the dual antiplatelet medications take effect. The bivalirudin infusion may be extended

Table 3.8

Comparison of Unfractionated Heparin and Bivalirudin		
	Unfractionated Heparin	**Bivalirudin**
Effect on clot-bound thrombin	None	Inactivation
Effect on thrombin	High-affinity interaction; inhibits thrombin and factor Xa	High-affinity interaction
Effect on factor Xa bound to platelets	None	Inactivation
Binding to endothelium and plasma proteins	High; results in less heparin availability to activate antithrombin	None
Risk of heparin-induced thrombocytopenia	High	None
Anticoagulant effects	Highly variable	Predictable
Laboratory monitoring	Essential	May be unnecessary with bivalirudin

at full dose for up to 4 hours after the procedure if antiplatelet agents are delayed, although the benefit of this approach on stent thrombosis rates remains unclear (MATRIX trial). Patients with femoral access, planned PCI, preprocedural P2Y12 inhibition, and high bleeding risk may benefit from bivalirudin.

IV infusion of argatroban is approved for treatment of HIT, with limited case reports of its use in PCI.

Table 3.8 compares UFH with direct thrombin inhibitors.

Oral Anticoagulants

Oral anticoagulants (OAC) are typically used for patients with conditions such as atrial fibrillation or prior venous thromboembolism (VTE). The concomitant use of OAC is a marker for high bleeding risk. Multiple contemporary randomized trials (WOEST, PIONEER-PCI, AUGUSTUS) have demonstrated that compared with triple therapy (warfarin + aspirin + clopidogrel), dual therapy with a P2Y12 inhibitor (usually clopidogrel) and an OAC reduces bleeding without increasing major adverse cardiovascular event (MACE) rates. These agents are best held before planned procedures because they increase the risk of bleeding from other anticoagulants for PCI.

Warfarin

Warfarin acts by inhibiting the gamma-carboxylation of glutamic acid residues in the clotting proteins II (prothrombin), VII, IX, and X. Despite the increasing use of direct OAC (DOACs), warfarin retains a role for patients with mechanical heart valves and active left ventricular or atrial thrombus.

Warfarin requires 4 to 7 days to produce a therapeutic level as measured by the international normalized ratio (INR). For femoral procedures, warfarin is held for several days to obtain a preprocedure INR of less than 1.8. Transradial procedures can often be safely performed regardless of the INR. The practice of "bridging" anticoagulation with LMWH or UFH before most surgical procedures is largely nonbeneficial and associated with higher bleeding rates. Bridging should be reserved for patients with mechanical heart valves or active VTE.

Oral Anti-Xa Inhibitors

The oral anti-Xa inhibitors (i.e., novel oral anticoagulants [NOAC] rivaroxaban, apixaban, and edoxaban) are replacing warfarin in many patients, but their role in PCI is uncertain currently. Rivaroxaban 2.5 mg twice daily has demonstrated a benefit in ACS patients after stabilization and revascularization (ATLAS ACS 2-TIMI 51 trial) and in the vascular disease patient in secondary prevention of MACE (COMPASS trial) but at the cost of increased bleeding.

The NOACs can generally be held 24 to 48 hours before planned procedures to minimize the risk of bleeding during PCI.

Antiplatelet Agents

Antiplatelet agents are required for stenting and are very useful for primary and secondary prevention of thrombotic cerebrovascular or cardiovascular disease. Antiplatelet drugs decrease platelet aggregation and inhibit thrombus formation to prevent both acute and chronic stent thrombosis. These drugs are highly effective in the arterial circulation, where anticoagulants have reduced effect. Coupled with antithrombin drugs (e.g., heparin or bivalirudin), the antiplatelet drugs are the mainstay of PCI pharmacology.

There are multiple classes of antiplatelet drugs, each with different mechanisms of action. Several drugs are often given together for synergistic inhibition of platelet activity (weighing the risk of bleeding against benefit of preventing thrombosis). The classes of antiplatelet drugs are:

- Cyclooxygenase inhibitors (aspirin)
- Adenosine diphosphate (ADP) receptor inhibitors (clopidogrel [Plavix], prasugrel [Effient], ticlopidine [Ticlid], ticagrelor [Brilinta], cangrelor [Kengreal])
- Phosphodiesterase inhibitors (cilostazol [Pletal])
- GPIs (abciximab [ReoPro], eptifibatide [Integrilin], tirofiban [Aggrastat])
- Adenosine reuptake inhibitors (dipyridamole [Persantine])
- Thrombin receptor (PAR-1) antagonist (Vorapaxar)

Aspirin

Aspirin acetylate irreversibly binds and inactivates platelet cyclooxygenase, inhibiting production of thromboxane A2 (TXA2), which is a potent inducer of platelet aggregation and vasoconstriction via the production of cyclic adenosine monophosphate. Aspirin 81 mg is considered effective for most indications, but 162 to 325 mg is indicated for ACS. After oral ingestion, rapid absorption occurs with peak plasma levels in 20 minutes. Aspirin is rapidly cleared, but its effects last for the lifetime of the platelet (7–10 days). The whole-blood bleeding time can be used to gauge aspirin's effect on platelet function, but this is rarely necessary. Aspirin should be used with caution in those with aspirin allergies (asthma), active peptic ulcer disease, or predisposition to bleeding. Platelet resistance to aspirin is rare.

Clopidogrel

Together with aspirin, clopidogrel, a thienopyridine, is the most used antiplatelet agent. The thienopyridine drug class affects the ADP-dependent activation of platelet aggregation and adhesion through the IIb/IIIa receptors (see Fig. 3.2).

Clopidogrel has a plasma half-life of 6 to 8 hours, but its onset of action is typically 2 hours with peak effect only occurring at 6 hours. An unidentified hepatic metabolite of clopidogrel interferes with platelet membrane function by inhibiting ADP-induced platelet-fibrinogen binding (via von Willebrand factor) and platelet-to-platelet interactions (via platelet receptor IIb/IIIa). Platelets exposed to the active metabolite are inhibited for their lifetime, about 7 to 10 days. Patients with variants of the CYP2C19 allele are poor metabolizers of clopidogrel and exhibit resistance to its effect. The dose of clopidogrel is a 300 to 600 mg per os (PO) load before or at the time of PCI, then 75 mg PO daily. Classic trials demonstrating the benefit of clopidogrel with aspirin in ACS include the CURE, CREDO, CLARITY, and COMMIT trials.

Prasugrel

Prasugrel is a thienopyridine prodrug whose metabolite irreversibly inhibits the ADP receptor. Like clopidogrel, it requires a two-step metabolism; however, one step is mediated by serum esterases, which results in prasugrel exhibiting a high degree of platelet inhibition regardless of cytochrome P450 (CYP) inhibitors or variants. Its onset of action is rapid at 30 minutes with effective inhibition at 2 hours in most cases. Its duration of effect is longer than clopidogrel at 5 to 10 days and thus should be discontinued 7 days before major surgery. Prasugrel is administered as a 60 mg oral load at the time of PCI and 10 mg daily thereafter. Preloading of prasugrel is not beneficial and caused more bleeding in the ACCOAST trial. The TRITON-TIMI 38 trial randomized 13,608 patients with ACS to either prasugrel or clopidogrel and showed that prasugrel reduced MACE but had a higher bleeding rate.

Prasugrel should be avoided in patients with a history of stroke or transient ischemic attack (TIA), age greater than 75 years, and patients with low body weight (<60kg) who had a higher risk for bleeding in clinical trials.

Ticagrelor

Ticagrelor is a newer ADP-receptor antagonist called a cyclopentyltriazolopyrimidine. It binds reversibly to the P2Y12 receptor and has a half-life of 12 hours. Ticagrelor requires no metabolism for activity, exhibits a rapid onset of action, and has high levels of platelet inhibition. Based on its shorter half-life and reversible inhibition, ticagrelor may be held for as little as 1 to 3 days before coronary artery bypass graft surgery (CABG). It must be administered twice daily at a dose of 90 mg after a 180-mg loading dose. There is also up to a 15% rate of dyspnea and an increase in heart block with ticagrelor, which may be complicating factors after myocardial infarction (MI).

Ticagrelor reduced MACE in ACS compared with clopidogrel without any difference in the rates of major bleeding from clopidogrel (11.2% vs. 11.6%, $p = 0.43$, PLATO trial). Ticagrelor was found to have an overall mortality benefit compared with clopidogrel (4.5% vs. 5.9%, $p < .01$), which was driven by reductions in cardiovascular death. Aside from ACS, ticagrelor has indications for patients with a history of MI and extended use (PEGASUS trial). It also has been tested as monotherapy without aspirin, which may reduce bleeding (TWILIGHT trial).

Although ticagrelor was presumed to be superior to prasugrel based on indirect comparisons with clopidogrel, in the only head-to-head trial comparing ticagrelor and prasugrel (ISAR-REACT5), 4018 patients with ACS (>80% undergoing PCI) were found to have higher 1-year MACE rates with ticagrelor compared with prasugrel, with no differences in major bleeding.

Glycoprotein IIb/IIIa Receptor Blockers

The most potent antiplatelet agents are the GPIs (abciximab [ReoPro], eptifibatide [Integrilin], tirofiban [Aggrastat]), which are administered intravenously. These agents exhibit rapid and high levels (>90%) of platelet inhibition because they act on the final step in platelet aggregation, the binding of the platelet to fibrinogen. As a group, these agents reduce ischemic complications (~9% relative risk reduction) but also increase the risk for bleeding.

Abciximab is a monoclonal antibody to the GPIIb/IIIa receptor, which has a prolonged effect (48 hours) and risks for thrombocytopenia; because of its relative expense, it has been largely supplanted by the small molecule inhibitors eptifibatide and tirofiban.

Eptifibatide is administered as a double IV bolus of 180 mcg/kg 10 minutes apart and an infusion of 2 mcg/kg/min for up to 24 hours after PCI.

Tirofiban is administered as a high dose bolus of 25 mcg/kg IV and 0.15 mcg/kg/min IV for up to 18 hours. Both tirofiban and eptifibatide have 2- to 2.5-hour plasma half-lives and shorter duration of effect of 4 to 6 hours. Platelet transfusion can reverse the effect of abciximab but not the small molecule inhibitors. Excess bleeding with GPIs can be potentially reduced with shorter post-PCI infusions, bolus-only regimens, and radial access.

GPIs have primarily demonstrated a benefit in ACS patients treated with an invasive approach, although the more commonly practiced use of oral dual-antiplatelet therapy has largely supplanted the routine administration of these agents. The benefits of GPIIb/IIIa inhibition are highest in those patients with elevated thrombolysis in myocardial infarction (TIMI) risk scores (>4), especially those with positive troponin assays. It is reasonable to delay the administration of GPIIb/IIIa agents until the time of PCI because the benefit of "upstream" treatment is nearly balanced by an increased risk for bleeding except in cases of STEMI.

Although the ischemic benefits of GPIIb/IIIa inhibitors were primarily demonstrated in the pre-clopidogrel era, they have been shown to persist in more contemporary studies. Their role in the era of potent oral P2Y12 inhibition with prasugrel and ticagrelor remains unclear. Nevertheless, in patients with STEMI or NSTEMI not pretreated with P2Y12 inhibitors, the onset of action of all oral P2Y12 inhibitors is delayed by 2 to 6 hours, putting the patient at

Table 3.9

Platelet Glycoprotein IIb/IIIa Antagonists for Percutaneous Coronary Intervention

	Abciximab	Eptifibatide	Tirofiban
Dose for PCI	0.25 mg/kg IV bolus plus 0.125 µg/kg/min (maximum 10 µg/min) IV infusion for 12 hr. Low-dose heparin and early sheath removal to minimize bleeding. For patients with unstable angina planning to undergo PCI within 24 hr, bolus plus infusion of abciximab (PCI dose) can be started up to 24 hr before PCI and continued at the same rate until 1 hr after the procedure.	*Acute coronary syndromes (PURSUIT dose):* 180 µg/kg IV bolus plus 2.0 µg/kg/min IV infusion. If arrive in cath lab >4 hr after initiating therapy, no additional bolus is required. *Percutaneous intervention (ESPRIT dose):* 2 × 180 µg/kg/min IV bolus 10 min apart, plus 2.0 µg/kg/min IV infusion for 18–24 hr.	25 mcg/kg IV bolus (over 5 min) followed by an infusion of 0.15 mcg/kg/min for 18 hr (high-dose bolus). Patients with creatinine clearances <60 mL/min should receive the same bolus but half the usual infusion rate.

ACT, Activated clotting time; *IV,* intravenous; *PCI,* percutaneous coronary intervention, *PO,* per os.

risk for stent thrombosis after PCI. As a result, IV antiplatelet agents or cangrelor might be needed. Table 3.9 summarizes the use of glycoprotein receptor blockers for PCI.

Cangrelor. Cangrelor is an IV P2Y12 antagonist with a rapid onset of action (2–3 minutes) and rapid recovery of platelet function after discontinuation. In the CHAMPION-PHOENIX trial, compared with oral clopidogrel at the time of or immediately after PCI, cangrelor-treated patients had a lower risk for recurrent MI or stent thrombosis at the cost of an increase in minor but not major bleeding. As a result, in patients who were not adequately pretreated with clopidogrel before PCI, cangrelor may provide sufficient platelet inhibition to conduct PCI safely.

The clinical efficacy of cangrelor compared with ticagrelor or prasugrel at the time of PCI is unclear but may persist given the known delays in absorption and activity of all oral P2Y12 inhibitors. Cangrelor provides less powerful platelet inhibition than tirofiban but faster onset of action compared with oral loading of prasugrel.

Cangrelor binds competitively with the P2Y12 receptor and prevents the binding of prasugrel or clopidogrel. Oral loading doses of these agents should be administered only after cangrelor is discontinued, making cangrelor less useful for bridging to the onset of absorption and action of these agents compared with the GPIs. The effect of ticagrelor is unchanged by the presence of cangrelor.

Duration of Dual Antiplatelet Therapy

Increasingly shorter durations of dual antiplatelet therapy (DAPT) have been studied for patients treated with the newest drug-eluting stents, in elective PCI, and in patients with high bleeding risk (Fig. 3.3). Longer durations of 6 to 12 months remain recommended for lower bleeding risk patients and all ACS patients, given the higher risk of MACE. Long-term DAPT (>1 year) with clopidogrel or ticagrelor has been shown to be potentially beneficial in secondary prevention in patients with a low risk for bleeding. The use of short or prolonged DAPT is best guided by validated risk scores, such as the PRECISE-DAPT (Predicting Bleeding Complications In Patients Undergoing Stent Implantation and Subsequent Dual Anti Platelet Therapy) and DAPT scores (Fig. 3.4)

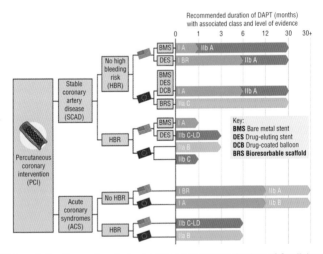

Figure 3.3 Comparison between US and European Society of Cardiology (ESC) guidelines regarding duration of antiplatelet therapy in patients after percutaneous coronary intervention (PCI) with and without acute coronary syndrome or high bleeding risk. From Capodanno D, Alfonso F, Levine GN, Valgimigli M, Angiolillo DJ. ACC/AHA versus ESC guidelines on dual antiplatelet therapy: JACC guideline comparison. *J Am Coll Cardiol.* 2018;72(23 Pt A):2915–2931, central illustration, with permission.

Time of use	PRECISE-DAPT score[18]						DAPT score[15]
	At the time of coronary stenting						After 12 months of uneventful DAPT
DAPT duration strategies assessed	Short DAPT (3–6 months) vs. Standard/long DAPT (12–24 months)						Standard DAPT (12 months) vs. Long DAPT (30 months)

Score calculation[a]	HB	≥12 11·5 11 10·5 ≤10					Age
							  ≥75 −2 pt
							  65 to <75 −1 pt
							  <65 0 pt
							Cigarette smoking +1 pt
							Diabetes mellitus +1 pt
							MI at presentation +1 pt
							Prior PCI or prior MI +1 pt
							Paclitaxel-eluting stent +1 pt
							Stent diameter <3 mm +1 pt
							CHF or LVEF <30% +2 pt
							Vein graft stent +2 pt

	WBC	≤5 8 10 12 14 16 18 ≥20					
	Age	≤50 60 70 80 ≥90					
	CrCl	≥100 80 60 40 20 0					
	Prior Bleeding	No / Yes					
	Score Points	0 2 4 6 8 10 12 14 16 18 20 22 24 26 28 30					
Score range	0 to 100 points						−2 to 10 points
Decision making cut-off suggested	Score ≥25 → Short DAPT Score <25 → Standard/long DAPT						Score ≥2 → Long DAPT Score <2 → Standard DAPT
Calculator	www.precisedaptscore.com						www.daptstudy.org

Figure 3.4 Use of the PRECISE-DAPT and DAPT scores to determine duration of dual antiplatelet therapy. *CHF,* Congestive heart failure; *CrCl,* creatinine clearance; *DAPT,* dual antiplatelet therapy; *Hb,* hemoglobin; *LVEF,* left ventricular ejection fraction; *MI,* myocardial infarction; *PCI,* percutaneous coronary intervention; *PRECISE-DAPT,* Predicting Bleeding Complications In Patients Undergoing Stent Implantation and Subsequent Dual Anti Platelet Therapy; *WBC,* white blood cell count. From Valgimigli M, Bueno H, Byrne RA, et al. 2017 ESC focused update on dual antiplatelet therapy in coronary artery disease developed in collaboration with EACTS: The Task Force for dual antiplatelet therapy in coronary artery disease of the European Society of Cardiology (ESC) and of the European Association for Cardio-Thoracic Surgery (EACTS). *Eur Heart J.* 2018;39(3):213–260, Table 3, with permission.

De-Escalation in the Intensity of Anticoagulants and Antiplatelet Therapy

Because the risk of stent thrombosis is highest in the first month after PCI or ACS but declines thereafter (Fig. 3.5), de-escalation from potent P2Y12 inhibitors such as ticagrelor or prasugrel with aspirin to clopidogrel may be a reasonable strategy in high-risk bleeding patients (TROPICAL-ACS, TOPIC trials).

Platelet Function Testing

Although there is considerable literature about platelet function testing and resistance, evidence linking posttreatment platelet reactivity to long-term ischemic events is weak. At this time, it is not justified to routinely test for platelet resistance in the clinical setting. Platelet function testing may be helpful in a patient with recent subacute stent thrombosis, although such patients should likely be changed to a potent antiplatelet agent in most cases. Patients with a recently implanted stent who require surgery may benefit from platelet function testing before the procedure to document residual platelet activity and minimize periprocedural bleeding. If platelet function is near normal, one can proceed with surgery as needed. If platelet function is greatly impaired, then the timing of surgery must be balanced against the timing of the P2Y12 inhibitor withdrawal.

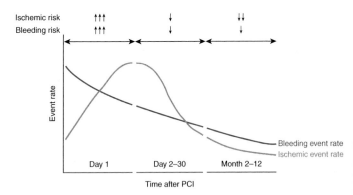

Figure 3.5 Conceptual risk of ischemic versus bleeding complications after percutaneous coronary intervention (PCI), demonstrating the potential benefits of short duration dual-antiplatelet therapy or de-escalation. From Kupka, D, Sibbing D. De-escalation of P2Y12 receptor inhibitor therapy after acute coronary syndromes in patients undergoing percutaneous coronary intervention. *Korean Circ J.* 2018;48(10): 863–872, Figure 1.

Thrombolytic Agents

Thrombolytic agents are proteins that convert a plasma proenzyme, plasminogen, to the active enzyme plasmin. Plasmin then solubilizes fibrin and degrades several other plasma proteins, most notably fibrinogen, ultimately producing clot lysis. All the currently available thrombolytic (fibrinolytic) agents are plasminogen activators. They all work enzymatically, directly, or indirectly to convert the single-chain plasminogen molecule to the double-chain plasmin (which has potent intrinsic fibrinolytic activity).

Tissue Plasminogen Activator

Derived by recombinant genetics from human DNA, tissue plasminogen activator (t-PA) is fibrin specific and activates plasminogen associated with fibrin directly by enzymatic action. The plasma half-life is 5 minutes, requiring an IV bolus and infusion.

TNKase

TNKase is a nonglycosylated deletion mutation of t-PA (contains 355 out of 527 of the amino acids that t-PA contains). It is given as a dose of 10 units and then again as a 10-unit double bolus injection. Each bolus is given intravenously over 2 minutes. The second bolus is given 30 minutes after the first (supplied as a kit of two single-use vials). Dosing is based on weight (<60 kg, 30 mg IV over 5 minutes, maximum 50 mg; weight 60 to 69 kg, 35 mg IV, maximum 50 mg; weight >70 kg, 40 mg IV, maximum 50 mg).

Precautions and Contraindications

See Table 3.10. Bleeding is the major complication of thrombolytic therapy. Consequently, absolute contraindications include dissecting aortic aneurysm, pericarditis, stroke, or neurosurgical procedures within 6 months of known intracranial neoplasm. Relative contraindications include major surgery or bleeding within 6 weeks, known bleeding diathesis, and severe uncontrolled hypertension. Allergic reactions are associated most with anisoylated plasminogen streptokinase activator complex. t-PA also induces antibody production, which makes treatment with either of these agents less effective.

Clinical Use

Thrombolytics are primarily used for urgent revascularization of patients with STEMI where primary PCI is unavailable or would be

Table 3.10

Contraindications and Precautions for Thrombolytic Use in Myocardial Infarction

Contraindications

- Previous hemorrhagic stroke at any time, other strokes, or cerebrovascular events within 1 year
- Known intracranial neoplasm
- Active internal bleeding (does not include menses)
- Suspected aortic dissection

Caution/Relative Contraindications

- Severe uncontrolled hypertension on presentation (blood pressure >180/110 mm Hg)[a]
- History of prior cerebrovascular accident or known intracerebral pathology not covered in contraindications
- Current use of anticoagulants in therapeutic doses (INR 2–3); known bleeding diathesis
- Recent trauma (within 2–4 wk) including head trauma or traumatic or prolonged (>10 min) CPR or major surgery (3 wk)
- Noncompressible vascular punctures
- Recent (within 2–4 wk) internal bleeding
- For streptokinase/anistreplase: prior exposure (especially within 5 days to 2 years) or prior allergic reaction
- Pregnancy
- Active peptic ulcer
- History of chronic severe hypertension

These contraindications and cautions are viewed as advisory for clinical decision making and may not be all-inclusive or definitive.
CPR, Cardiopulmonary resuscitation; *INR,* international normalized ratio.
[a]Could be an absolute contraindication in low-risk patients with myocardial infarction.
Reproduced with permission from Ryan TJ, Antman EM, Brooks NH, et al. ACC/AHA guidelines for the management of patients with acute myocardial infarction: A report of the American College of Cardiology/American Heart Association Task Force on Practice Guidelines (Committee on Management of Acute Myocardial Infarction). *J Am Coll Cardiol* 1999;34:890–911.

delayed by longer than 60 minutes. They are effective in approximately 70% of cases of STEMI, at the cost of an increased risk for bleeding. Urgent transfer to a PCI-capable center is indicated for the possible rescue PCI. The routine use of thrombolytics as part of a planned pharmacoinvasive approach has not been found to be beneficial. Similarly, intracoronary administration of thrombolytics is discouraged.

Thrombolytics are used widely for venous and peripheral arterial procedures, including for deep venous thrombosis, pulmonary embolism, and acute leg ischemia. They have also been reported to have been given intracoronary for treatment of intracoronary thrombus that has been resistant to other mechanical and pharmacologic therapies.

Vasodilators

Adenosine

Adenosine, an endogenous nucleoside, is the most used vasodilatory agent for hyperemia induction (Table 3.11). Stimulation of the adenosine A2a receptor causes vasodilatation and hyperemia (increased flow) in the coronary circulation, and the A1 receptor causes bradycardia. The A2b receptor causes bronchoconstriction. Adenosine is rapidly inactivated by adenosine deaminases in red blood cells and endothelium, resulting in a short duration of action.

Exogenous adenosine for coronary hemodynamic measurements has a short half-life and relatively few persistent side effects.

Table 3.11

Vasodilatory Agents for Hyperemia Induction			
Agent	**Route**	**Dose**	**Comments**
Adenosine	IV	140 mcg/kg/min	Reference standard used in trials. Side effects of dyspnea, chest pain, bradycardia. Inconsistently causes sustained hyperemia.
Adenosine	IC	60–100 mcg (RCA) 100–200 mcg (LCA)	Fewer systemic side effects than IV, rapid onset of hyperemia that lasts 15–20 seconds. Rapidly repeatable. Requires guide catheter engagement that may risk dampening.
Regadenoson	IC	0.4 mg	Expensive. Variable duration of hyperemia, potentially prolonged.
Nitroprusside	IC	0.6 mcg/kg	Easy to use but causes significant hypotension.
Nicorandil	IC	2 mg	Fewer side effects than adenosine. Not available in United States.
Papaverine	IC	10–20 mg	Rare side effect of polymorphic VT (2%–3%).

IC, Intravenous cannula; *IV*, intravenous; *LCA*, left coronary artery; *RCA*, right coronary artery; *VT*, ventricular tachycardia

It is injected via the IV (typically 140 mcg/kg/min) or intracoronary (IC) route (40–200 mcg). IC adenosine (50–200 mg) may be helpful in resolving cases of slow- or no-refill after PCI. Adenosine is administered in larger doses (6–12mg IV) for suppression of atrioventricular node conduction, which is a diagnostic and therapeutic maneuver in the treatment of supraventricular tachycardia. Adenosine should be used with caution in patients at risk for bronchospasm and is contraindicated in patients on dipyramidole. Recent ingestion of caffeine at high doses may inhibit the response to IV adenosine, but the effect is modest at clinically relevant doses.

Nitroglycerin

Nitroglycerin is an arterial and venous vasodilator with multiple uses in the cath lab. It is administered via the intraarterial route to relieve coronary spasm and prevent spasm from IC tools, such as intravascular ultrasound catheters or coronary wires. Nitroglycerin relieves angina and heart failure by causing coronary dilatation and reducing preload and afterload.

Nitroglycerin can be administered via the IC, IV, transdermal, and sublingual routes. Typical doses range from 50 to 300 mcg IC, 20 to 200 mcg/min IV, and 0.3 to 0.4 mg sublingual. Doses can be repeated until the desired effect is generated or hypotension develops. Tachyphylaxis can occur with chronic nitroglycerine use.

Papaverine

Papaverine is a vasodilator opioid derivative that inhibits phosphodiesterase, resulting in elevated cyclic adenosine monophosphate (AMP) levels. It is a direct smooth muscle vasodilator that affects both the coronary and peripheral circulation. It is approved to treat spasms of the gastrointestinal tract and is also used to treat erectile dysfunction and migraine headaches. IC papaverine produces consistent vasodilatation and hyperemia (lasting about 2 minutes), making it useful for fractional flow reserve measurements. Nevertheless, it is associated with QT prolongation and occasional polymorphic ventricular tachycardia (VT) and ventricular fibrillation (2–3%), constipation, hypotension, and tachycardia.

Calcium Channel Blockers

Calcium channel blockers dilate vascular smooth muscle and reduce heart muscle contractility, and some agents block atrioventricular nodal conduction. Calcium channel blockers are used to reduce peripheral vascular resistance, decrease blood pressure, block coronary spasm, and increase coronary blood flow. Acute use in the cardiac catheterization laboratory is limited to treating arrhythmias and no-reflow of coronary interventions or to treat radial artery spasm when the transradial approach is used. Because of variable absorption, sublingual administration is not recommended.

Verapamil is a nondihydropyridine calcium channel blocker used in supraventricular tachycardia and vasodilator for radial artery procedures. Although compared with dihydropyridines it has minimal vasodilatory effects, in patients with no-reflow or slow-reflow after PCI, verapamil is effective in improving distal perfusion. The typical dose ranges from 100 mcg to 1000 mcg IC, with heart block and bradycardia as the main side effects. Other routes for verapamil are orally (120 mg) or intravenously (2.5–5 mg IV; for coronary no-reflow, intracoronary bolus of verapamil, 200 μg, to be repeated for two to four doses if needed). Doses for diltiazem are 30 to 60 mg orally, 10 mg IV.

Nicorandil

Nicorandil is an antianginal medication with properties of nitrates and K+-ATPase agonist. It is not available in the US. Nicorandil stimulates guanylate cyclase to increase cGMP formation, which increases protein kinase G to cause increased activity of the K+ ATPase, resulting in hyperpolarization and inhibition of smooth muscle constriction. It causes dilatation of the epicardial coronary arteries at low concentrations and reductions in coronary vascular resistance at high concentrations. It has been demonstrated to be safe and potentially cardioprotective during PCI. Nicorandil (2 mg IC) is administered for hyperemia for hemodynamic measurements and has fewer side effects (heart block) compared with adenosine. Nicorandil may be useful to prevent and treat no-reflow.

Nitroprusside

Nitroprusside is a direct arterial vasodilator, acting by supplying nitric oxide to the arteriole smooth muscle. It is used for patients with hypertensive crisis as a continuous infusion. IC nitroprusside (0.6 mcg/kg IC bolus) acts as a hyperemic agent for hemodynamic measurements but is infrequently used because it causes significant hypotension in higher doses.

Nitroprusside may be beneficial in patients with no-reflow, typically at a dose of 100 mcg IC, but this benefit was not confirmed in a larger trial. Nitroprusside is inactivated by light and

Table 3.12

Agents for Treatment of No-Reflow	
First-line	Adenosine (10–100 mcg intracoronary [IC] for treatment; 24–48 mcg IC for prevention)
	Verapamil (100 mcg IC, up to 1500 mcg total)
	Nitroprusside (100 mcg IC, repeated boluses)
	Nicorandil (2 mg IC, single dose)
Second-line	Diltiazem (0.5–2.5 mg IC bolus, up to 5–10 mg)
	Papaverine (10 mg IC)
	Nicardipine (200 mcg IC, mean dose 460 mcg)
Controversial, probably ineffective	Glycoprotein inhibitors (Effective in prevention but unclear benefit in treatment)
	Forceful injection of saline
Ineffective	Nitroglycerin (but can resolve superimposed spasm)
	Stenting, bypass surgery
	Thrombolytics

must be stored in protective (dark) IV bags. It has a very short onset and duration of action of less than 3 minutes. Cyanide toxicity can occur in patients with renal insufficiency with prolonged use.

Nicardipine

Nicardipine is a dihydropyridine IV calcium channel blocker that causes arteriolar vasodilation with minimal inotropic or chronotropic effects. It is used in hypertensive crisis, where it can be infused at up to 15 mg/hour. It may be helpful in prevention or treatment of no-reflow.

Table 3.12 lists the vasodilators used in the treatment of coronary no-reflow during PCI.

Inotropes

Dobutamine

Dobutamine is an exogenous inotropic agent that stimulates the adrenergic beta-1 and beta-2 receptors with no peripheral vasoconstrictor effects. It increases cardiac inotropy and chronotropy, making it useful in congestive heart failure, cardiogenic shock, and bradycardia. Dobutamine should be started at a low rate (0.5–1.0 mcg/kg/min) and titrated by the patient's systemic blood pressure, urine flow, frequency of ectopic activity, heart rate, pulmonary capillary wedge pressure, and cardiac output. Dobutamine may be used in conjunction with a potent vasodilator, such as nitroprusside, in patients with markedly elevated filling pressures and poor cardiac output. In the cath lab, dobutamine is used to differentiate true low-flow, low-gradient aortic stenosis from pseudostenosis.

Vasoconstrictors

Dopamine

Dopamine is an endogenous amine with multiple actions. In normal subjects, dopamine stimulates the dopamine receptor at low doses (3–5 mcg/kg/min IV), the beta receptor at intermediate doses (5–10 mcg/kg/min), and the alpha receptor at high doses (10–20 mcg/kg/min). The specific action of dopamine may vary with the dose and the patient's particular condition. At low doses, dopamine increases renal perfusion, but the effect is not clinically meaningful. Dopamine is readily available and useful for shock but, because of its various actions, has been largely supplanted by norepinephrine.

Norepinephrine

Norepinephrine (also known as levophed) is a neurotransmitter synthesized from dopamine. It is released from the adrenal medulla into the blood as a hormone. It activates the sympathetic nervous system via the binding to adrenergic receptors when it is released from noradrenergic neurons. Norepinephrine is a potent vasopressor for patients with critical hypotension. It is given intravenously and acts on both alpha-1 and alpha-2 adrenergic receptors to cause vasoconstriction. It increases blood pressure through the increase in peripheral vascular resistance. At high doses, and especially when it is combined with other vasopressors, it can lead to limb ischemia and limb death. Norepinephrine is mainly used to treat patients in vasodilatory shock states such as septic shock and neurogenic shock and has shown a survival benefit over dopamine. Dosing of norepinephrine begins at 2 to 4 mcg/min for an initial bolus with a maintenance dose of 1 to 12 mcg/min.

Epinephrine

Epinephrine (1:10,000) is a naturally occurring catecholamine that stimulates cardiac function. It is administered only during cardiac emergencies. This medicine increases heart rate and blood pressure immediately, sometimes to very high levels. Epinephrine should be reserved for patients needing cardiac resuscitation, patients in whom refractory hypotension is present and not responding to peripheral vasoconstrictors, or patients with ana-phylactic reactions. Transthoracic administration of epinephrine through a long needle is no longer performed. IV or intraarterial administration of 1 mL of 1:10,000 dilution can increase systemic pressure transiently during hypotension to a safe level until IV vasopressors have been prepared. This dose of epinephrine has a duration of action of 5 to 10 minutes. For management of cardiac arrest, an IV dose of 1:10,000 (0.1 mg/mL) solution at 0.1 to 1 mg (1–10 mL), repeated every 5 minutes, as necessary, is recommended. Alternatively, in intubated patients, epinephrine can be injected via the endotracheal tube directly into the bronchial tree at the same dose as for IV injection. Epinephrine is life saving for patients in anaphylactic shock.

Phenylephrine

Phenylephrine is a selective alpha-adrenergic agonist that causes arterial vasoconstriction. Phenylephrine increases cardiac afterload without increasing inotropy, potentially reducing cardiac output. It is useful as a resuscitative agent because it provides a rapid increase in blood pressure when given as an IV bolus (100 mcg). It is less effective and should be avoided in cardiogenic shock because systemic vascular resistance is typically elevated.

Phenylephrine increases the blood pressure without increasing the heart rate or contractility. Rarely, reflex bradycardia may accompany the blood pressure increase. This response is especially useful if the heart is already tachycardic and/or has a cardiomyopathy. Phenylephrine is dosed at 0.2 mg/dose (range: 0.1–0.5 mg/dose) every 10 to 15 minutes as needed (initial dose should not exceed 0.5 mg). The IV infusion rate is 100 to 180 mcg/min initially. The usual maintenance dose is 40 to 60 mcg/min. The elimination half-life of phenylephrine is about 2.5 to 3 hours.

Table 3.13 lists the relative receptor activity of the commonly used catecholamines.

Anticholinergics for Vagal Reactions

Atropine

Atropine is used to block vagally induced slowing of the heart rate and hypotension. Doses of 0.6 to 1.2 mg IV can be given immediately and reverse bradycardia and hypotension within 2 minutes. In elderly patients and patients who have pacemakers, the heart

Table 3.13

Activity of Catecholamines					
	Activity at receptors				
Agent	**α1**	**α2**	**β1**	**β2**	**Dopamine**
Dobutamine	+	−	+++	+	−
Dopamine	++	+	++	+++	++++
Norepinephrine	+++	+++	+	−	−
Epinephrine	+++	++	+++	++	−
Phenylephrine	+++	+	−	−	−

rate may not slow during vagal episodes in which the only manifestation is low blood pressure. This low blood pressure can be alleviated by the administration of IV atropine and normal saline. In the rare patient in whom IV access is not immediately available, intraaortic atropine can be administered. Vasoconstrictors are reserved for persistent hypotension after recovery of heart rate.

Antiarrhythmic Drugs

Amiodarone

Amiodarone is used to treat poorly controlled atrial fibrillation and VT. In the catheterization laboratory, amiodarone is indicated for recurrent ventricular fibrillation or recurrent hemodynamically unstable VT. The loading dose is 150 mg IV over 10 minutes (15 mg/min), then 360 mg IV over the next 6 hours (1 mg/min), followed by 540 mg IV over the next 18 hours (0.5 mg/min). After the first 24 hours, a maintenance IV infusion of 720 mg/24 hr (0.5 mg/min) is continued.

In the catheterization laboratory, amiodarone has been associated with bradycardia, hypotension, arrhythmias, heart failure, heart block, sinus arrest, and edema. Amiodarone may reduce hepatic or renal clearance of certain antiarrhythmics (especially flecainide, procainamide, and quinidine). Use of amiodarone with other antiarrhythmics (especially mexiletine, propafenone, quinidine, disopyramide, and procainamide) may induce torsades de pointes. Amiodarone should be used cautiously with antihypertensives, beta-blockers, and calcium channel blockers because of increased cardiac depressant effects and slowing of sinoatrial node and atrioventricular conduction. Amiodarone may potentiate anticoagulant response with the potential for serious or fatal bleeding.

The warfarin dose should be decreased by 33% to 50% when amiodarone is initiated.

Amiodarone is contraindicated in cardiogenic shock, second-degree or third-degree atrioventricular block, and severe sinoatrial node disease resulting in preexisting bradycardia unless a pacemaker is present.

References

Amsterdam EA, Wenger NK, Brindis RG, et al. 2014 AHA/ACC Guideline for the management of patients with Non-ST-Elevation acute coronary syndromes: a report of the American College of Cardiology/American Heart Association Task Force on Practice Guidelines. *J Am Coll Cardiol.* 2014;64(24):e139-e228.

Bhogal S, Mukherjee D, Bagai J, et al. Bivalirudin versus heparin during intervention in acute coronary syndrome: a systematic review of randomized trials. *Cardiovasc Hematol Disord Drug Targets.* 2020;20(1):3-15.

Capodanno D, Alfonso F, Levine GN, Valgimigli M, Angiolillo DJ. ACC/AHA versus ESC guidelines on dual antiplatelet therapy: JACC guideline comparison. *J Am Coll Cardiol.* 2018;72(23 Pt A):2915-2931.

Valgimigli M, Bueno H, Byrne RA, et al. 2017 ESC focused update on dual antiplatelet therapy in coronary artery disease developed in collaboration with EACTS: the Task Force for dual antiplatelet therapy in coronary artery disease of the European Society of Cardiology (ESC) and of the European Association for Cardio-Thoracic Surgery (EACTS). *Eur Heart J.* 2018;39(3):213-260.

Guide Catheters, Guide Extenders, Guidewires, Balloons, and Stents

YOUSEFF AYATT • MEGAN TOOLE • ADHIR SHROFF

KEY POINTS

- Guiding catheter selection remains one of the essential pieces enabling a successful coronary intervention procedure in the cath lab.

- Alternatives, such as using sheathless guides and guide catheter extensions, are now available to facilitate interventional procedures.

- Numerous coronary guidewires are available today for operators to choose from, including several workhorse wires, hydrophilic coated wires, and specialty wires that have niche applications.

- Coronary balloon catheters range from compliant to non-compliant and specialty balloons, and each has a specific role during a specific interventional procedure.

- Currently available stents include bare metal stents, drug-eluting stents, and covered stents, with present-day procedures almost always employing the deployment of third- and fourth-generation drug-eluting stents.

Introduction

Guide catheters, guidewires, balloons, and stents represent the foundation upon which all percutaneous coronary interventions (PCIs) are built. For many of us, we became familiar with these tools during fellowship and have not "expanded our horizons" since, using the same "go-to" guide catheters and guidewires whenever possible. Each of these devices undergo continuous refinements and adaptations that have made PCI easier, safer, and applicable to more patients. In this chapter, we cannot extensively discuss the engineering and details of all these tools for use in the lab; instead, we have tried to put together a general overview. Recognizing that new products are introduced frequently for clinical practice, we have focused on the "theory" that defines and differentiates the equipment rather than the specific brand names.

Guide Catheters

One of the most vital steps in performing a successful PCI is choosing an appropriate guide catheter. Without adequate guide support, device delivery and PCI can be very challenging and even dangerous. There are many characteristics that should be considered when selecting a guide catheter. Size, backup support, coaxial engagement, and trackability are several of the characteristics one should have in mind when choosing a guide catheter (Fig. 4.1).

Construction

Guide catheters generally have three layers:

1. The outer layer is usually nylon and contributes to the stiffness of the catheter.
2. The middle layer is a braided wire mesh layer, which gives the torque control and radiopacity to a catheter. It also helps to provide the required stiffness to the catheter while preserving a larger inner diameter compared with a similar sized diagnostic catheter.
3. The inner layer is hydrophilic coated to allow smooth passage for device delivery.

Choosing the Optimal Guide Catheter

Operators typically have default guide catheters for left and right coronary interventions and internal mammary artery (IMA) and graft interventions based on personal experience and training. Nevertheless, on occasion, one needs to select an alternate guide catheter shape because of anatomic considerations, particular device-related concerns, or inventory supply issues. Support, size, length, presence of ostial disease, access site (right/left transradial or transfemoral), need to access bypass grafts versus native arteries, anomalous origins, and aortic root size are some of the important factors in choosing a guide catheter.

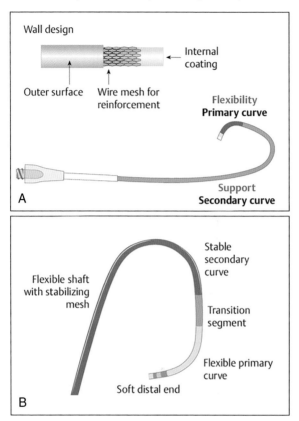

Figure 4.1 (A) Below is a typical JL-4 guiding catheter and above that the elements of the construction of the catheter are illustrated. (B) Relative features of the guiding catheter are shown, with the shaft of the catheter meant to be somewhat flexible; the end of the catheter has a soft portion that seats into the coronary artery. The primary curve allows a coaxial position within the coronary artery, with the secondary curve providing support against the aortic wall. From Percutaneous coronary intervention and coronary stent implantation. *Thoracic Key. https://thoracickey.com/percutaneous-coronary-intervention-and-coronary-stent-implantation-2/*

Backup Support

When discussing guide support (backup) we mainly refer to two types of support: active and passive backup. Active backup uses the aortic root to assist in the development of a desired guide catheter shape and requires more manipulation. With the transradial approach, active support of the guiding catheter plays a more important role than with the femoral approach. Deep-seating the guide beyond the ostium of the vessel for easier deliverability of devices is an example of active support. On the other hand, passive backup is related to the catheter's shape, size, and shaft length. This support relies on the composition and thickness of the walls of the guide shaft and tip of the catheter to engage the coronary ostium in a coaxial manner. This is inherent to the physical characteristics of the guide. In general, larger diameter guides provide more support. As one can imagine, active and passive approaches are used in combination.

Size

The majority of coronary diagnostic and interventional procedures can be performed with 6F guiding catheters (Fig. 4.2). Nevertheless, certain techniques and rare devices require large-diameter guiding catheters. Appropriate case planning includes anticipating such considerations. Larger French catheters provide better support and better visualization at the risk of vascular complications, a longer recovery period, and increased contrast use. Thus current recommendations encourage the use of the smallest possible system that can provide the desired therapy for that individual patient. Catheter diameters or gauge are measured in French (F) sizes.

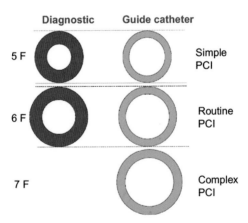

Figure 4.2 Picture demonstrating the relative sizes of diagnostic catheters and guide catheters and potential differential uses. Adapted from Prashant PU. Current and emerging catheter technologies for percutaneous transluminal coronary angioplasty. *Res Rep Clin Cardiol.* 2014;5:213–226, Fig. 4.

(F size is calculated by multiplying the diameter in millimeters by 3; to calculate the diameter of a catheter in millimeters, multiply the F size by 0.33.)

Length

The standard length of a guiding catheter is 100 cm, although a length of greater than 100 cm can be used for a tortuous aorta or a very tall person. For distal lesion sites (saphenous vein graft, tortuous internal mammary artery) or chronic total occlusion cases where a retrograde approach is used, an operator may select a shorter length guide catheter (e.g., 90 cm) to allow devices to reach the intended target.

Side Holes

Side hole–guiding catheters have been used in the presence of ostial lesions, which lead to changes in pressure waveforms (dampened waveforms or "ventricularization") during engagement. This suggests that the catheter is occluding the entire effective orifice of the coronary ostia. With the ostia occluded with the catheter, coronary perfusion may be impeded; furthermore, powerful injection may result in coronary dissection. Side holes *may* allow blood flow through the catheter tip to perfuse the artery. Although the presence of side holes will yield a normal-appearing waveform, it is unclear that it decreases adverse patient outcomes. Catheters with side holes have their own disadvantages. There is an increase in contrast use from catheters with side holes because contrast is extruded from the side holes in addition to the main lumen. There may also be a false sense of security because the aortic pressure rather than the coronary pressure is being monitored that operators should be mindful of during a procedure with one of these guides.

Influence of Access Site

Transradial (TR) intervention has several advantages compared with transfemoral (TF) intervention. The TR route is more convenient for patients because the period of immobilization is less, the risk for bleeding is lower, and the overall hospital stay is shorter. Nevertheless, TR intervention has taken time to become adopted in the US because of misconceptions surrounding backup support from traditional TF guide catheters. Clinical trials have consistently demonstrated similar PCI success rates regardless of the access site.

In terms of guide catheter support, investigators have suggested that the angle between the primary curve of the guide catheter and the contralateral wall of the aorta helps to determine the amount of "support" a guide catheter can provide. In theory, these investigators suggest that slightly different catheter sizes would provide improve support for radial procedures compared with traditional TF guides; however, many radial operators use the same guiding catheter shapes regardless of access site. Given the relatively small caliber of the radial artery compared with the femoral artery, catheter size is generally limited to up to 7F with the advent of thin-walled sheaths.

Sheathless Guide Catheters

Sheathless guide catheters are a newer innovation to overcome the size limitations of the radial artery. Traditionally, a guide catheter is inserted through a vascular access sheath. A 6F sheath refers to the inner diameter (ID) of the sheath, which will accommodate the outer diameter (OD) of a 6F guiding catheter. In reality, the OD of the access sheath is approximately 1.5F to 2F sizes larger than its ID (Fig. 4.3). A sheathless guiding catheter (Eaucath, Asahi Intecc USA, Inc; Fig. 4.4) takes advantage of that fact by eliminating

Relative Size

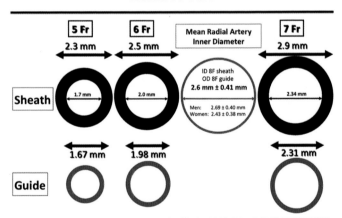

Adapted from From AM, Gulati R, Prasad A, Rihal CS. CCI 2010. 76: 911-916.

Figure 4.3 Relative size of 5, 6, and 7 French sheaths and guiding catheters. Note the increase in size of the inner diameter (ID) and outer diameter (OD) for both sheath and guide with increasing French size and the amount of room that the guiding catheter takes in the sheath. From From AM, Gulati R, Prasad A, Rihal CS. Sheathless transradial intervention using standard guide catheters. *Cathet Cardiovasc Interv.* 2010;76:911–916, Fig. 3.

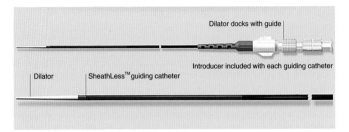

Figure 4.4 Sheathless Eaucath System (from Asahi Intecc Co Ltd). The sheathless guiding catheter is inserted with the dilator "locked" in place over a wire, and once positioned, the dilator is then removed from the "dock" and the catheter is connected to a hemostatic valve or Y-connector in the standard fashion to perform angiography and subsequent delivery of any wire or percutaneous coronary intervention (PCI) equipment.

the need for an access sheath, thereby allowing a guiding catheter with a much larger ID. For example, a 7F guiding catheter has a similar OD to a traditional 5F sheath. This advance makes it possible to undertake complex procedures requiring large bore vascular access. Complications such as vasospasm, radial artery occlusion, and coronary artery dissections are possible, however. In a related manner, a tapered dilator (Railway Sheathless Access System, Cordis) can be used in a more universal fashion to facilitate sheathless insertion of any guide catheter.

Universal Guiding Catheter

A universal catheter has a specialized curve or curves, usually meant for use from a right radial approach, recognizing the greater tortuosity and leveraging the increased contact points with the large vessels of the arm and the aorta in coming from a right radial (versus a left) radial approach. A universal catheter (e.g., Tiger) is meant to cannulate multiple vessels in a single use, whereas most femoral catheters are meant for a single, dedicated application, such as a catheter for the native left system, a catheter for the native right coronary artery, and different catheters for various types of bypass grafts. With a universal catheter, an operator can cannulate multiple vessels with a single catheter, which allows for efficiencies during the procedure. Some operators use universal guiding catheters for primary PCI for ST-segment elevation myocardial infarction (STEMI). Use of a universal guiding catheter from the radial approach minimizes the number of passes through the arm and therefore has the potential for lessening the incidence of radial spasm.

Guide Catheter Extensions

Guide catheter extensions are very helpful tools that have been added to the armamentarium of interventional cardiologists. In the US, there are three commercially available guide extensions (Table 4.1). Guide catheter extensions allow an operator to telescope a smaller catheter from inside a larger guiding catheter; some also refer to this as a "parent-child" concept.

These devices are particularly helpful in the coaxial engagement of coronary ostia with unusual takeoffs, which are not easily accessible with traditional guide catheter shapes. They offer a significant advantage in the delivery of interventional devices into significantly tortuous and calcified coronary segments where additional support is required and upsizing the guiding catheter system is not desired or possible. They also play a role in complex interventions involving supraannular aortic valve prostheses that extend above the coronary ostia. Engagement of the coronary arteries through the struts of the valve frame is difficult. A common technique is for the guiding catheter to be placed inside the frame and then telescoping the extension catheter through the struts of the valve frame to the coronary ostium. Careful low injection rate and selective coronary branch angiography are feasible, which can improve visualization and substantially decreases contrast volume.

It is crucial to understand the dynamic interaction of these devices with the guiding catheter, coronary artery wall, and various coronary interventional devices to avoid complications. The most important concern is the potential for arterial wall dissection, which can happen because of (1) noncentered advancement of a guide catheter extension into tortuous, diseased, and calcified coronary artery branches; (2) inadvertent advancement of a nonsecured guide catheter extension into a coronary artery branch during a vigorous contrast injection through the guiding catheter;

Table 4.1

Currently Available Guide Extending Catheters		
Guide Extension Catheter	**Sizes (ID)**	**Manufacturer**
Guidezilla	6(0.056), 7(0.062), 8(0.071)	Boston Scientific Corp.
Telescope	6, (0.056), 7 (0.062)	Medtronic
Guideliner	≥ 0.056 (5 F); ≥ 0.066, ≥ 0.070 (6F); ≥ 0.078 (7 F); ≥ 0.088 (8 F)	Teleflex

or (3) injection of contrast while the guide catheter extension is parked in a noncoaxial position relative to the axis of the intubated coronary artery branch, especially when there is slight dampening of the pressure waveform. Prolonged pressure dampening during the intubation of a small to intermediate-sized target vessel can lead to worsening myocardial ischemia. Finally, a complication that is much less likely to occur with the most recent iterations of the extension catheter designs involves longitudinal stent deformation and stent/balloon separation that occurs during the interaction of the stent delivery system with the proximal port of the extension catheter system.

Coronary Guidewires

Coronary guidewires are an essential component of every PCI procedure. Key characteristics of a coronary guidewire include the ability to be steerable, visible, flexible, and allow device delivery. Discussion of the "best" guidewire for PCI can often generate passionate debate among interventional operators. All operators must have a working knowledge of the construction, strengths, and limitations of coronary guidewires that they plan to use during PCI procedures.

Guidewires come with specific terminology that is important to understand for an operator to communicate effectively (Table 4.2).

The next step in learning about coronary guidewires is to understand some of the core concepts regarding their construction (Fig. 4.5). Guidewires commonly come in 180 to 195 cm for rapid exchange (RX) or 300 cm for over-the-wire (OTW) use.

Table 4.2

Guidewire Features	
"Workhorse"	Wire with a gentle-tip, less likely to traumatize the vessel or cause a perforation
Tip load (Gram-tip)	Measure of force needed to buckle the tip
Penetration power	Tip load divided by cross-sectional area of the tip
Jacketed	Hydrophilic coating over the body and tip of the wire
Hydrophilic	Water-avid coating that provides a feeling of lubricity or slipperiness
Hydrophobic	Water-repelling coating that provides better control
Support	Ability to deliver equipment through tortuous, calcified, or narrow lumens

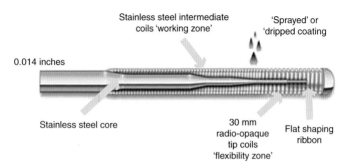

Figure 4.5 The typical construction elements for coronary guide wires (focusing on the distal tip of the wire). Note the inner core element that tapers from proximal to distal. Also note the coils at the tip denoting the "working zone" of the wire that are typically radio-opaque to be easily seen on fluoroscopy. Also depicted is the presence of a "shaping ribbon" on some wires, specifically designed to maintain the shape given to the wire by the operator. From Ali R, Greenbaum AB, Kugelmass AD. A review of the available angioplasty guiding catheters, wires, and balloons – making the right choice. *Interv Cardiol.* 2012;7:100–103, Fig. 3.

Wires consist of four components: the core, the wire tip, the body, and the coating.

1. The *core* is the inner part of the wire. The proximal portion is commonly made of steel or another alloy. The distal portion of the core can be a continuation of the same material or another material, such as a nickel-titanium alloy (nitinol). The material that makes up the core, its thickness, and length of distal tapering determines the wire's flexibility, support, trackability, and steerability.

2. The *wire tip* can be an extension of the core, which provides good tactile feedback and torquability. If the core does not extend to the tip, a metal ribbon makes up the tip. Such ribbons are often more shapeable, but there is a sacrifice in tip control. For certain specialty wires, the tip may be tapered or larger in diameter than the body of the wire.

3. The *body* of the wire surrounds the core and can be made of coils or plastic. The entire wire can be covered by a polymer (covered) or the entire wire can be covered except the tip (sleeved). A covered wire is more trackable but less likely to retain its shape, whereas the sleeved wires are less trackable but allow better shape retention.

4. As for the *coating*, the body of the wire can be overlaid with a hydrophilic material that attracts water and gives a slippery

performance to the wire. Alternatively, wires can be coated with hydrophobic material that repel water and give more tactile feedback. Hybrid wires with both types of coating are common as well.

Wire Selection Process for Nonchronic Total Occlusion Lesions

Operators will begin with their workhorse wire of choice based on prior experience, local practices, and availability. Workhorse wires are typically hydrophobic with a low-gram tip and a spring coil (Table 4.3). In experienced hands, these wires are successful in a majority of cases. Hydrophilic wires are not recommended for routine use because their lubricious coating can slide under a plaque or into a false lumen. Also, if the operator does not keep a close eye on the distal tip of the wire, it can cause a perforation.

Common scenarios where workhorse wires are not successful include excessive vessel tortuosity, calcification, severe stenosis, long stenosis, and jailed side-branches. Based on the operator's suspicion for the cause of the failure, secondary wires can be used to address the issue. Excessive vessel tortuosity may respond better to a polymer-jacketed hydrophilic wire (Table 4.4) because this type of wire may generate less friction with the vessel wall. Long lesions may also benefit from a low-gram tip hydrophilic wire.

Table 4.3

Common Workhorse Wires	
Wire	**Manufacturer**
HT Balance Middleweight Universal	Abbott
Prowater Flex, Sion Blue	Asahi Intecc USA, Inc.
Luge, Samurai	Boston Scientific Corp
Cougar LS, XT	Medtronic
Runthrough NS Extra Floppy	Terumo Interventional Systems

Table 4.4

Common Polymer-Jacketed/Hydrophilic Wires	
Wire	**Manufacturer**
Pilot 50	Abbott
Whisper	Abbott
Sion Black	Asahi Intecc USA, Inc.
PT2 Light Support Guidewire	Boston Scientific Corporation

Table 4.5

Common Stiff or Support Wires	
Wire	**Manufacturer**
Ironman	Abbott
Mailman	Boston Scientific Corporation
Grandslam	Asahi Intecc USA, Inc.
Thunder	Medtronic
Wiggle	Abbott

Long lesions and calcified lesions may require more force for device delivery. More supportive or stiff wires are useful for these applications (Table 4.5). The initial crossing of a lesion with stiff wires is difficult. A common approach is to cross the lesion with a workhorse or polymer-jacketed wire, then exchange for the stiff wire over a microcatheter or OTW balloon. The Wiggle wire (Abbott) has a unique construction involving sinusoidal curves along the distal end of the wire.

Changing Wire Lengths

In certain scenarios, such as atherectomy cases, an operator may want to change from a short (190 cm) to a long (300 cm) wire without losing wire position. Use of a wire extension is a common way to do this. These extensions (DOC, Abbott or Extension, Asahi) connect to the back of the short wire and extend the total wire length to 300 cm. In another approach, a short-shafted balloon (Trapper Exchange Device, Boston Scientific) can be inserted in the guide catheter but adjacent to the wire and advanced to the end of the guide catheter. With this balloon inflated, the wire is controlled between the balloon and the inner wall of the guiding catheter (Fig. 4.6). OTW devices can now be advanced/removed over the short wire.

For the converse scenario, there are at least a few ways to exchange a long wire for a short wire. If there is an OTW catheter in place, the long wire can be removed using a short wire with an extension. Once the OTW catheter is "walked" out, the extension is disconnected. The less conventional option is to "hydroplane" the catheter over the short wire. This involves exchanging the long wire for the short wire via an OTW catheter, then withdrawing the catheter back until just a few inches of the wire can be seen exiting the back of the catheter. At this point, the operator can connect a syringe or an insufflator device (being careful to maintain a liquid to liquid interface) to the back of the catheter. While holding the Tuohy open, the operator either injects contrast from the syringe or

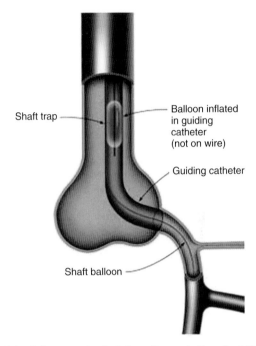

Figure 4.6 Balloon trapping technique. Demonstration of a guiding catheter in a coronary artery with wire and balloon shaft advanced down a coronary artery. The "trap" balloon is shown inflated within the guiding catheter to "pinch" the equipment against the wall of the guiding catheter and not allow it to move while other equipment may be safely retrieved. Wilson W, Spratt JC. Advances in procedural techniques—antegrade. *Curr Cardiol Rev.* 2014;10(2):127-144. doi:10.2174/1573403x10666140331142016

begins to "inflate" the insufflator while pulling the catheter out. This maneuver take practice and should not be performed when loss of wire position would impair the success of the procedure.

Specialty/Functional Wires

Pressure Wires, Flow Wires

See Chapter 5 for more detail. With the advent of miniaturized pressure transducers, a class of functional wires that measure pressure are commonly used in modern practice. These wires can assess

Table 4.6

Common Pressure/Doppler Flow Wire	
Wire	**Manufacturer**
PressureWire X Guidewire	Abbott
Comet II Pressure Guidewire	Boston Scientific
OptoWire	Opsens Medical
Verrata Plus Pressure Guidewire	Philips
FloWire Doppler Guidewire	Philips
ComboWire Guidewire	Philips

intracoronary pressure and flow through a transducer mounted on the distal end of the wire. Through the use of these specialized wires, assessment of fractional flow reserve and all its iterations are common in current practice. Performance of these wires is not equivalent to workhorse wires but has improved dramatically with time. There are several wires and systems on the market in the US currently (Table 4.6).

Atherectomy Wires

There are currently two coronary atherectomy systems available in the US. Boston Scientific (Marlborough, MA) produces a rotational atherectomy system with Rotawire as part of its Rotapro system. The Rotawire wire has a 0.009 inch core with a varied distal, tapered length between the Floppy and Extra support versions of the wire. The tip is a 0.014 platinum coil that helps to present the atherectomy burr from advancing beyond the end of the wire.

Cardiovascular Systems, Inc (St. Paul, MN) supplies an orbital atherectomy system with ViperWire Advance with FlexTip wire to accompany the Diamondback 360 system. This wire is made with a nitinol core and a shapeable floppy tip. The body is also constructed of nitinol to reduce wire bias. Because of the interaction between the rotating element of the atherectomy system that occurs over the wire, the coatings and covers are not possible. (See Chapter 6 for further details and descriptions of atherectomy.)

Coronary Balloons for Angioplasty

There are a variety of balloons available for PCI, the use of which is predicated on characteristics of coronary lesion/stenosis, such as whether the lesion is heavily calcified, soft plaque, or in-stent restenosis.

Percutaneous Transluminal Coronary Angioplasty

The backbone of endovascular interventions continues to be the coronary balloon. There are many available types, including both noncompliant and compliant balloons. The main purpose of coronary balloon angioplasty is to provide coronary lumen gain by inflation. Balloon angioplasty aims to expand the coronary lumen by stretching and tearing the vessel wall and atherosclerotic plaque, in the process redistributing the plaque along its longitudinal axis. This additional space allows for delivery of other specialized equipment, in particular a coronary stent, with the goal of maintaining a patent vessel and allowing blood flow past a previous area of stenosis to the myocardium. Other purposes of balloon angioplasty during contemporary PCI include assessing vessel compliance, assessing lesion length and diameter, furthering stent expansion, and delivering specific therapy, such as radiation or sonic waves.

Compliant Balloon

A wide variety of compliant balloons are available by multiple different manufacturers (Table 4.7). Compliant balloons are often used before stent delivery in coronary interventions to allow space for eventual delivery of additional devices used in endovascular intervention. The compliant balloon has the capacity to expand and conform to the vessel anatomy with inflation. Compliant balloons are usually composed of silicone or polyurethane.

Table 4.7

Coronary Balloon Dilation Catheters	
Compliant Balloon	**Manufacturer**
Mini Trek RX Coronary Dilation Catheter	Abbott
Pantera Pro	Biotronik, Inc.
Emerge Monorail PTCA Dilatation Catheter	Boston Scientific Corporation
Sapphire II Pro Coronary Dilation Catheter	Cardiovascular Systems, Inc. (manufactured by OrbusNeich)
Empira RX PTCA Balloon Dilatation Catheter	Cordis
Euphora	Medtronic
RX Takeru PTCA Balloon Dilation Catheter	Terumo Interventional Systems

Noncompliant Balloon

Noncompliant balloons are typically less flexible compared with compliant balloons. They are primarily used during coronary interventions to deliver high-pressure balloon inflations to discrete segments of the vasculature. In addition, noncompliant balloons are routinely used to deliver high-pressure balloon inflations within a stent that has been deployed to expand and provide maximal stent apposition to the vessel wall. Noncompliant balloons are typically composed of nylon or polyester. As with compliant balloons, there are a wide variety of manufacturers of noncompliant balloons with similar names to their compliant balloon product line. Noncompliant and compliant balloons are available to use as OTW or as RX delivery systems.

Specialty Balloons

Specialty balloons, such as the cutting balloon and the scoring balloon, are available from a wide variety of manufacturers (Table 4.8). There are special considerations with use of scoring and cutting balloons. Scoring and cutting balloons are primarily used to prevent the balloon migration "watermelon seed effect" in the setting of in-stent restenosis (ISR) or intervention on difficult-to-dilate lesions. Some believe that cutting balloons are simple atherectomy tools to treat calcific lesions. Finally, some have advocated the use of cutting balloons to treat ostial disease of branch vessels when the parent vessel is intact, arguing that this balloon is less likely to migrate into the parent vessel. The Chocolate balloon (Fig. 4.7) is constructed with a metallic cage that create grooves in the balloon to distribute the force more focally while providing areas where less force is delivered. This modification may limit propagation of dissections.

Intravascular Lithotripsy

See Chapter 6 for more detail. A more recent development in coronary angioplasty focused on improving stent delivery and expansion

Table 4.8

Specialty Balloon Dilation Catheters	
Specialty Balloon	**Manufacturer**
Wolverine Monorail Cutting Balloon Dilation Device	Boston Scientific Corporation
AngioSculpt RX PTCA Scoring Balloon Catheter	Philips
Chocolate PTCA Balloon Catheter	TriReme Medical LLC

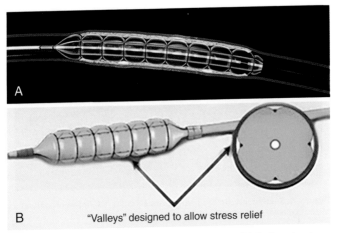

A

B   "Valleys" designed to allow stress relief

Figure 4.7 (A), Chocolate balloon (TriReme Medical). This balloon has been designed with rings that are along the length of the balloon. (B), Schematic diagram showing that these rings allow "valleys" to form to minimize outward trauma on the vessel wall.

in the setting of heavily calcified lesion is intravascular lithotripsy (IVL). A specialized balloon catheter "delivers acoustic pressure waves to modify calcium, enhancing vessel compliance and optimizing stent deployment" (Fig. 4.8). More investigation is warranted; however, the recently published Disrupt CAD III study suggests that IVL is both a safe and effective intervention to facilitate stent deployment in severely calcified lesions.

Coronary Stents

Coronary artery stents were developed in an effort to maintain both short-term and long-term patency of a vessel after percutaneous transluminal coronary angioplasty (PTCA). Similar to coronary balloons, there are a variety of coronary stents now available for use during PCI. Modern "third-generation" drug-eluting stents (DES) are balloon expandable and are made up of stainless steel or metal alloys, such as cobalt-chromium or platinum-chromium.

Bare Metal Stents

Bare metal stents (BMS), the earliest iteration of the intracoronary stents, were developed as a treatment for flow limiting dissection,

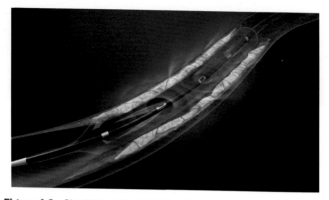

Figure 4.8 ShockWave Medical (Santa Barbara, CA) intracoronary lithoplasty balloon.

an early complication of PTCA. As noted previously, the first implanted coronary stents were self-expanding, implanted in 1986 by Ulrich Sigwart and colleagues. With the introduction of coronary stents in late 1980s, the rates of acute vessel closure after PCI declined somewhat, but ISR remained a significant limitation. In the peak of the BMS era, rates of restenosis ranged from 20% to 40% at 6 to 12 months in clinical trials. By reducing the rate of ISR, DES quickly replaced BMS as the dominant stent platform in clinical practice. Until recently, BMS continued to be used in clinical practice primarily for patients who were ineligible for prolonged dual antiplatelet therapy (DAPT) or were unable to afford DES. With recent clinical trials demonstrating the safety of shorter duration DAPT with DES, the clinical utility of BMS has diminished further.

Drug-Eluting Stents

DES successfully built on the success of BMS by reducing ISR at the cost of prolonging DAPT. DES may be made up of metal or metal alloys (cobalt-chromium, stainless steel, or platinum-chromium), a polymer coating to control drug delivery, and an antiproliferative drug. The stent struts for modern DES are thin (60–80 μm) compared with earlier-generation DES and BMS (127–140 μm), yet they maintain the radial and longitudinal strength necessary to maintain cross-sectional area (Fig. 4.9). The delivery of drug therapy (antiproliferative or antiinflammatory agents) to the vessel wall is meant to inhibit the mechanisms of cellular proliferation, thereby limiting neointimal hyperplasia and stent restenosis. A variety of antiproliferative agents have been

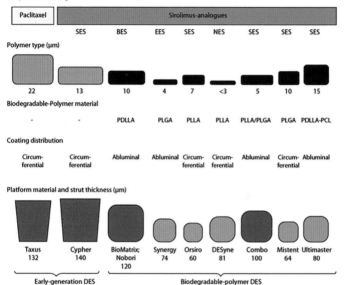

Figure 4.9 Comparison of the general features of drug-eluting stents, including the antiproliferative drug, polymer type and thickness, and coating, as well as stent thickness. From Piccolo R, Giustino G, Mehran R, Windecker S. Stable coronary artery disease: Revascularisation and invasive strategies. *Lancet.* 2015;386:702–713.

studied in clinical trials with the most used antiproliferative agents in modern stents now being sirolimus and its analogs (zotarolimus, or everolimus; Table 4.9).

The implantation of DES represents the mainstay of current PCI in the cath lab. Nevertheless, operators have multiple competing factors involved in making decisions about which one may be best for their patient. These include the current economics, in which DES are frequently purchased through larger cooperative buying groups that individual operators may not have much influence on. Furthermore, the issues of late stent thrombosis, restenosis, bleeding issues brought on by prolonged DAPT, and late stent fractures or neointimal plaque formation all create the impetus for further refinement in DES design and development. Some of these issues have been thought to arise from the polymer that was applied to the metal struts and allows the drug to "elute" over

Table 4.9

Common Coronary Stent Platforms

Stent	Manufacturer	Stent Metal Alloy	Drug/ Coating	Stent Strut Thickness (μm)
BMS				
Multi-Link Coronary Stent System	Abbott	Cobalt chromium or stainless steel		81.3 μm
Pro-Kinetic Energy	Biotronik	Cobalt-Chromium		60 μm
Rebel	Boston Scientific	Platinum-Chromium		81 μm
Integrity	Medtronic	Cobalt-Chromium		91 μm
DES (Durable Polymer)				
Xience	Abbott	Cobalt-Chromium	Everolimus	81 μm
Resolute	Medtronic	Cobalt-Chromium	Zotarolimus	81–91 μm
Promus Elite Everolimus-Eluting Platinum Chromium Coronary Stent System	Boston Scientific Corporation	Platinum chromium	Everolimus	81–86 μm
Synergy Bioabsorbable Polymer Drug-Eluting Stent System	Boston Scientific Corporation	Platinum chromium	Everolimus	74 μm
DES (Bioabsorbable Polymer)				
Orsiro	Biotronik	Cobalt-Chromium	Sirolimus	60–80 μm
Synergy	Boston Scientific	Platinum-Chromium	Everolimus	79–81 μm
Other Stent: Covered stent or Bifurcation stent				
PK Papyrus	Biotronik	Cobalt-Chromium	Nonwoven, electrospun polyurethane	60 μm

Table 4.9

Common Coronary Stent Platforms (Continued)				
Stent	**Manufacturer**	**Stent Metal Alloy**	**Drug/ Coating**	**Stent Strut Thickness (μm)**
Graftmaster	Abbott	Stainless steel	Expandable Polytetrafluoroethylene (ePTFE) sandwiched between two identical stents	520 μm
Tryton Side Branch Stent	Cordis	Cobalt-Chromium	None	85 μm
Retired Stents (First-generation DES)				
Taxus	Boston Scientific	Stainless steel	Paclitaxel	132 μm (later generation 81 μm)
Cypher	Cordis	Stainless steel	Sirolimus	140 μm

BMS, Bare metal stent; *DES*, drug-eluting stent

time, and some stents now have been developed with a bioabsorbable polymer (e.g., Synergy) or without a polymer entirely (e.g., BioFreedom).

Presently, two main factors drive stent choice by the operator: (1) DAPT duration and (2) the ability to expand the stent without deformation. From the standpoint of DAPT, many patients have higher bleeding risks, and operators should be aware of the available stents and associated studies allowing a shorter period of time needed to continue these agents safely (Table 4.10). PCI of the left main often requires poststent inflations with sequentially larger balloons and the thinner-strut DES platforms have been reported to change their conformation during some of these inflations, which has worried some operators. A newer DES has now been developed to fit this purpose, the Synergy Megatron stent (Boston Scientific, Galway, Ireland; Fig. 4.10), and many operators have now started to preferentially chose this platform for their left main PCI procedures.

Although bioabsorbable stents were eagerly awaited for routine clinical use given that the entire stent platform would no longer be present in the coronary artery within 2 years after implantation, the clinical studies that were ongoing to lead to approval of

Table 4.10

Drug-Eluting Stent Platforms Studied With Short-DAPT in High-Bleeding-Risk Patients

Study	Stent	DAPT Duration	N	Design
EVOLVE Short DAPT NCT02605447	Synergy	3 months	2000	Registry
POEM NCT03112707	Synergy	1 month	1023	Registry
SENIOR NCT02099617	Synergy	1 month (SIHD) 6 months (ACS)	1200	Randomized (Synergy vs. BMS)
XIENCE 90 NCT03218787	Xience	3 months	2000	Registry
XIENCE 28 Global and USA NCT03355742 and NCT03815175	Xience	1 month	960 and 640–800	Registry
STOP-DAPT2 NCT02619760	Xience	1 month	3009	Randomized (1 vs. 12 mo DAPT)
MASTER-DAPAT NCT03023020	Ultimaster	1 month	4300	Randomized (1 vs. 12 mo DAPT)
Onyx ONE CLEAR NCT03647475	Onyx Resolute	1 month	1506	Registry
Onyx ONE Global RCT NCT03344653	Onyx Resolute	1 month	2000	Randomized (Onyx vs. Bio-Freedom)

ACS, Acute coronary syndrome; BMS; bare metal stent; DAPT, dual antiplatelet therapy; SIHD, stable ischemic heart disease

use showed a higher rate of adverse events compared with the standard DES platforms, and bioabsorbable platforms have moved back to preclinical development.

Covered Stents

These stents have struts that are coated in polytetrafluoroethylene (PTFE) or sandwiched between two layers of stent. These devices are exclusively to be used to treat coronary perforations of native vessels. Both devices are considered "Humanitarian Use Devices" and require institutional review board approval for use in the US.

Stent Designs

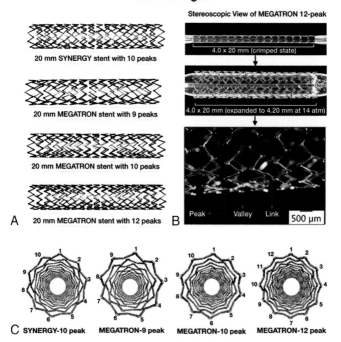

Figure 4.10 Overall design elements that make up the Synergy Megatron stent. From Samant S, Wu W, Zhao S, et al. Computational and experimental mechanical performance of a new everolimus-eluting stent purpose-built for left main interventions. *Sci Rep.* 2021;11:8728, Fig. 2.

Key References

McKavanagh P, Zawadowski G, Ahmed N, Kutryk M. The evolution of coronary stents. *Expert Rev Cardiovasc Ther.* 2018;16:219-228.

Shroff AR, Fernandez C, Vidovich MI, et al. Contemporary transradial access practices: Results of the second international survey. *Catheter Cardiovasc Interv.* 2019; 93:1276-1287.

Toth GG, Yamane M, Heyndrickx GR. How to select a guidewire: technical features and key characteristics. *Heart.* 2015;101:645-652.

References

Aminian A, Iglesias JF, Van Mieghem C, et al. First prospective multicenter experience with the 7 French Glidesheath slender for complex transradial coronary interventions. *Catheter Cardiovasc Interv.* 2017;89:1014-1020.

Dangas GD, Di Mario C, Kipshidze N. *Interventional Cardiology: Principles and Practice*. 2nd ed. Hoboken, New Jersey: Wiley Blackwell; 2017:1 online resource.

Griffin BP, Menon V. *Manual of Cardiovascular Medicine*. 5th ed. Lippincott Williams & Wilkins (LWW); 2018.

Hill JM, Kereiakes DJ, Shlofmitz RA, et al. Intravascular lithotripsy for treatment of severely calcified coronary artery disease. *J Am Coll Cardiol*. 2020;76:2635-2646.

Horie K, Tada N, Isawa T, et al. A randomised comparison of incidence of radial artery occlusion and symptomatic radial artery spasm associated with elective transradial coronary intervention using 6.5 Fr SheathLess Eaucath Guiding Catheter vs. 6.0 Fr Glidesheath Slender. *EuroIntervention*. 2018;13:2018-2025.

Ikari Y, Nagaoka M, Kim JY, Morino Y, Tanabe T. The physics of guiding catheters for the left coronary artery in transfemoral and transradial interventions. *J Invasive Cardiol*. 2005;17:636-641.

Mann D, Libby P, Bonow R. *Braunwald's Heart Disease: A Textbook of Cardiovascular Medicine*, Section 3. Saunders; 2014.

Tan C, Schatz RA. The history of coronary stenting. *Interv Cardiol Clin*. 2016;5:271-280.

Tonino PAL, Keulards DCJ, Pijls NHJ. Invasive physiological assessment of coronary disease. In: *Percutaneous Interventional Cardiovascular Medicine: The EAPCI Textbook*. 2012. Available at: https://www.pcronline.com/eurointervention/textbook/pcrtextbook/ table-of-contents/.

Urban P, Meredith IT, Abizaid A, et al. Polymer-free drug-coated coronary stents in patients at high bleeding risk. *N Engl J Med*. 2015;373:2038-2047.

Waterbury TM, Sorajja P, Bell MR, et al. Experience and complications associated with use of guide extension catheters in percutaneous coronary intervention. *Catheter Cardiovasc Interv*. 2016;88:1057-1065.

Intravascular Lesion Assessment: Physiology and Imaging

MORTON J. KERN • MICHAEL J. LIM

KEY POINTS

- Angiographic determination of the significance for a given coronary lesion remains limited.

- Numerous physiologic indexes are now available that rely on coronary hyperemia (fractional flow reserve [FFR]) and nonhyperemic indexes [aka NHPR] (e.g., instantaneous wave-free pressure ratio [iFR], mean distal coronary divided by mean proximal aortic pressure [Pd/Pa], resting full-cycle ratio [RFR], diastolic hyperemia-free ratio [DFR]), which can all reliably assess the significance of a coronary lesion.

- FFR remains the most studied physiologic index to date in terms of validation and patient outcomes.

- Operators should become facile with using a nonhyperemic index in today's cath lab and have the ability to perform FFR when critical decision making is not supported by complementary clinical data.

Introduction

The techniques for coronary lesion assessment are divided into physiologic (i.e., those identifying abnormal coronary flow) and anatomic (i.e., those displaying the coronary lumen/vessel wall/plaque morphology).

For physiology, there are several pressure sensor coronary pressure wires and microcatheters now available to measure pressure (and flow). Myocardial perfusion is the net result of blood flow transiting the epicardial arteries, microcirculation, and myocardial bed (Fig. 5.1). Different intracoronary physiologic tools are used to measure each of these subdivisions of blood flow. Although coronary flow reserve (CFR) encompasses both the macrocirculation and microcirculation, other indexes have been developed to evaluate specific domains of the heart circulation.

For intravascular imaging, catheters developed to visualize the cross-sections of vessels use ultrasound (IVUS) or light (optical coherence tomography [OCT]) to provide unique information that complements physiology and further improves decision making by providing stenosis and reference vessel dimensions and plaque composition to refine device selection and percutaneous coronary intervention (PCI) strategy.

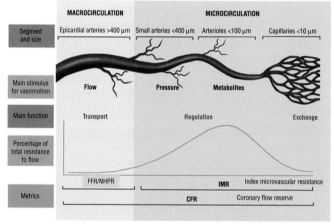

Figure 5.1 The Macrocirculation and Microcirculation. The normal structure and function of coronary macrocirculation and microcirculation are depicted with the regions of physiologic measurement techniques. Myocardial perfusion is the net result of blood flow transiting the epicardial arteries, microcirculation, and myocardial bed. Different intracoronary physiologic tools are used to measure each of these subdivisions of blood flow. Although coronary flow reserve (CFR) encompasses both the macrocirculation and microcirculation, other indexes have been developed to evaluate specific domains of the heart circulation. *CFR*, Coronary flow reserve; *FFR*, fractional flow reserve; *IMR*, index of microvascular resistance; *NHPR*, nonhyperemic pressure ratio. (Adapted with permission from De Bruyne B, Oldroyd KG, Pijls NHJ. Microvascular (Dys)Function and Clinical Outcome in Stable Coronary Disease*. *JACC* 2016;67:1170.)

Rationale for Lesion Assessment Tools

There are three major goals in using intravascular lesion assessment tools: (1) to avoid unnecessary revascularization procedures; (2) to improve periprocedural and long-term PCI outcomes in coronary artery disease (CAD) patients; and (3) to diagnose microvascular dysfunction in patients with symptoms but no CAD.

Revascularization (via PCI or coronary artery bypass graft [CABG]) is indicated with the presence of ischemia, which depends on the hemodynamic significance of a lesion. Unfortunately, the coronary angiogram frequently cannot reliably identify the hemodynamic significance of coronary stenoses, mostly but not exclusively in the intermediately narrowed (between 30% and 80% diameter stenosis) range. This limitation of angiography is attributed to the anatomic eccentric complexity of the atherosclerotic lumen and repeatedly demonstrated by poor correlations to stress testing and intracoronary translesional physiology.

Coronary angiography, which produces a two-dimensional (2D) silhouette of the three-dimensional (3D) vascular lumen, is also unable to differentiate diffusely "diseased" and "normal" vessel segments showing patent lumenograms. In addition, unlike intravascular imaging (IVUS or OCT), angiography does not provide much specific vascular wall information to characterize plaque size, length, and tissue composition (e.g., lipid, fibrofatty, calcium).

The angiographic appearance of an eccentric lumen, when viewed from different angulations, presents conflicting images (Fig. 5.2): one with a large lumen, the other with a severely narrowed lumen, leaving the operator with uncertainty as to its impact on coronary blood flow and ischemic potential. In addition to the eccentric shape, there are at least six morphologic features that determine resistance to flow, few of which can be measured from the angiogram or even IVUS/OCT (Fig. 5.3). Additional angiographic artifacts interfering with lesion interpretation include contrast streaming, branch overlap, vessel foreshortening, calcifications, and ostial origins, all of which contribute to ambiguous angiographic lesion interpretation.

Coronary Physiology for the Cath Lab

Translesional Pressure Ratios

Translesional physiology is the term given to the intracoronary wire-based pressure or flow measurements obtained proximal

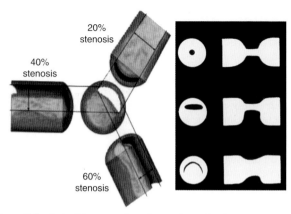

Figure 5.2 *Left,* Diagram of angiographic projections demonstrating markedly different diameter narrowings illustrating the greatest limitation of angiography for eccentric lesions. *Right,* Orthogonal projections of different orifice configurations that complicate determination of physiologic impact of narrowing.

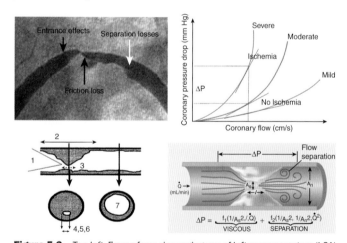

Figure 5.3 *Top left,* Frame from cineangiogram of left coronary artery (LCA) with an intermediate left anterior descending (LAD) lesion. *Bottom right,* Diagram of regions of stenosis resistance causing poststenotic pressure loss (1, entrance angle; 2, length of disease; 3, length of stenosis; 4, minimal lumen diameter; 5, minimal lumen area; 6, eccentricity of lesion; 7, area of reference vessel segment). *Top right,* Pressure gradient–coronary flow curves demonstrating effect of increasing hemodynamic severity. Straight lines indicate portion of curves where pressure and flow are linearly related, permitting the derivation of fraction flow reserve (FFR) to function.

(usually aortic pressure from the guide catheter [P_{aortic} or Pa]) and distal to a stenosis (from a pressure wire or microcatheter [P_{distal} or Pa]). Translesional pressure measurements are most often used to assess a stenosis for appropriateness of stenting during PCI. Translesional pressure indices include resting or nonhyperemic pressure ratios (NHPR, such as mean distal coronary divided by mean proximal aortic pressure [Pd/Pa] and instantaneous wave-free pressure ratio [iFR]; Fig. 5.4) and hyperemic pressure ratios (e.g., fractional flow reserve [FFR] or contrast FFR [cFFR]).

Physiologic lesion assessment is indicated when clinical ischemia is not documented by objective data like electrocardiogram (ECG) changes or ischemic stress testing. Many patients require physiologic assessment because less than half of stable angina CAD patients have documented ischemia by ECG changes or stress testing before undergoing elective procedures. Moreover, unlike nuclear imaging studies, which cannot precisely identify a culprit ischemic vessel, direct translesional pressure measurement can specify which vessel/lesion may be responsible for symptoms in patients with multivessel CAD and hence benefit from PCI. This feature is particularly important for lesions narrowed between 50% to 90% diameter stenosis by visual estimation.

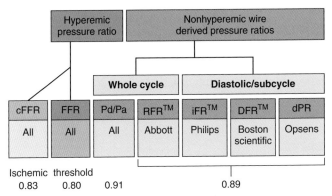

Figure 5.4 Summary of translesional pressure indices at rest and hyperemia. dPR is average Pd/Pa during entire diastole. DFR is average Pd/Pa during Pa less than mean Pa with negative slope. RFR is defined as the lowest filtered mean Pd/Pa during the entire cardiac cycle. Threshold cut points for ischemia are shown below each index. *cFFR*, Contrast fractional flow reserve; *DFR*, diastolic hyperemia-free ratio; *dPR*, diastolic pressure ratio; *FFR*, fractional flow reserve; *iFR*, instantaneous wave free ratio; *Pd/Pa*, pressure distal/pressure aortic; *RFR*, resting full-cycle ratio. (Modified from Kogame N, Ono M, Kawashima H, et al. The impact of coronary physiology on contemporary clinical decision making. *JACC Cardiovasc Interv.* 2020;13:1617–1638.)

Hyperemic Pressure Ratios

Pijls and De Bruyne first validated a translesional pressure derived index for determining the physiologic impact of coronary stenoses called the *fractional flow reserve (FFR)*. FFR is defined as the coronary flow across a lesion as a percent of normal flow in the same vessel in the theoretical absence of the lesion.

FFR is measured as the ratio of mean distal coronary pressure divided by the mean proximal aortic pressure (Pd/Pa) during maximal hyperemia. The coronary pressure beyond the stenosis is measured with a 0.014-inch pressure sensor guidewire with a high-fidelity pressure transducer mounted 3 cm from the tip of the wire at the junction of the radiopaque and radiolucent segments. (A microcatheter with an optical pressure sensor can be used as well.) The foundational concept of FFR is the linear coronary pressure-flow relationship during maximal hyperemia; thus the ratios of translesional pressure at maximal hyperemia (i.e., minimal vascular resistance) are equivalent to the ratios of hyperemic flows (poststenotic flow [Qs] divided by normal flow [Qn]). Thus FFR expresses the percentage (Qs/Qn) of a coronary flow across the stenosis and degree of myocardial flow impairment. Table 5.1 lists the calculations for FFR. A full discussion of the FFR method and results can be found elsewhere (see suggested readings).

FFR was developed as a pressure-only method of computing coronary flow reserve of a stenosis independent of the microvascular bed. CFR (maximal flow/basal flow) was thought to reflect the stenosis severity, initially observed in canine models. When CFR was tested in patients undergoing coronary bypass surgery with

Table 5.1

Calculations of Fractional Flow Reserve

Myocardial fraction flow reserve (FFR_{myo}):
$$FFR\_myo = 1 - \Delta P/Pa - Pv = Pd - Pv/Pa - Pv = Pd/Pa$$
Coronary fractional flow reserve (FFR_{cor}): $FFR_{cor} = 1 - \Delta P(Pa - Pw)$
Collateral fractional flow reserve (FFR_{coll}): $FFR_{coll} = FFR_{myo} - FFR_{cor}$

Note: All measurements are made during hyperemia except Pw. *Pa,* Mean aortic pressure; *Pd,* distal coronary pressure; *ΔP,* mean translesional pressure gradient; *Pv,* mean right atrial pressure; *Pw,* mean coronary wedge pressure or distal coronary pressure during balloon inflation.

(From Pijls NHJ, van Som AM, Kirkeeide RL, et al. Experimental basis of determining maximum coronary, myocardial, and collateral blood flow by pressure measurements for assessing functional stenosis severity before and after percutaneous transluminal coronary angioplasty. *Circulation.* 1993;87:454–467.)

Doppler flow meters, however, the relationship between angiographic narrowing (% diameter) and CFR was weak. Some patients had impaired CFR because of microvascular disease, and some angiographically severe lesions (e.g., lesion eccentricity) did not reduce CFR at all. Because a normal CFR cannot exclude a stenosis as the cause of a reduced CFR, FFR was developed to be specific for epicardial stenosis narrowing. Table 5.2 shows comparative features of FFR and CFR.

Technique of Translesional Pressure Measurements

See Fig. 5.5. Pressure across a stenosis can be easily measured using a 0.014-inch pressure sensor wire through a 5 French (5F) or 6F guide catheter. There are several commercially available pressure wire/microcatheter systems. Resting NHPR and/or hyperemic pressure ratios (FFR) are obtained after diagnostic angiography is completed.

The steps to measure translesional pressure at rest and during hyperemia are as follows:

1. The pressure wire is connected to the system's pressure analyzer, calibrated, and zeroed to ambient atmosphere on the table, outside the body.

2. Anticoagulation (intravenous [IV] heparin, usually 70 u/kg) and intracoronary (IC) nitroglycerin (100–200 mcg bolus) are administered.

3. The wire is advanced through the 'Y' connector on the guide to the coronary artery. Before crossing the stenosis, the pressure wire signal and the guide catheter pressure are matched (i.e.,

Table 5.2

Comparative Features of FFR and CFR			
	FFR	**CFR**	**Comment**
Normal Value	1.0	Range >2.0	CFR age related.
Change with Hemodynamics	No	Yes	Basal flow changes with demand.
Detects microcirculation	No	Yes	
Specific for epicardial vessel	Yes	No	CFR measures sum flow response of both epicardial and microvasculature.

CFR, Coronary flow reserve; *FFR*, fractional flow reserve.

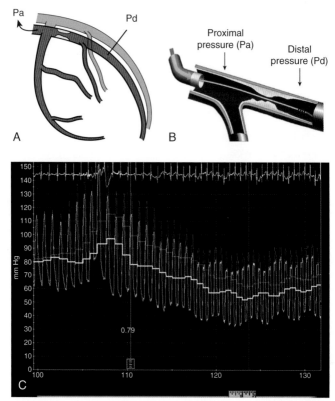

Figure 5.5 (A) Diagrams of the theory of fractional flow reserve (FFR). FFR is the ratio of maximal myocardial perfusion in the stenotic territory divided by maximal hyperemic flow in that same region in the hypothetical case that the lesion is not present (the faint pink artery is the hypothetical normal artery without the stenosis.). FFR represents that fraction of hyperemic flow that persists despite the presence of the stenosis. FFR is defined as myocardial flow (Qs) across stenosis/myocardial flow (Qn) without stenosis. (B) Diagram of pressure wire inside guide catheter across a target lesion. (C) These are the pressure signals used to calculate FFR. Mean aortic pressure (*red*) and distal coronary pressure (*yellow*) are recorded at rest and then during hyperemia induced by adenosine. The nadir of Pd/Pa pressures (*green line*) is used for the FFR calculation, which is 0.79.

equalized, also called *normalized*). By early convention, the guidewire transducer was positioned at the end of the guide catheter. In fact, it does not matter exactly where the wire is in relation to the guide catheter or coronary ostium except that at a minimum, the guide pressure should not be damped in the coronary ostium and the guide wire should not be beyond a narrowed left main artery before crossing the target lesion.

4. The wire is then advanced across the stenosis about 2 cm distal to the coronary lesion (at least 10 artery diameters distal to the lesion).

5. After waiting for the effect of flushing contrast out of the guide (>1 min), resting NHPR (e.g., Pd/Pa or iFR, or other NHPRs) are measured in duplicate. For FFR, maximal hyperemia is induced with IV adenosine (140 mcg/kg/min) or IC bolus adenosine (50–100 mcg for the right coronary artery [RCA], 100–200 mcg for the left coronary artery [LCA]). Alternative hyperemic agents are rarely used but include nitroprusside (50–100 mcg) or adenosine triphosphate (ATP; 50–100 mcg). FFR is measured at the lowest Pd/Pa ratio after the onset of hyperemia, usually within 2 minutes for IV adenosine and at 15 to 20 seconds after IC adenosine.

6. FFR is calculated as the ratio of the mean distal guidewire pressure to mean proximal guide catheter pressure (Pd/Pa) during maximal hyperemia. An FFR of less than 0.80 is associated with a hemodynamically significant lesion that benefits from PCI/CABG. NHPR is calculated according to the algorithm selected (Pd/Pa during the diastolic period or fraction thereof).

7. If a lesion is hemodynamically significant, and PCI is deemed necessary, it can be performed using the pressure wire as the angioplasty guidewire. After the stent implantation, FFR and pressure pullback can be measured along the course of the vessel to assess the adequacy of the intervention and impact of any residual disease or hidden lesions in the target or other vessels.

8. Finally, at the end of the procedure, check for pressure signal drift. The pressure wire should be pulled back into the guide to confirm equal pressure readings and the lack of pressure signal drift. Signal drift can occur because of changes in the electrical signals from either the wire transducer or the fluid-filled guide catheter pressure transducer. Drift shifts the zero setting of the tracings producing a false reading. On occasion the drift is large, and the last measurements will need to be repeated after re-equalization of pressures in the guide catheter.

Pharmacologic Hyperemic Agents

Maximal coronary hyperemia is required for accurate FFR. Table 5.3 lists available pharmacologic agents suitable for inducing hyperemia. The most common in use today is adenosine.

Adenosine is the most used hyperemic agent. IV adenosine is weight-based, operator-independent, and the preferred method used for ostial lesion assessment and pressure pullbacks for serial lesions or diffuse disease assessment. By providing a sustained hyperemic stimulus, IV adenosine allows for a slow pullback of the pressure wire, useful to identify the exact location of a pressure drop or the gradual slope of increasing pressure associated with diffuse disease. IV adenosine is often required for the assessment of aorto-ostial narrowings without the guide catheter in place to permit maximal coronary flow without coronary obstruction. Nevertheless, pressures may fluctuate with IV adenosine, such that, at times, no stable period of pressure can be seen. Johnson et al. and Seto et al. reported various fluctuation patterns of pressure changes during IV adenosine infusion (Fig. 5.6). Johnson et al. demonstrated that the lowest Pd/Pa, called a *smart minimum,* during the adenosine infusion is the FFR value with the highest reproducibility on repeat infusions. The smart minimum FFR is the lowest Pd/Pa without pressure wave artifact that occurs any time after the adenosine effect has begun. Current FFR signal monitors have incorporated software that automatically computes and displays the FFR as the lowest Pd/Pa. The operator and team must continue to view the pressure recordings to ensure that FFR is the smart minimum value and not just "a value" that might be artificial.

IC adenosine is equivalent to IV infusion for determination of FFR. Although IV adenosine has been the standard for FFR for more than three decades and was used successfully to generate the data sets that demonstrated superior FFR-guided outcomes in the FAME (FFR Versus Angiography for Multivessel Evaluation) trial and other studies, recent examinations of hemodynamic variability during IV adenosine have prompted a return to using IC adenosine.

There are many reports of different doses of IC adenosine, ranging from 16 mcg to more than 700 mcg. The optimal doses appear to be 50 to 100 mcg for the RCA and 100 to 200 mcg for the LCA. These doses will eliminate any uncertainty that the operator achieved maximal hyperemia or did not give enough adenosine to get the most accurate FFR. Heart block in more than 10% of patients is observed with RCA IC adenosine in doses greater than 50 mcg. The concentration of IC adenosine should be mixed to provide 10 to 30 mcg/mL. One liter of the adenosine/saline mix can supply the entire lab's needs for the day. A stopcock and flush

Table 5.3

Pharmacologic Agents Used to Induce Maximal Coronary Hyperemia in the Cath Lab	Adenosine	Adenosine	Papaverine	NTP	Regadenoson
Route	IV	IC	IC	IC	IV
Dosage	140 mcg/kg/min	100–200 mcg LCA, 50–100 mcg RCA	15 mg LCA, 10 mg RCA	50–100 mcg	0.4 mg
Half-life	1–2 min	30–60 sec	2 min	1–2 min	2–4 min (up to 30 min)
Time to max hyperemia	<1–2 min	5–10 sec	20–60 sec	10–20 sec	1–4 min
Advantage	Gold standard	Short action	Short action	Short action	IV bolus
Disadvantage	↓BP, chest burning	AV Block, ↓BP	Torsades, ↓BP	↓BP	↑HR, ? redose, long action

AV, Atrioventricular; *BP,* blood pressure; *HR,* heart rate; *IC,* intracoronary; *IV,* intravenous; *LCA,* left coronary artery; *NTP,* nitroprusside; *RCA,* right coronary artery.

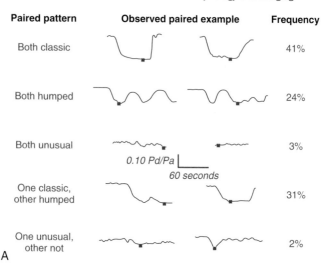

Figure 5.6 (A) Adenosine variability. Paired patterns of pressure distal/pressure aortic (Pd/Pa) during hyperemia. Each lesion underwent repeat study separated by 2 minutes of rest, producing five observed paired patterns of varying frequency. For each observed example, the red dot marks the smart minimum fractional flow reserve (FFR). The blue scale for Pd/Pa and time applies to the example tracings. Even with the same patient/lesion, the two paired tracings differ 31% of the time. (From Johnson NP, Johnson DT, Kirkeeide RL, et al. Repeatability of fractional flow reserve despite variations in systemic and coronary hemodynamics. *JACC Cardiovasc Interv.* 2015;8[8]:1018–1027.)

syringe connected to the adenosine syringe make delivery of the drug easy (Fig. 5.7).

Submaximal Hyperemia and Contrast FFR

Radiographic contrast injection causes submaximal coronary hyperemia. Intracoronary contrast media provides an easy and inexpensive tool for predicting FFR. Johnson et al. evaluated cFFR to adenosine FFR and found that approximately an injected bolus contrast volume of 8 mL (give or take 2 mL) per measurement showed less variability for cFFR than resting Pd/Pa and iFR, which had equivalent performance against FFR less than 0.8 (78.5% vs. 79.9% accuracy; $p = .78$). cFFR improved both metrics (85.8% accuracy and 0.930 area under the curve [AUC]; $p < .001$ for each) with an optimal binary threshold of 0.83. Leone et al. compared cFFR, Pd/Pa, and FFR (Fig. 5.8). A binary cutoff of 0.83 for cFFR was

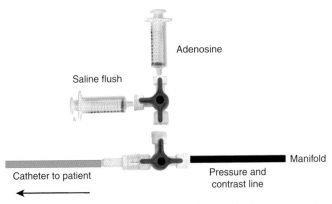

Figure 5.7 Syringe and stopcock assembly for rapid intracoronary adenosine injection.

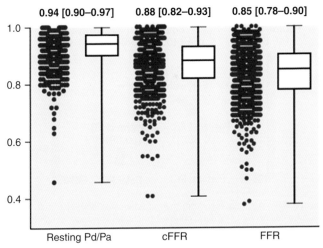

Figure 5.8 cFFR median values (interquartile ranges) of resting pressure distal/pressure aortic (Pd/Pa), contrast fractional flow reserve (cFFR), and fractional flow reserve (FFR). (From Leone AM, Martin-Reyes R, Baptista SB, et al. The Multicenter Evaluation of the Accuracy of the Contrast MEdium INduced Pd/Pa RaTiO in Predicting FFR (MEMENTO-FFR) Study. *EuroIntervention.* 2016;12:708–715.)

the best for prediction of FFR and more accurate than resting Pd/Pa (cutoff of 0.92) and iFR (cutoff of 0.90) in predicting FFR, with resting Pd/Pa and iFR providing equivalent diagnostic accuracy. To maximize the accuracy of cFFR, a hybrid approach has been proposed deferring revascularization when cFFR is greater than 0.88 and stenting when cFFR is up to 0.83 (Fig. 5.9). Advantages of cFFR include universal availability with any FFR system, no additional expense, and minimal side effects related to those of contrast media. Because of the short half-life of contrast hyperemia, cFFR is not suitable for pressure pullback curves. cFFR provides diagnostic performance superior to that of Pd/Pa or iFR for predicting FFR and may be useful in clinical scenarios or health care systems in which adenosine is contraindicated or prohibitively expensive.

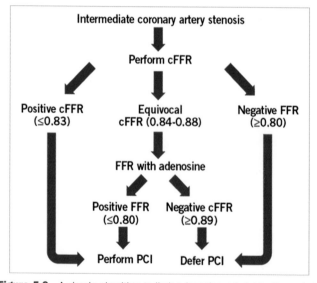

Figure 5.9 A simple algorithm to limit adenosine administration only to doubtful cases. We consider a contrast fractional flow reserve (cFFR) value ≤ 0.83 significant (consequently we suggest performing percutaneous coronary intervention [PCI]), a cFFR value ≥ 0.89 not significant (consequently we suggest deferring PCI), and inducing maximal hyperemia using adenosine for FFR assessment when cFFR is between 0.84 and 0.88. After that, PCI would be performed when FFR is ≤ 0.80 and deferred when FFR is > 0.80. (From Leone AM, Martin-Reyes R, Baptista SB, et al. The Multicenter Evaluation of the Accuracy of the Contrast MEdium INduced Pd/Pa RaTiO in Predicting FFR (MEMENTO-FFR) Study. *EuroIntervention*. 2016; 12:708–715.)

Pitfalls of Translesional Pressure Measurement

The three most common pitfalls of accurate FFR/NHPR are guide pressure damping, failure to capture the smart minimum Pd/Pa (for FFR), and signal drift. Tables 5.4 and 5.5 list factors that can reduce the accuracy of FFR and NHPR. Fig. 5.10 shows some of the artifacts that may produce false FFR readings.

Guide catheters that produced obstruction with pressure signal damping are at times substituted with catheters having side holes permitting coronary perfusion despite catheter obstruction. These

Table 5.4

Hemodynamic Artifacts or Errors

1. *Signal drift.* Identified by unmatched Pd and Pa on pullback to guide catheter. Also can be seen in distal artery pressure waveform by shifted waveform with preserved dichrotic notch. If suspicious, check with re-matching of signals on pullback to aortic location.
2. *Incorrect height of pressure transducer.*
3. *Loss of pressure because of guidewire introducer or loose connections.* Remove and tighten Touhey-Borst valve.
4. *Damping of pressure by guiding catheter.* Flat diastolic aortic pressure waveform resembling left ventricle (LV). Solution: use intravenous (IV) adenosine, remove guide catheter from coronary ostium. Flush guide catheter with saline to clear bubbles.
5. *Guiding catheters with side holes* produce pseudostenosis across the catheter into the coronary ostium. (see #4)
6. *Pressure damping with 4F or 5F catheters because of* contrast media viscosity. Flush with saline before accepting pressure.

Failure to Induce Hyperemia

A. Adenosine, intracoronary bolus administration
   1. *Submaximum stimulus in some patients because of residual caffeine or idiosyncratic response (*very rare); if suspected, select alternative agent (e.g., nitroprusside, papaverine, adenosine triphosphate [ATP]).
   2. *Failure to capture pressure change at peak hyperemia.* Use smart minimum fractional flow reserve (FFR).
   3. *Guiding catheter not seated and fails to deliver drug.*
   4. *Guide catheter flow is obstructed.*
   5. *Incorrect dose mix or dilution.*
B. Adenosine, IV Adenosine
   1. Check infusion, pump system, and lines.
   2. Infuse through large central vein.
   3. Avoid Valsalva maneuver during infusion.
   4. *Transient side effects include hypotension, burning or angina-like chest pain during infusion are* harmless and do not indicate ischemia. IV adenosine is not to be used in patients with severe obstructive lung disease (bronchospasm).

Table 5.5

Confounding Technical Factors for Translesional Pressure Measurements

1. Equipment factors
   Erroneous zero
   Incomplete pressure transmission (tubing/connector leaks)
   Faulty electric wire connection
   Pressure signal drift
   Hemodynamics recorder miscalibration
2. Procedural factors
   Guide catheter damping
   Incorrect placement of pressure sensor
   Inadequate hyperemia (fractional flow reserve [FFR])
3. Physiologic factors
   Serial lesion
   Reduced myocardial bed
   Acute myocardial infarction
4. Theoretical conditions that might influence FFR
   Severe left ventricular hypertrophy
   Exuberant collateral supply
   Adenosine insensitivity (FFR)

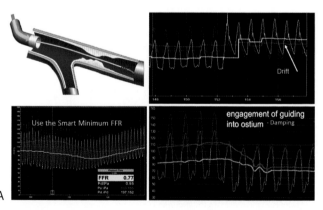

Figure 5.10 (A) *Top left,* The guide catheter and pressure wire across a lesion. Artifacts and errors are principally related to the malposition of the guide catheter (*lower right,* damping) or signal drift (*upper right*). Correct FFR (i.e., the lowest Pd/Pa during hyperemia) is also a source of error (*lower left*).

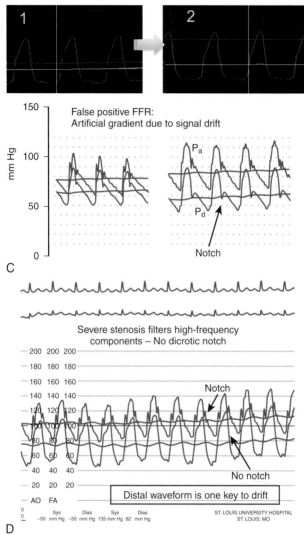

Figure 5.10, cont'd (B) Example of pressure signals during damping (*left*) and after withdrawal of guide catheter (*right*). (C) Example of pressure signal drift as a cause for false-positive fractional flow reserve (FFR). Note preservation of dichrotic notch on distal pressure indicating normal transmission of pressure. (D) Example of distal pressure across severe stenosis. Note distal pressure wave configuration with wide pulse pressure and loss of dichrotic notch indicative of severe stenosis.

catheters should be avoided because side holes do not eliminate the catheter obstruction but rather create an artificial stenosis through the holes. Removing the guide catheter from the coronary ostium after giving the hyperemic agent will avoid this pitfall.

Nonhyperemic Pressure Ratios

Procedural cost and time and the need to administer adenosine to achieve maximal hyperemia are thought to have been barriers to the use of FFR. Adenosine-free pressure ratios or NHPRs have been developed as alternatives to FFR and appear to be clinically noninferior to FFR in initial large multicenter trials. All NHPRs use the ratio between distal coronary pressure and aortic pressure. They differ principally in the portion of the diastolic period of the cardiac cycle that is measured. NHPRs are divided into diastolic only (iFR, diastolic pressure ratio [dPR], diastolic hyperemia-free ratio [DFR]) or whole-cycle indices (Pd/Pa, resting full-cycle ratio [RFR]; Fig. 5.11). NHPR reproducibility depends on stable resting coronary

Resting (i.e. no adenosine) instantaneous pressure during wave free period = iFR

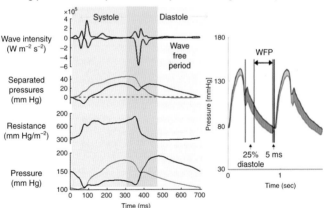

Davies JE et al. Circulation 2006;113:1767-1778

Davies JE et al. JACC 2012;59:1392-402

Figure 5.11 *Left,* Instantaneous wave-free ratio (iFR) is defined as average pressure diastolic/pressure aortic (Pd/Pa) during the wave-free period (WFP; *pink shaded area*). The WFP was calculated beginning 25% of the way into diastole and ending 5 ms before the end of diastole. *Right,* Diastolic pressure ratio (dPR) is defined as average Pd/Pa during entire diastole. Diastolic hyperemia-free ratio (DFR) is defined as average Pd/Pa during Pa less than mean Pa with negative slope. Resting full-cycle ratio (RFR) is defined as the lowest filtered mean Pd/Pa during the entire cardiac cycle. (Modified from *Davies J et al, JACC 2012.*

blood flow. Measurements made close in time to saline flushing, contrast, or nitroglycerin administration may differ because of alteration of resting flow related to residual minimal hyperemia. Other factors and pressure wave artifacts altering reproducibility of NHPRs are the same as those discussed for FFR. Advantages and limitations of hyperemic ratios and NHPRs in the cath lab are summarized in Table 5.6.

Instantaneous Wave-Free Ratio

For pressures to be linear with coronary flow ratios, FFR must be measured during minimal and stable coronary resistance, usually achieved during adenosine-induced hyperemia. Sen et al. determined from wave intensity analysis that there is a period in diastole in which the reflected pressure waves from the aorta and distal microcirculatory bed are quiescent and called this a "wave-free period" (WFP). The WFP has a fixed resistance and thus the resting Pd/Pa over this interval could be equivalent to FFR (Fig. 5.12). The ratio of Pd/Pa during the wave-free period was called the iFR and was found to correlate with FFR ($r = 0.90$) with an approximately 80% concordance. After the completion of the two major iFR outcome studies, Define-Flair and iFR Swedeheart (see later), the iFR dichotomous threshold for treatment decisions is 0.89. Overall correspondence between iFR and FFR is approximately 80% to 85%.

Since the introduction of iFR, four other NHPRs have been introduced that are all relatively similar and dependent on the company that manufactured the pressure measuring device. dPR is defined as average Pd/Pa during entire diastole. DFR is defined as average Pd/Pa during Pa less than mean Pa with negative slope. RFR is defined as the lowest filtered mean Pd/Pa during the entire cardiac cycle (Fig. 5.13). Several algorithms exist for calculating dPR, the resting ratio of mean Pd/mean Pa during diastole, with no significant advantage to any calculation. Compared with iFR, dPR is numerically equivalent. One algorithm uses the automatically delineated diastolic period based on the dP/dt curve of the aortic pressure with the flat line of the dP/dt tracing detecting the diastolic WFP. The resting Pd/Pa ratio is available for every translesional pressure measure and is calculated as the ratio of the mean continuous Pd and Pa over the entire cardiac cycle. Numerous studies demonstrated equivalent diagnostic performance of Pd/Pa to iFR noting the higher ischemic threshold of 0.92 for resting Pd/Pa used in most comparative clinical studies. Pd/Pa suffers from the same limitations of other NHPRs in that it has lower reproducibility and higher susceptibility to hemodynamic variability compared with FFR.

Table 5.6

Advantages and Limitations of Physiologic Assessment in the Catheterization Laboratory

Wire-Based Physiologic Assessment			
Hyperemic Index		**NHPR**	
FFR	**iFR**	**Novel NHPRs (DFR, dPR, RFR)**	**Pd/Pa**
ADVANTAGES			
• Evidence for outcomes up to 15 yrs (vs. angiography guided PCI, OMT alone) • Well validated with noninvasive functional tests in various clinical settings • Cost-effectiveness was demonstrated against angiography guided PCI • Available with all pressure wires	• Evidence for outcomes up to 2 yrs (vs. FFR-guided PCI) • Validated with noninvasive functional tests in several clinical settings • Well validated with FFR in various clinical settings • Hyperemia independent • Quicker than FFR • Ability with potential to assess serial lesions • Coregistration with angiography available	• Validated with FFR and iFR in limited clinical settings (retrospective) • Hyperemia independent • Quicker than FFR	• Validated with FFR and iFR in limited clinical settings • Hyperemia independent • Quicker than FFR • Available with all pressure wires

LIMITATIONS

• Hyperemia required (additional cost and hyperemic agent related side effect)	• Pressure wire required (additional cost and wire-related complication)	• No evidence for outcomes	• No evidence for outcomes
• Pressure wire required (additional cost and wire-related complication)	• Precise acquisition of coronary pressure required	• Validation data with noninvasive functional tests are limited	• Validation data with noninvasive functional tests are limited
• Precise acquisition of coronary pressure required	• Proprietary and the software of specific vendor required	• Pressure wire required (additional cost and wire-related complication)	• Pressure wire required (additional cost and wire-related complication)
• Prolonged procedure		• Precise acquisition of coronary pressure required	• Precise acquisition of coronary pressure required
		• Proprietary and the software of specific vendor required	• Susceptible to miscalculation from pressure-wire drift
		• No coregistration with angiography available	• No coregistration with angiography available

DFR, Diastolic hyperemia-free ratio; *dPR,* diastolic pressure ratio; *FFR,* fractional flow reserve; *iFR,* instantaneous wave-free pressure ratio; *NHPR,* nonhyperemic pressure ratios; *OMT,* optimal anti-ischemic medications; *PCI,* percutaneous coronary intervention; *RFR,* resting full-cycle ratio.
(From Kogame N, Ono M, Kawashima H, et al. The impact of coronary physiology on contemporary clinical decision making. *JACC Cardiovasc Interv.* 2020;13:1617–1638.)

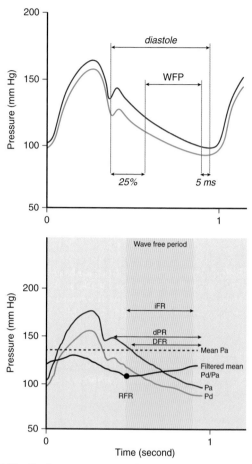

Figure 5.12 The instantaneous wave-free ratio (iFR). Wave-intensity analysis demonstrates the proximal and microcirculatory (distal) originating waves generated during the cardiac cycle. A wave-free period can be seen in diastole when no new waves are generated (*shaded*). This corresponds to a time in which there is minimal microcirculatory (distal)–originating pressure, minimal and constant resistance, and a nearly constant rate of change in flow velocity. Separated pressure above diastole is the residual pulsatile separated pressure component after subtraction of the diastolic pressure. (Top, From Sen S, Escaned J, Malik IS, et al. Development and validation of a new adenosine-independent index of stenosis severity from coronary wave–intensity analysis results of the ADVISE [ADenosine Vasodilator Independent Stenosis Evaluation] Study. *J Am Coll Cardiol.* 2012;59:1234.) Bottom from From Kogame N, Ono M, Kawashima H, et al. The impact of coronary physiology on contemporary clinical decision making. JACC Cardiovasc Interv. 2020;13:1617–1638.)

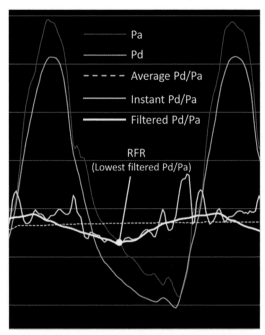

Figure 5.13 Hemodynamic tracings showing aortic pressure (Pa – *red*) and coronary pressure (Pd – *green*). Nonhyperemic ratios can be derived from these pressures, including the instantaneous or average Pd/Pa (*yellow*) and resting full-cycle ratio (RFR; *white*).

Clinical Applications of Translesional Pressure Assessment: Specific Angiographic Subsets

The use of translesional pressure ratios at rest (NHPR) or during hyperemia (cFFR and adenosine FFR) have been studied in a variety of angiographic substrates and clinical presentations. FFR has been available and has more than 25 years of studies, whereas NHPRs are relatively recent with more than 5 years of outcome studies.

The Intermediate Coronary Lesion

For patients with stable ischemic heart disease, the decision to treat or not treat coronary lesions should be based on ischemia from ECG changes, stress testing, or FFR/NHPR. It is a common but erroneous belief that not stenting an angiographically intermediate but hemodynamically insignificant lesions will result in harm to the patient later. This concern is unsupported by many studies (Table 5.7). The exemplar of such studies is the 15-year outcome of the DEFER study, which found that patients having an intermediate lesion (>50% narrowing) with an FFR greater than 0.75 could be safely treated medically with a low event rate over 15-year follow-up, which was no greater than any patient having stable ischemic heart disease treated medically (about 4%/year). In patients with intermediate lesions who were stented despite an FFR greater than 0.75 and in patients with FFR less than 0.75, both groups had significantly higher event rates over the same time. Stenting lesions with FFR greater than 0.75 gives the patient new problems related to the stent procedure acutely or late adverse events (subacute thrombosis, bleeding risk from dual antiplatelet medications). The composite rate of cardiac death and acute myocardial infarction (MI) in the deferred, performed, and reference groups was 3%, 8%, and 16%, respectively (p = .21 for deferred vs. performed and p = .003 for reference vs. both the deferred and performed groups; Fig. 5.14). The percentage of patients free from chest pain on follow-up was not different between the deferred and performed groups. The 5-year risk of cardiac death or MI in patients with a normal FFR is less than 1% per year and not decreased by stenting. Fig. 5.15 is an example of FFR for intermediate lesion assessment.

Instantaneous Wave-Free Ratio

In clinical practice the outcomes of treating intermediate stenosis based on iFR were identified in two large randomized trials, the DEFINE-FLAIR (Functional Lesion Assessment of Intermediate Stenosis to Guide Revascularization, n = 2492) and iFR SWEDE-HEART (Evaluation of iFR vs. FFR in Stable Angina or Acute Coronary Syndrome, n = 2042) studies, and found that iFR-guided PCI was noninferior to FFR-guided PCI for either deferral or treatment of stenoses based on iFR threshold of 0.89 (Fig. 5.16). Although major adverse events were similar, long-term prognostic data for iFR is limited. After iFR SWEDEHEART and DEFINE-FLAIR, the European Society of Cardiology (ESC) guidelines gave a Class I (Level of Evidence: A) recommendation for guiding PCI in both iFR and FFR. Some advantages of iFR over FFR include shorter procedure time, less patient discomfort, and easy pull back, especially for evaluation of serial lesions.

FFR, iFR, or Other NHPR Compared

With the availability of multiple indexes that have been shown to be accurate and easy to perform, there now becomes a question on which index to use. The following are some general considerations:

Table 5.7

Fractional Flow Reserve Studies on Long-Term Outcomes

FFR Outcome Studies	N =	Study Design	Question	Outcome	Journal
DEFER (2007)	325	Prospective MC RCT	Is it safe to defer FFR normal intermediate lesions?	Less MACE in FFR >0.75 when rx'd medically	JACC
FAME (2009)	750	Prospective MC RCT	Does FFR-guided PCI vs. angio-guided for MVD improve outcomes?	Less MACE, lower cost w FFR	NEJM
FAME II (2012)	1220	Prospective MC RCT	Does FFR-guided PCI + OMT vs. OMT alone improve outcomes?	Less MACE w FFR, cost effective	NEJM
FAMOUS-NSTEMI (2014)	350	Prospective MC Randomized (UK)	Does FFR-guided PCI in NSTEMI change angio decisions for revasc? Outcomes?	FFR reclass revasc decision in 22%. Less revasc w FFR	EHJ
DANAMI3-PRIMULTI (2015)	600	Prospective MC Randomized (Denmark)	Dose FFR-guided PCI in MV STEMI vs. IRA only revasc improve outcomes?	Less MACE with FFR	Lancet
Mayo (2013)	7358	Retrospective SC Registry	Does FFR-guided vs. angio-guided PCI improve outcomes in routine practice?	Less MACE with FFR	EHJ
R3F (2014)	1.075	Prospective MC Registry (France)	Does FFR change angio decisions for revasc?	FFR reclass revasc decision in 47%, similar outcomes	Circulation
POST-IT (2015)	918	Prospective MC Registry (Portugal)	Does FFR change angio decisions for revasc? Outcomes?	FFR reclass revasc decision in 44% (follow-up data in press)	In press
Asan registry (2013)		Prospective SC Registry	Does FFR-guided vs. angio-guided PCI improve outcomes in routine practice?	Fewer stents and less MACE with FFR	EJHJ

Angio, Angiography; *FFR,* fractional flow reserve; *MACE,* major adverse cardiac event; *MC,* multicenter; *PCI,* percutaneous coronary intervention; *RCT,* randomized controlled trial; *revasc,* revascularization; *rx'd,* prescribed; *SC,* single center.

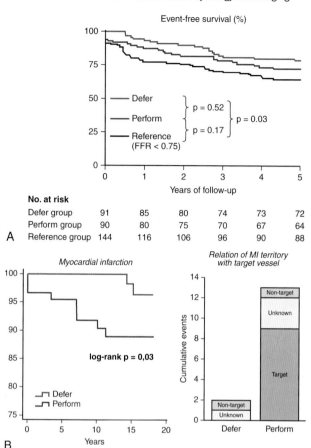

Figure 5.14 (A) Adverse cardiac events during 5-year follow-up for the defer group (*blue line*), treatment group (*red line*), and reference group (*yellow line*). (B, *lower panel*) DEFER 15-year outcomes. Kaplan-Meier of myocardial infarction (MI) (B, *lower right*) and relation of myocardial infarction with study vessel territory (B). The rate of MI was significantly lower in the DEFER group (2.2%) compared with the Perform group (10.0%), *p* = .03. This was almost exclusively because of less target vessel–related infarctions. Patients with a baseline fractional flow reserve (FFR) of 0.75 or higher had a significantly lower rate of MI compared with patients with an FFR of less than 0.75 (6.1 vs. 12.5%, *p* = .044). (A is from Pijls NHJ, Van Schaardenburgh P, Manoharan G, et al. Percutaneous coronary intervention of functionally non-significant stenoses: 5-year follow-up of the DEFER study. *J Am Coll Cardiol.* 2007;49:2105–2111; B is from Zimmermann FM, Ferrera A, Johnson NP, et al. The deferral vs. performance of percutaneous coronary intervention of functionally non-significant coronary stenosis: 15-year follow-up of the DEFER trial. *Eur Heart J.* 2015;36[45]:3182–3188.)

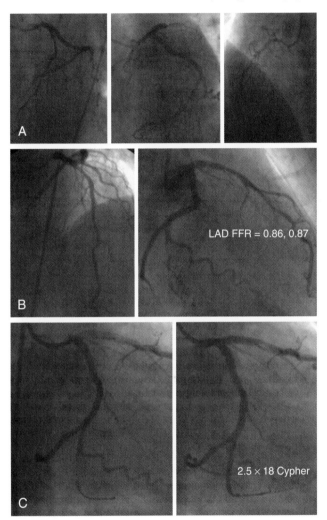

Figure 5.15 Angiograms of patient with intermediate left anterior descending (LAD) and severe OM1 branch lesion. (A) *Left panel,* left anterior oblique (LAO) view of LAD, middle LAO caudal view of left coronary artery (LCA), and *right panel,* occluded right coronary artery (RCA) of 2 years ago. (B) *Left panel,* RAO cranial shows intermediate LAD; *right panel,* severe OM1 branch stenoses. Fractional flow reserve (FFR) of LAD is 0.86, 0.87. (C) *Left panel,* pre-percutaneous coronary intervention (PCI) of OM1 and post-PCI. Patient became pain free and did well.

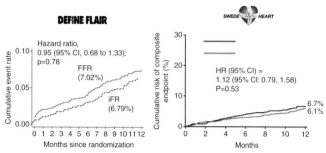

Figure 5.16   iFR SWEDEHEART (Evaluation of iFR vs FFR in Stable Angina or Acute Coronary Syndrome) and DEFINE-FLAIR (Functional Lesion Assessment of Intermediate Stenosis to Guide Revascularization) both demonstrated that instantaneous wave-free ratio (iFR)–guided percutaneous coronary intervention (PCI) was noninferior to fractional flow reserve (FFR)–guided PCI with similar low event rates of major adverse cardiac events (MACE) at 12 months and that the incidence of MACE in both arms did not differ up to 2 years in both trials. (left panel, From Davies JE, Sen S, Dehbi HM, et al. Use of the instantaneous wave-free ratio or fractional flow reserve in PCI. *N Engl J Med.* 2017;376:1824–1834); (right panel, Gotberg M, Christiansen EH, Gudmundsdottir IJ, et al. Instantaneous wave-free ratio versus fractional flow reserve to guide PCI. *N Engl J Med.* 2017;376:1813–1823.)

- Use of any physiologic index to further assess an intermediate angiographic coronary lesion is superior to using angiography alone.
- FFR remains the best-studied physiologic index in terms of number of patients studied, variety of clinical scenarios in which it was used, and prediction of clinical outcomes.
- iFR has been shown to be noninferior from a clinical outcome standpoint to FFR-guided revascularization.
- Other NHPR indices do not have clinical outcome data and their use is reliant on strong correlations with either FFR or iFR.
- Developing a hybrid algorithm for use in the lab probably makes most sense, depending on the available equipment in the lab. Labs will not likely have the equipment to perform each and every index.
  - Suggested hybrid algorithm:
    - Perform a resting NHPR after crossing the lesion.

- If index above is at the "cut-off" for that index or if uncertainty exists regarding the clinical patient scenario then – proceed with performing FFR by administering IV or IC adenosine (as previously described).
- If index is clearly nonischemic, proceed with next steps of caring for patient (usually medical therapy).

- Routine performance of both FFR and an NHPR for the same lesion is not recommended unless for specific predefined research interest.

The Borderline FFR/NHPR: A Cautionary Note

Operators must base all decisions on specific clinical indications, patient presentations, risks, and benefits of treatment as well as all objective data. A positive FFR/NHPR in the absence of symptoms, clinical findings, or other indications should not automatically require a stent. This situation is particularly troubling when the FFR/NHPR value is close to or on the border of the ischemic threshold. In these situations, judgment on whether to proceed or stop must be guided by a complete clinical evaluation. Borderline FFR/NHPR values are equivalent to a "yellow light" when driving your car. Decisions should be based on safety for the passengers (or patients).

Multivessel Disease PCI

The use of FFR to guide multivessel PCI demonstrated better reduction in major adverse cardiac events (MACE) than the conventional angiographically guided approach. Among the first multivessel FFR PCI-guided studies was the FAME trial by Tonino et al. FAME compared a physiologically guided PCI approach (FFR-PCI) to a conventional angiographic-guided PCI (angio-PCI) in 1005 patients with multivessel CAD undergoing PCI with drug-eluting stents (DES). By visual angiographic appearance, patients with lesions with more than 50% diameter stenosis to be treated were randomized to a stenting strategy guided by FFR or angiography alone. For the FFR-PCI group ($n = 496$), only those stenoses with an FFR less than 0.80 were stented. For the angio-PCI group ($n = 509$), all lesions identified were stented. Clinical characteristics and angiographic findings were similar in both groups, with average SYNTAX scores of 14.5 (indicating low- to intermediate-risk patients).

Compared with the angio-PCI group, the FFR-PCI group used fewer stents per patient (1.9 ± 1.3 vs. 2.7 ± 1.2; $p < .001$) and less contrast (272 mL vs. 302 mL; $p < .001$), had a lower procedure cost ($5332 vs. $6007; $p < .001$) and shorter hospital stay (3.4 vs. 3.7 days; $p = .05$). More importantly, the 2-year rates of mortality or MI were 13% in the angio-PCI group compared with 8% in the FFR-PCI group

(p = .02). Composite rates of death/nonfatal MI or revascularization were 22% and 18%, respectively (p = .08). For lesions deferred based on an FFR of more than 0.80, the rate of MI was only 0.2% and the rate of revascularization was 3.2% after 2 years (Fig. 5.17).

The most impactful FFR study was the Fractional Flow Reserve-Guided PCI Versus Medical Therapy in Stable Coronary Disease (FAME 2) trial, which compared optimal medical therapy with optimal medical therapy with PCI in patients who had proven ischemia by FFR. Patients with multivessel CAD and at least one stenosis with an FFR of less than 0.80 were randomized to be treated with optimal anti-ischemic medications (OMT) or treated with OMT and stenting. Those patients with stenoses that did not undergo PCI for an FFR greater than 0.80 were entered into a registry and followed. Medically treated registry patients had a low rate of the primary endpoint of death (0), MI (1.8%), or urgent revascularization (2.4%) over the follow-up 12 months, thus reproducing the findings of the pre-DES era DEFER trial (Fig. 5.18). For patients with FFR less than 0.80, revascularization reduced unstable anginal hospitalizations and MIs despite no reduction in mortality.

Together these data are the initial foundational support for the use of FFR for CAD patients. Over the last two decades, continued studies strongly support the concept that patients benefit from coronary revascularization guided by FFR results with rare exceptions (Table 5.8).

Left Main Stenosis

Decisions about whether to revascularize the patient with a left main (LM) coronary stenosis are of critical importance. Because of the inherent limitations, angiography alone is particularly unreliable in LM stenoses. Translesional physiology is valuable for LM decision making.

Among numerous studies of FFR in equivocal LM disease (Table 5.9), the largest is that of Hamilos et al. who reported 5-year outcomes in 213 patients with an angiographically equivocal LM coronary artery stenosis who were treated medically if the FFR was greater than 0.80 (nonsurgical group; n = 138) and if the FFR less than 0.80 were revascularized (surgical group; n = 75). The 5-year survival estimates were 90% in the nonsurgical (FFR > 0.80) group and 85% in the surgical (FFR < 0.80) group (p = .48). The 5-year event-free survival estimates were 74% and 82% in the two groups, respectively (p = .50; Fig. 5.19A). Of note, only 23% of patients with a diameter stenosis of greater than 50% had a hemodynamically significant LM by FFR. For iFR and the LMCA stenosis, the DEFINE LM registry observed patients with LM stenoses that were treated or deferred based on iFR of approximately 0.89 and found that decisions based on iFR were safe with low composite clinical endpoints at 30 months (see Fig. 5.19B).

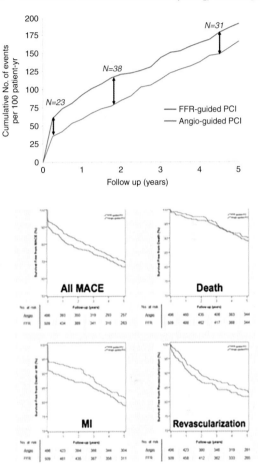

Figure 5.17 (A) The FAME (FFR Versus Angiography for Multivessel Evaluation) study results and Kaplan-Meier survival curves according to study group. Results confirm the long-term safety of fractional flow reserve (FFR)-guided percutaneous coronary intervention (PCI) in patients with multivessel disease. A strategy of FFR-guided PCI resulted in a significant decrease of major adverse cardiac events (MACE) for up to 2 years. From 2 years to 5 years, the risks for both groups developed similarly. This clinical outcome in the FFR-guided group was achieved with a lower number of stented arteries and less resource use. These results indicate that FFR guidance of multivessel PCI should be the standard of care in most patients. (From van Nunen LX, Zimmermann FM, Tonino PAL, et al. Fractional flow reserve versus angiography for guidance of PCI in patients with multivessel coronary artery disease (FAME): 5-year follow-up of a randomized controlled trial. *Lancet* 2015;386:1853–1860.)

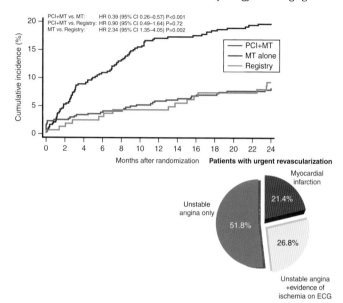

Figure 5.18 FAME 2 (Fractional Flow Reserve-Guided PCI Versus Medical Therapy in Stable Coronary Disease) study results. Kaplan-Meier curve for primary endpoint of death, myocardial infarction (MI), or urgent revascularization at 12 months in the group assigned to percutaneous coronary intervention (PCI) and optimal medical therapy (*blue*) versus optimal medical therapy alone (*red*) versus those who did not undergo revascularization (*green*). The pie chart shows the events prompting revascularization with about 50% unstable angina, 25% MI, and 25% unstable angina (UA) with electrocardiogram (ECG) changes. (Modified from De Bruyne B, Pijls NHJ, Kalesan B, et al. Fractional flow reserve-guided PCI versus medical therapy in stable coronary disease. *N Engl J Med.* 2012;367(11):991–1001.)

LM With Downstream Disease

The assessment of an isolated LM is straightforward. The pressure wire can be put into either the left anterior descending (LAD) artery or the circumflex artery (CFX) and FFR measured. For distal LM, FFR is measured twice, once in each branch. The LM FFR assessment becomes more complex, however, when there is additional potentially significant LAD disease that may reduce flow to the anterior wall, thus creating a falsely elevated LM FFR.

Fearon et al. demonstrated that the LM FFR measured in the setting of downstream LAD disease was only affected when the FFR of both the LM and LAD was less than 0.45. In 25 patients,

Table 5.8

Hard Endpoints Between FFR- and Angio-Guided PCI in Large Clinical Trials

1st Author, Yr	Trail Outline	Pts	F-up (yrs)	Events	FFR (%)	Angio (%)	P Value
Pijls 2010	RCT	1,005 MVD 33% ACS	2	All mort	2.6	3.8	.25
				MI	6.1	9.9	.03
				Death/MI	8.4	12.9	.02
Völz 2020	Cohort	23,860 SCAD	4.7	All mort	8.2	14.2	<.001
				No MI data			
Parikh 2020	Cohort	17,989 SCAD	1	All mort	2.8	5.9	<.0001
				MI	0.64	0.79	.31
Fröhlich 2014	Cohort	41,688 CAD; no STEMI	3.3	Unadj mort	-	-	<.001
				Adj mort			.37
Iannaccone 2019	Meta-Anal	69,150 CAD; 52% ACS	3	All mort, MI	-	-	-
Omran 2019	Cohort	304,548 ACS	-	In-hosp mort	1.1	3.1	<.01
Park 2013	Propensity-	4,356 CAD no STEMI	1	All mort	1.0	1.1	.89
				MI	2.3	3.9	.003
				Death/MI	3.3	5.0	.007
Li 2013	Cohort	7,358 CAD	7	All mort, MI	-	-	.28
				Death/MI			.12
				Death/MI*			.02
De Backer 2016	Propensity	1,716 SCAD	4	All mort	-	-	.346
				MI			.015
				Death/MI			.011

Table 5.8

Hard Endpoints Between FFR- and Angio-Guided PCI in Large Clinical Trials (Continued)

1st Author, Yr	Trail Outline	Pts	F-up (yrs)	Events	FFR (%)	Angio (%)	P Value
Zimmermann	Meta-analysis	2,400 SCAD	5	All mort	7.0	-	.89
				MI	8.5		.03
				Death/MI	13.9		.04
Xaplanteris 2018	RCT	888 SCAD	5	All mort	5.1	-	.98 (.55–1.75)
				All MI	8.1		.66 (.43–1.00)
				Spont MI	6.5		.62 (.39–.99)
				Death/MI	11.9		.72 (.50–1.03)

FFR, Fractional flow reserve; *MI,* myocardial infarction; *mort,* mortality; *PCI,* percutaneous coronary intervention; *RCT,* randomized controlled trial.
(From Fearon WF, Arashi H. Fractional flow reserve and "hard" endpoints. *JACC.* 2020;22:2800–2803.)

Table 5.9

Fractional Flow Reserve Studies Assessing Intermediate Left Main Stenosis

Study	FFR Threshold	N	Medical Therapy			Surgical Therapy			Follow-Up Time
			N (%)	MACE	Death	n (%)	MACE	Death	
Hamilos (2009)	0.8	213	136 (65%)	26%	9 (6.5%)	73 (35%)	17%	7 (9.6%)	35 ± 25
Courtis (2009)	0.75 surg; >0.80 med	142	82 (58%)	13%	3 (3.6%)	60 (42%)	7%	3 (5%)	14 ± 11
Lindstaedt (2006)	0.75 surg; >0.80 med	51	24 (47%)	31%	0	27 (53%)	34%	5 (19%)	29 ± 16
Suemaru (2005)	0.75	15	8 (53%)	0	0	7 (47%)	29%	0	33 ± 10
Legutko (2005)	0.75	38	20 (53%)	10%	0	18 (46%)	11%	2	24 mean
Jimenez-Navarro (2004)	0.75	27	20 (74%)	10%	0	7 (26%)	29%	2	2 ± 12
Bech (2001)	0.75	54	24 (44%)	24%	0	30 (56%)	17%	1	29 ± 15

FFR, Fractional flow reserve; *MACE,* major adverse cardiac event.
(From Lokhandwala J, Hodgson J. Assessing intermediate left main lesions with IVUS or FFR. *Cardiac Interventions Today.* 2009.)

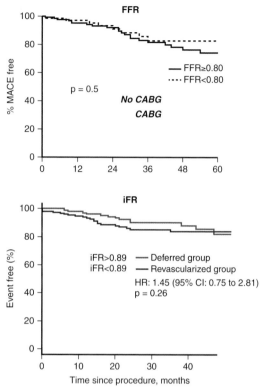

Figure 5.19 *Left,* The left main (LM) fraction flow reserve (FFR) 5-year outcome study and (*Right*) instantaneous wave-free ratio (iFR) LM outcome study showing similar rates of major adverse cardiac event-free survival in patients deferred for revascularization based on FFR > 0.80. (From Hamilos M, Muller O, Cuisset T, et al. Long-term clinical outcome after fractional flow reserve–guided treatment in patients with angiographically equivocal left main coronary artery stenosis. *Circulation.* 2009;120:1505–1512.) (*Right* from Warisawa T, Cook CM, Rajkumar C, et al. Safety of revascularization deferral of left main stenosis based on instantaneous wave-free ratio evaluation. *JACC Cardiovasc Interv.* 2020;13[14]:1655–1664.)

Fearon et al. created an intermediate narrowing in the LM with a balloon catheter after stenting the LAD or the left circumflex (LCx) or both. FFR was measured in the LAD and LCx coronary arteries before and after creation of "downstream" stenosis by inflating an angioplasty balloon within the newly placed stent, thus mimicking the LM/LAD anatomy. The true FFR (FFR$_{true}$) of the LM, measured in the nondiseased downstream vessel in the absence of stenosis in the other vessel, was compared with the apparent FFR (FFR_{app}) measured in the presence of stenosis. LM FFR was significantly lower than apparent FFR (FFR_{app}, 0.81 ± 0.08 vs. 0.83 ± 0.08, $p < .001$), although the numerical difference was small. This difference correlated with the severity of downstream disease ($r = 0.35, p < .001$). In all cases in which FFR_{app} was greater than 0.85, FFR_{true} was greater than 0.80. In most cases, downstream disease does not have a clinically significant impact on the assessment of FFR across an intermediate LMCA stenosis with the pressure wire positioned in the nondiseased vessel (Fig. 5.20).

Ostial and Side Branch Lesions

Ostial narrowings of side branches or newly produced narrowings inside branches within stents ("jailed" branches) are particularly

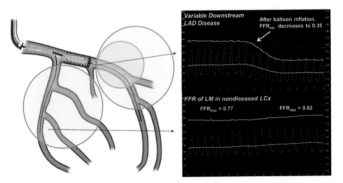

Figure 5.20 *Left,* Cartoon of experimental layout to test relationship between left main (LM) and left anterior descending (LAD) lesions of increasing severity. There is a deflated ("winged") balloon in the LM coronary artery with a variably inflated balloon within the newly placed LAD coronary artery stent and pressure wires down the LAD and the left circumflex (CFX) coronary artery. The circles represent changing bedside when the LAD balloon is inflated. Only when the LAD lesion is very severe does the fractional flow reserve (FFR) apparent in the CFX rise. (H) *Left,* Bland-Altman plot demonstrating the relationship between the difference in FFR_{true} and FFR_{app} based on the severity of downstream disease as assessed by FFR of the left middle coronary artery (LMCA) and the downstream stenosis (FFR_{epi}). *Right,* Chart demonstrating the average difference between the FFR_{true} and FFR_{app} depending on the severity of the downstream stenosis (FFR_{epi}). (From Fearon W, Yong AS, Lenders G, et al. The impact of downstream coronary stenosis on FFR assessment of intermediate left main CAD: Human validation. *JACC Cardiovasc Interv.* 2015;8[3]:398–403.)

difficult to assess by angiography because of their overlapping orientation relative to the parent branch, stent struts across the branch, and image foreshortening (Fig. 5.21A). Koo et al. compared FFR to angiography in 97 "jailed" side branch lesions (vessel size > 2.0 mm, percent stenosis > 50% by visual estimation) after stent implantation. No lesion with less than 75% stenosis had an FFR of less than 0.75. Among 73 lesions with at least 75% stenosis, only 20 lesions (27%) were functionally significant. Of 91 patients, side branch intervention was performed in 26 of 28 patients with an FFR of less than 0.75. In this subgroup, FFR increased to greater than 0.75 despite residual stenosis of 69% (plus or minus 10%). At 9 months, functional restenosis was 8% (5/65) with no difference in events compared with 110 side branches treated by angiography alone (4.6% vs. 3.7%, p = .7; see Fig. 5.21B). Measurement of FFR for ostial and side branch assessment thus identifies the minority of lesions that are functionally significant, reducing the need for complex, time-consuming, and potentially detrimental side-branch interventions.

Saphenous Vein Graft Lesions

When assessing a lesion in a saphenous vein graft (SVG), recall that there are three sources of coronary blood flow to the myocardium: the epicardial artery, the bypass conduit, and collateral flow (Fig. 5.22). The FFR is the summed responses of three competing flows (and pressure) from (1) the native vessel, (2) the CABG conduit, and (3) the collateral flow induced from long-standing native coronary occlusion. In the most uncomplicated situation of an occluded native vessel with minimal distal collateral supply, the theory of FFR will apply just as much to a lesion in an SVG as to a native right coronary artery feeding a normal myocardial bed. For more complex situations, the FFR will reflect the summed responses of the three supply sources and yield a net FFR indicating potential ischemia in that region.

For surgical decisions, coronary bypass conduit patency is reduced in those implanted distal to hemodynamically insignificant lesions. Although most surgeon consultants typically recommend bypassing all lesions with greater than 50% diameter narrowing in patients with multivessel disease, the patency rate of SVGs on vessels with hemodynamically nonsignificant lesions should be questioned. Data from FFR CABG studies have suggested limited evidence on the benefit of using of FFR to guide CABG. The most recent data have shown that FFR might simplify CABG procedures and optimize patency of arterial grafts without any clear impact on clinical outcomes (Fig. 5.23). In patients requiring CABG for multivessel revascularization, angiographic

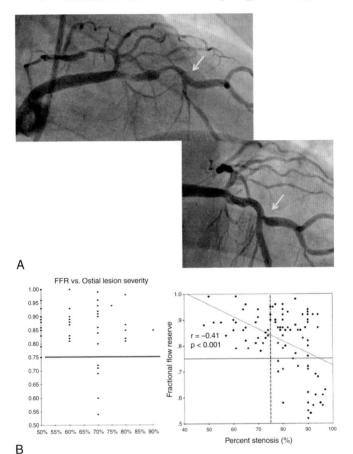

Figure 5.21 (A) Angiographic frames showing jailed side branch before (*left*) and after (*right*) left anterior descending (LAD) artery stenting. (B) *Left,* Comparison of fractional flow reserve (FFR) and percent stenosis for ostial lesions. (From Zaiee A, Parham A, Herrmann SC, et al. FFR vs ostial lesion severity. *Am J Cardiol.* 2004;93:1404–1407; and *right* Koo B-K, Kang H-J, Youn T-J, et al. Physiologic assessment of jailed side branch lesions using fractional flow reserve. *J Am Coll Cardiol.* 2005;46: 633–637.)

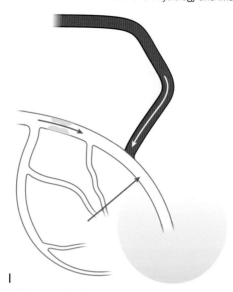

Figure 5.22 Diagram of saphenous vein graft (SVG; *red*) to left anterior descending (LAD). Blood flow to distal bed (*blue circle*) is result of three flows: native LAD, collaterals from other native vessels (*red arrow*), and flow from SVG.

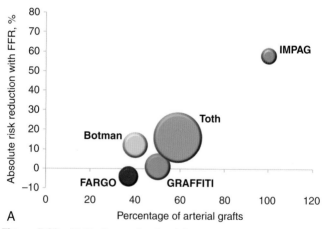

Figure 5.23 (A) Studies on fractional flow reserve (FFR) and coronary artery bypass graft (CABG) patency. The size of circles represents the study population. The proportion of arterial grafts in the study are plotted on the x-axis and absolute proportion risk reduction using fractional flow reserve on the y-axis.

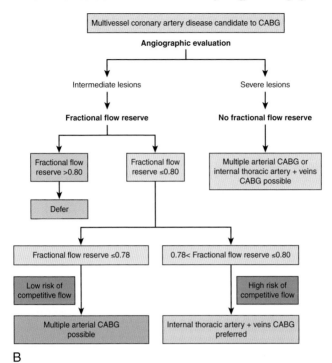

B

Figure 5.23, cont'd (B) Proposed algorithm to guide surgical revascularization strategy based on the angiographic and functional evaluation of the lesion. *FARGO*, Fractional Flow Reserve Versus Angiography Randomization for Graft Optimization; *GRAFFITI*, GRAft patency after FFR-guided versus angiography-guided CABG; *IMPAG*, Impact of Preoperative FFR on Arterial Bypass Graft Functionality. (From Spadaccio C, Glineur D, Barbato E, et al. Fractional flow reserve–based coronary artery bypass surgery. *JACC Cardiovasc Interv.* 2020;13[9]:1086–1096.)

lesions of uncertain significance may benefit from FFR assessment, providing prognosis of graft patency and potentially reducing unnecessary graft placement.

Nonculprit Vessel in Acute Coronary Syndrome

In acute coronary syndrome (ACS) settings and especially in acute MI (AMI), the pathophysiology of the infarcted artery and its subtended microvascular bed is both dynamic and complex. The predictive ability of FFR in ACS has several limitations: (1) the microvascular bed in the infarct zone may not have uniform, constant, or minimal resistance; (2) the severity of stenosis may evolve as thrombus and vasoconstriction abate; and (3) FFR measurements are not meaningful when normal perfusion has not been achieved. Thus FFR has limited utility in the infarct-related artery during the first 24 to 48 hours after ACS. Nevertheless, FFR has demonstrated value in remote lesion assessment and in target lesion assessment during the recovery phase of MI (see Table 5.7).

ST-Elevation Myocardial Infarction and FFR. In the target ST-elevation myocardial infarction (STEMI) vessel territory, FFR is not used because of changing myocardial blood flow to a myocardium in the recuperation phase after an acute infarction. FFR can be used in a culprit artery 4 to 6 days after the event, when myocardial function is believed to stabilize. For the noninfarct-related artery (non-IRA or nonculprit [NC] artery) in STEMI/NSTEMI patients, the zone of myocardial injury of the culprit vessel is unknown but may extend close to the region supplied by the non-IRA. Most non-IRA FFR values remain stable over a 3-month follow-up comparison. In some patients, however, a normal NC FFR at the time of STEMI might be lower several days later if the myocardial flow improves to the remote non-IRA zone, changing the initial treatment decision based on a high FFR.

Given the results of the FFR for non-IRA PCI, wherein long-term outcomes remain durable and a function of the FFR, the use of FFR for decisions about treating non-IRA is emerging as a dominant strategy for the revascularization of multivessel disease in the ACS patient.

Serial (Multiple) Lesions in a Single Vessel

When more than one discrete stenosis separated by greater than 20 mm is present in the same vessel, the hyperemic flow and pressure through the first lesion will be attenuated by the second and vice versa (Fig. 5.24), making FFR a technical challenge. One stenosis will mask the true effect of its serial counterpart. The interaction between two stenoses is such that the FFR of each individual lesion cannot be calculated by the simple equation for isolated stenoses applied to each separately but can be predicted by more complete equations considering Pa, Pm, Pd, and coronary occlusion pressure (Pw). The requirement for the coronary occlusion pressure makes this approach unsuitable for most diagnostic purposes.

In clinical practice, the use of a pressure pullback recording is particularly well suited to identify the specific regions of a vessel with large pressure gradients that may benefit from treatment. The one stenosis with the largest gradient can be treated first and the FFR remeasured for the remaining stenoses to determine the need for further treatment.

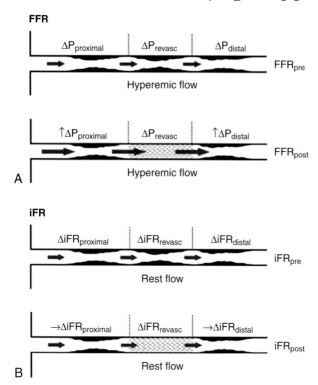

Figure 5.24 Serial lesion fractional flow reserve (FFR) diagram during hyperemia (A, FFR) or at rest (B, instantaneous wave-free ratio [iFR]). Individual lesion FFR cannot be determined without a coronary occlusion wedge pressure since either the proximal or distal lesion impairs maximal hyperemia producing a falsely high FFR. In addition, the result after stenting is unpredictable based on hyperemia. In practice, treatment of largest translesional gradient is performed, then reassessment of remaining lesion will determine treatment approach. Nevertheless, resting flow velocity remains stable post-stenting, leaving trans-stenotic pressure gradients in remaining lesions unchanged. *FFR,* Fractional flow reserve; *iFR,* instantaneous wave-free ratio; *Pa,* aortic pressure; *PCI,* percutaneous coronary intervention; *Pd,* distal (coronary) pressure. (From Kikuta Y, Cook CM, Sharp ASP, et al. Pre-angioplasty instantaneous wave-free ratio pullback predicts hemodynamic outcome in humans with coronary artery disease primary results of the international multicenter iFR GRADIENT registry. *JACC Cardiovasc Interv.* 2018;11:757–767.)

A simpler and perhaps more accurate method is the iFR pressure pullback coregistered to the angiogram (Fig. 5.25). Resting flow, in theory, does not produce lesion interaction. Lesions with significant gradients can be treated and assessed afterward as to the predicted iFR improvement. Outcome studies for serial lesions treated in this way are in progress.

Diffuse Coronary Disease

Using continuous pressure wire pullback from a distal to a proximal location, the impact of diffuse atherosclerosis can be documented. Diffuse atherosclerosis, rather than a focal narrowing, is characterized by a continuous and gradual pressure recovery during pullback, without any abrupt increase in pressure related to a focal region. The pressure pullback recording at maximum hyperemia or at rest will provide the necessary information to decide if and where stent implantation may be useful (Fig. 5.26). The location of a focal pressure drop superimposed on diffuse disease can also be identified as an appropriate location for treatment.

Post-PCI FFR/NHPR and Prognosis

Most operators do not remeasure FFR/NHPR at the end of the procedure, often accepting the angiographic result. The final FFR after stenting has important prognostic implications. FFR post-PCI identifies suboptimal results and can be improved by "functional optimization" of the vessel/stent regions based on further physiologic assessment. Post-PCI FFR is an independent predictor of long-term outcomes. Most studies evaluating post-PCI FFR find more than 50% patients had post-PCI FFR less than 0.90. Samady et al. noted that LAD location, pre-PCI FFR value, and vessel diameter were independently predictive of suboptimal post-PCI FFR (<0.90). In another study of DES, diffuse disease, LAD location, and use of IV adenosine for post-PCI FFR were also independent predictors of low FFR.

Treatable causes of low post-PCI FFR include suboptimally deployed stent, stent edge dissection, and/or new previously unsuspected CAD either distal or proximal to the stent. Diffuse disease beyond the stent may ultimately be the cause of the low FFR, a condition not amenable to more stenting. Pressure pullback and IVUS become critical tools in understanding the low post-PCI FFR (Fig. 5.27). The accumulated evidence suggests that post-PCI FFR be incorporated into routine practice in those patients having undergone pre-PCI FFR as part of clinical decision making.

Safety of Intracoronary Sensor-Wire Measurements

The use of intracoronary sensor wires is associated with an exceptionally low rate of complications such as dissection, thrombus, or

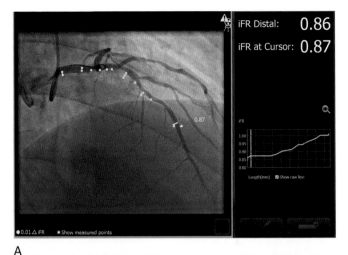

A

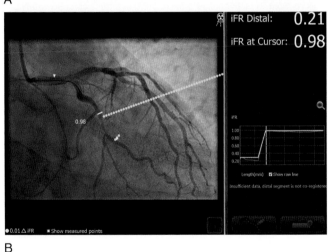

B

Figure 5.25 Left anterior descending (LAD; A) and circumflex (CFX; B) instantaneous wave-free ratio (iFR) pullback coregistered with the angiogram. Each dot represents 0.01 pressure units. Diffuse disease in the LAD is noted with no focal pressure gradient > 3 units, whereas in the CFX the severe mid lesion is confirmed by large focal pressure drop without other lesions evident. Ostial CFX disease is excluded as a contributor to the net gradient as well.

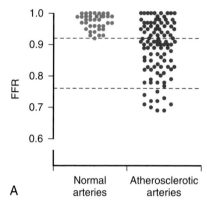

Figure 5.26 Fractional flow reserve (FFR) in diffuse coronary artery disease (CAD). (A) Graphs of individual values of FFR in normal arteries and in atherosclerotic coronary arteries without focal stenosis on arteriogram. The upper dotted line indicates the lowest value of FFR in normal coronary arteries. The lower dotted line indicates the 0.75 threshold level. (From De Bruyne B, Hersbach F, Pijls NH, et al. Abnormal epicardial coronary resistance in patients with diffuse atherosclerosis but "normal" coronary angiography. *Circulation*. 2001;104:2401–2406.)

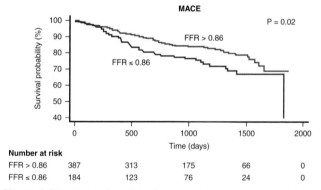

Figure 5.27 Prognostic value of post-percutaneous coronary intervention (PCI) fractional flow reserve (FFR). *Top left,* Kaplan–Meier curve showing significantly higher survival free of major adverse cardiac events (MACE) in the patients with final FFR > 0.86 in comparison with the final FFR ≤ 0.86 group.

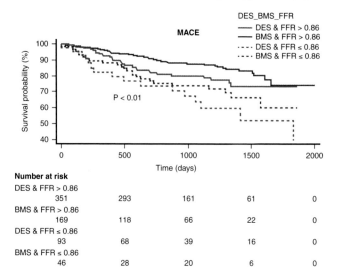

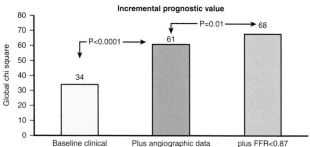

Figure 5.27, cont'd *Top right*, Kaplan–Meier curve showing significantly higher survival free of MACE in the patients with drug-eluting stents (DES) and final FFR > 0.86 followed by patients with bare-metal stents (BMS) and final FFR > 0.86, followed by patients with DES and final FFR ≤ 0.86 and followed by patients with BMS and final FFR ≤ 0.86, respectively. *Bottom*, Incremental prognostic value of final FFR. The addition of final FFR < 0.87 added incremental value for prediction of MACE over baseline clinical and angiographic data (all *P* < .05). (Adapted from Agarwal, SK, Kasula, S, Hacioglu, Y, Ahmed, Z, Uretsky, BF, Hakeem, A. Utilizing post-intervention fractional flow reserve to optimize acute results and the relationship to long-term outcomes. *JACC Cardiovasc Interv.* 2016;9:1022–1031. doi: 10.1016/j.jcin.2016.01.046.)

spasm. The rate is estimated to be lower than the complication rate of diagnostic catheters with ostial injury, emboli, and so on. Because most lesions undergoing assessment by sensor wires are intermediate, the risk of the wire producing lesion activation or injury remains low. Of course, operators should be experienced in handling angioplasty guidewires and using the systems, anticoagulation, antivasospasm medications, and safe catheter handling used in daily PCI practice.

The safety of intracoronary Doppler wire measurements was demonstrated by Quin et al. in 906 patients. Nine patients (1%) had coronary spasm during passage of the Doppler guidewire, and two patients (0.2%) had ventricular fibrillation during the procedure. Hypotension with bradycardia and ventricular asystole occurred in one patient (adenosine related). Transplant recipients were more sensitive to IC adenosine bradycardia and hypotension. All complications could be managed medically. Overall, the four decades of angioplasty sensor wire use support the safety of the methods.

Intravascular Imaging: Ultrasound and Optical Coherence Tomography

Intravascular visualization of the stent determines a successful and complete implantation with the absence of dissections, thrombus, and strut malposition and is critical to understanding the anatomic substrate, composition of the stenosis, and surrounding vascular tissue. Intravascular imaging is performed with either ultrasound (IVUS) or laser light with OCT.

IVUS

Intravascular ultrasound imaging (IVUS) characterizes the plaque, lesion length, and lumen dimensions. It is complementary to both angiography and physiology, allowing a thorough investigation of the disease within the vessel wall. By determining plaque characteristics, IVUS aids in selection of the interventional approach, such as use of atherectomy for plaque debulking. The expert consensus recommendations from the Society of Cardiovascular Angiography and Interventions for coronary IVUS and optical coherence tomography (OCT) are shown in Table 5.10.

Rotational or Solid-State IVUS

Two types of IVUS systems exist, both using 20 to 40 MHz silicon piezoelectric crystals: (1) a rotational transducer mechanical system with a rotating internal cable and (2) a solid-state system externally mounted on a catheter and controlled electronically.

Table 5.10

Advantages and Disadvantages of IVUS and OCT			
	IVUS (40–45 MHz)1–53, 1–5	IVUS (50–60 MHz)	OCT Frequency Domain
Wave source	Ultrasound	Ultrasound	Near-infrared light
Axial resolution, μm§	38–46	20–40	15–20
Penetration depth in soft tissue, mm	>5	3–8	1–2
Distance between adjacent frames, mm	0.02–0.03	0.02–0.17	0.1–0.25
Maximum pullback length, mm	100–150	100–150	75–150
Blood issue	Moderate backscatter from blood	Strong backscatter from blood	Requires clearance of blood
Aorto-ostial lesion visualization	+	+	-
Cross-sectional calcium evaluation	Angle only	Angle only	Thickness, angle
Lipidic plaque evaluation	Attenuated plaque	Attenuated plaque	Lipidic plaque and cap thickness
Plaque burden at lesion site	+	+	-

IVUS, Intravascular ultrasound; *OCT*, optical coherence tomography.

With the mechanical systems, the imaging core rotates via a flexible drive shaft to sweep the transducer continuously through a 360-degree arc in the vessel. The rotation rate is 1800 rpm, generating 30 images per second. The solid-state catheter (Philips, Einthoven, NL) has 64 ultrasound transducers arranged circumferentially around the catheter tip and sequentially activated to produce a 360-degree image. Both IVUS catheters range in size from 3.2F to 3.5F and have a tapered tip and shaft. They are designed to fit through a 6F guide catheter. The IVUS catheter connects to a console, which displays and records the images digitally. Images from both systems are displayed in a tomographic, real-time video format. Currently IVUS has a resolution of approximately 100 to 150 microns.

Technique of Intravascular Imaging Catheter Use

The technique of inserting the IVUS/OCT catheter is identical to PCI stent catheter placement. After administration of heparin and IC nitroglycerin (to avoid vasospasm), the IVUS/OCT catheter is then advanced over the guidewire, until the imaging transducer is beyond the region of interest. The IVUS/OCT catheter can then be pulled back (manually with IVUS or with an automated pullback device for OCT). An accurate pullback run is necessary to determine lesion length and volumetric analyses.

The mechanical IVUS and OCT catheters requires an initial flush of saline (or contrast for OCT) to remove microbubbles from the plastic sheath housing the rotating imaging cores and reduce image artifacts. For example, nonuniform rotational distortion (NURD) of the IVUS image can occur because of uneven drag on the catheter driveshaft, leading to changes in the rotational speed. This artifact most commonly occurs in tortuous vessels and manifests as a smearing of one side of the image. A ring-down artifact, seen with the solid-state system, results in white circles surrounding the ultrasound catheter and precluding near-field imaging and is because of acoustic oscillations in the transducer resulting in high-amplitude signals. Adjustments can now be made on the newer solid-state systems to minimize this problem.

Setup

Integration of the imaging tools into the laboratory's daily routine is critical for optimal use. To minimize problems, it is important for several members of the support staff to take specialized training and assume responsibility for the equipment. Current imaging systems can be fully integrated into the angiographic imaging system and do not require separate consoles (compared with the "stand-alone" units that must be wheeled into the lab). The following preparations make the most efficient use of IVUS/OCT:

1. Specialized support staff familiar with operation of the equipment and image interpretation

2. Use of an automated pullback device, which standardizes the procedure to prevent too rapid scanning and eliminates much of the physician operator effect on image quality

3. A system of maintenance for IVUS/OCT-related records, videotapes, and CD-ROMs

4. An image review station that is separate from the IVUS/OCT machine itself; direct transfer of the DICOM images to an image-archival network allows review at many stations

IVUS Image Features

There are six basic image features. From the center outward, a IVUS image will show the following (Fig. 5.28):

1. *Dead zone and ringdown artifact of the imaging catheter.* The black circular ring in the middle of the image is caused by the space occupied by the catheter. The *ringdown catheter artifact* is a "halo" around the catheter. It may also encroach onto the signals transmitted from the vessel wall. These artifacts are a property of the ultrasonic transducer producing disorganized near-field echo signals.

2. *Lumen.* The dark, echolucent area between the catheter and vessel wall. With some higher-frequency scanners or under conditions of slow blood velocity, a fine speckle pattern may be seen in the lumen.

3. *Vessel wall: Inner layer of the intima.* In a normal artery, the first layer of the vessel wall is the intima. Because it is so thin, it is not reliably seen. The thin inner echogenic layer surrounding the lumen usually represents the internal elastic lamina. In a diseased coronary artery, the atheromatous intima is seen as a

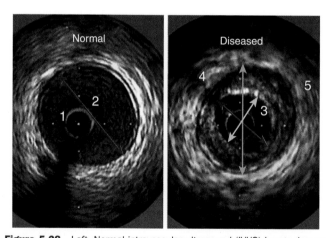

Figure 5.28 Left, Normal intravascular ultrasound (IVUS) image demonstrating the three normal layers of the coronary artery—the adventitia is the outermost, separated by a dark echolucent line from the media. The lumen and media border defines the intima. Right, This artery has an eccentric plaque from 11 o'clock to 4 o'clock. IVUS image anatomy. (1) Catheter and ringdown artifact, (2) lumen, (3) intima, (4) media, and (5) adventitia. In the disease artery, atherosclerotic plaque is measured between the intima and the adventitia.

thick echogenic layer surrounding the lumen. In vessels with mild to moderate atherosclerosis, a thin echodense layer at the intima–media interface can be seen, correlating histologically to the internal elastic lamina. This may be obscured in severely diseased atherosclerotic arteries.

4. *Vessel wall: Middle hypoechoic layer.* The medium, packed with smooth muscle cells and a few elastin fibers, appears as an echolucent area. The external elastic lamina (EEL) may appear as an echodense layer at the media–adventitia interface.

5. *Adventitia: Outer echogenic layer.* The adventitia is an echodense layer surrounding the hypoechoic media. The increased echodensity is because of both the inhomogeneous tissue with high elastin and the collagen content. This structure has the most intense echoes in normal arteries. Echoes that are more intense than the adventitia are therefore abnormal. Adjacent to the adventitia other structures may also be observed (i.e., veins and pericardium).

Dimensional Measurements

IVUS provides more precise measurements than angiography with superior accuracy in measuring lumen size and wall thickness. Correlations with histologic measurements have been uniformly high, although measurements of the dimensions of the layers and overall wall thickness are less accurate than lumen area determinations. The lumen–intima and media–adventitia interfaces are generally accurate. At this interface, however, there is a "trailing-edge" effect that can result in the spreading or blooming of the intimal image with the transition between layers obscured. The intima appears thicker than its histologic determination, and the media appears correspondingly thinner. Nevertheless, wall thickness using the combined intima and media corresponds closely to the histologic dimensions.

All ultrasound or OCT measurements are performed on *end-diastolic images* unless specified otherwise. Artery lumen dimensions are quantified from images of proximal, distal, or reference vessel segments and within the target lesion(s) or stent. The following measurements are routinely obtained.

1. *Lumen and vessel diameters:* Minimal, maximal, and mean diameters may be obtained.

2. *Percentage diameter or area stenosis* is the lumen diameter or area within the lesion segment divided by the lumen diameter or area within the reference segment. This is like the measures made by angiography.

3. *Total vessel area:* The vessel cross-sectional area is the area confined within the EEL or the media–adventitia interface.

4. *Lumen area* is the integrated area central to the leading-edge echo. The area is confined within the lumen–intima interface. If the catheter is tangential, the lumen area is slightly overestimated.

5. *Wall area* (intima and media) equals total area minus lumen area. In abnormal vessels, this is the plaque area (also called *plaque plus media area*).

6. *Percentage plaque area* (also called *plaque burden or percentage cross-sectional narrowing* [%CSN]) equals total vessel area minus lumen area divided by total vessel area:

> Percentage plaque area
>
> $$= (\text{total area-(lumen area)}/(\text{total area})) \times 100$$

Plaque distribution is classified into three categories:

1. *Concentric plaque:* Maximum plaque thickness (leading-edge plus sonolucent zone) of less than 1.3 times minimum plaque thickness

2. *Moderately eccentric plaque:* Maximum plaque thickness (leading edge plus sonolucent zone) 1.3 to 1.7 times minimum plaque thickness

3. *Severely eccentric plaque:* Maximum plaque thickness (leading edge plus sonolucent zone) greater than 1.7 times minimum plaque thickness

Plaque Morphology

In general, plaque may be classified as "soft" or "hard" based on whether the echodensity is less than or like the adventitia, respectively. Fig. 5.29 shows a general algorithm useful for interpreting IVUS images. Fig. 5.30 shows a general algorithm useful for interpretation of OCT images.

Soft plaque: More than 80% of the plaque area in an integrated pullback throughout the lesion is composed of thickened intimal echoes with homogeneous echo density less than that seen in adventitia

Fibrous plaque: More than 80% of plaque in an integrated pullback throughout the lesion is composed of thick and dense echoes involving the intimal leading edge, with homogeneous echo density greater than or equal to that seen for adventitia.

Calcified plaque: Bright echoes within a plaque demonstrate acoustic shadowing and occupy more than 90% of the vessel wall circumference in at least one cross-sectional image

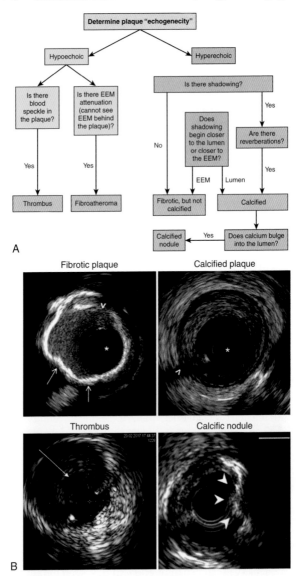

Figure 5.29 (A) General algorithm that can be used to interpret intravascular ultrasound (IVUS) images (as taught by Dr. Gary Mintz, Cardiovascular Research Foundation, New York). (B) Corresponding IVUS still-frame images representative of pathology seen in the algorithm.

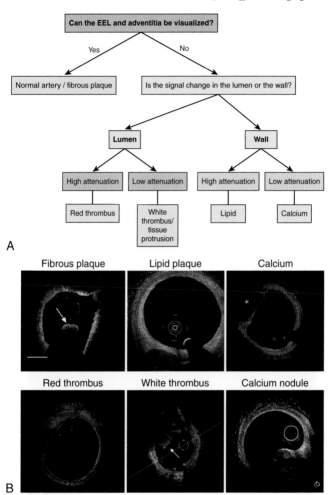

Figure 5.30 (A) General algorithm that can be used to interpret optical coherence tomography (OCT) images (as taught by Dr. Ziad Ali, Cardiovascular Research Foundation, New York). (B) Corresponding OCT still-frame images representative of pathology seen in the algorithm.

of the lesion. The extent of calcification, defined as the presence of any hyperechogenic structure that shadows underlying ultrasound anatomy, is reported as the degree of circumference in which shadowing is present. Calcium is also classified as deep or superficial. Detection of calcium using IVUS can guide appropriate device selection, such as the need for high-speed rotational atherectomy.

Mixed plaque: Bright echoes with acoustic shadowing encompass less than 90% of the vessel wall circumference, or a mixture of soft and fibrous plaque is seen with each component occupying less than 80% of the plaque area in an integrated pullback through the lesion.

Subintimal thickening: Subintimal thickening involving reference vessel segments is defined as a concentric prominent leading-edge echo and a widened subintimal echolucent zone with a combined thickness of more than 500 microns.

Additional Plaque Features

Stent edge dissection, stent malapposition, and tissue protrusion through stent struts can be easily seen by OCT or IVUS (Fig. 5.31). Intimal flap or dissection is seen as a linear structure with or without a free edge. True and false channels can also be visualized. The characteristic motion of an intimal flap may be seen within the lumen. Radiographic contrast injection can assist in defining the lumen and indicating whether there is communication of the lumen with an echo-free area below a flap. In some systems, blood flow can be colorized and may assist in defining dissections.

Thrombus: Fresh thrombus is a low to moderately echogenic or granular mass that occupies part of the lumen and adjoins the adjacent wall; often it is mobile and has an irregular border. Edge definition is possible with contrast injection (Fig. 5.32).

Aneurysm: Aneurysmal areas are expanded, thin-walled structures adjoining the lumen. They can be mistaken for branches, which have a similar appearance.

Side branches: Side branches appear as "buds" with a loss of the intimal border. The location of the lesion in relation to branch vessels and in relation to the coronary ostium can be well visualized with IVUS, which can aid decisions regarding stent placement.

"Vulnerable plaque" or atherosclerotic lesions at high risk for rupture: IVUS studies suggest that lesion eccentricity and the presence of echolucent zones within the plaque (representing

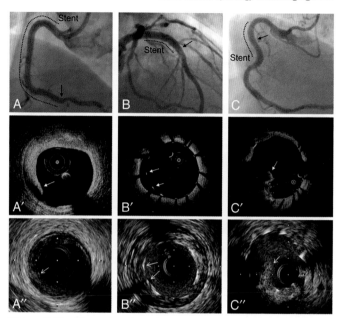

Figure 5.31 Stent edge dissection, stent malapposition, and tissue protrusion through stent struts by optical coherence tomography (OCT) and intravascular ultrasound (IVUS). Matched OCT and IVUS images are shown. The site corresponding to an OCT or IVUS cross-section is indicated as a black arrow in the angiogram (A, B, C), with the black dotted line showing the stent segment. OCT (A') and IVUS (A") show a medial dissection flap (*arrow*). OCT (B') and IVUS (B") show stent malapposition (*arrows*). Stent area measured 8.03 mm^2 by OCT and 8.15 mm^2 by IVUS. OCT (C') and IVUS (C") show tissue protrusion with attenuation indicating lipidic plaque (*arrows*) through the stent strut. (From Maehara A, Matsumura M, Ali ZA, Mintz GS, and Stone GW. IVUS-guided versus OCT-guided coronary stent implantation: A critical appraisal. *JACC Cardiovasc Imaging.* 2017;10:1487–1503.)

large necrotic lipid pools) are major determinants of plaque vulnerability and increased propensity for rupture (Fig. 5.33). The limited resolution of IVUS makes it unable to directly detect the thin (<65 microns) fibrous caps; thus the presence of a necrotic core in contact with the lumen (no IVUS evidence of a fibrous cap) has been used to identify vulnerable plaques. Unstable lesions may demonstrate ulceration or thin mobile dissection flaps by IVUS. In addition, the presence of "positive remodeling" or compensatory enlargement of the vessel to accommodate plaque and maintain lumen has also been

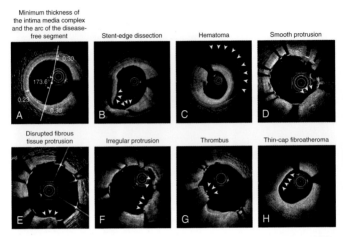

Figure 5.32 Representative optical frequency domain imaging (OFDI) images. (A) Measurement of minimum thickness of the intima-media complex and arc of the disease-free segment. (B) Stent-edge dissection. (C) Hematoma. (D) Smooth protrusion. (E) Disrupted fibrous tissue protrusion. (F) Irregular protrusion. (G) Thrombus. (H) Thin cap fibroatheroma. (From Hiromasa Otake et al. *JACC Cardiovasc Imaging. 2018 Q5 Jan;11(1):111-123.*

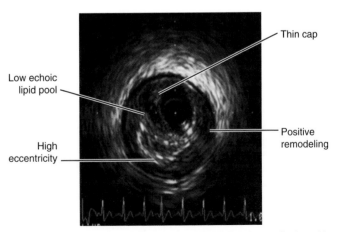

Figure 5.33 Intravascular ultrasound (IVUS) characteristics of vulnerable plaque.

found more commonly in unstable than in stable coronary lesions.

IVUS/OCT Versus FFR

Presently, determining the physiologic significance of a lesion should be done by using a physiologic index, and intravascular imaging by IVUS or OCT should not be used in its place. The one clinical situation in which this is not applied universally is that of the intermediate left main stenosis. Interrogating intermediate LM coronary lesions is another area where IVUS is commonly employed and a lesion with an IVUS MLA of less than 6.0 mm^2 has been generally considered a significant stenosis. The most common comparison of IVUS-derived parameters to FFR for assessing intermediate LM lesions found that an MLA area of 5.9 mm^2 correlated best with an FFR of less than 0.75. For all other lesions, modern PCI practice includes both intravascular physiologic and anatomic procedural guidance. IVUS and OCT imaging improves the clinical outcomes of patients undergoing PCI through several mechanisms: (1) lesion characterization for appropriate preparation (e.g., calcific lesion needing rotoablation); (2) appropriate stent sizing; (3) selecting the optimal stent length to minimize geographic miss; (4) facilitating optimal stent expansion; (5) demonstrating PCI-related complications (e.g., edge dissection, stent malapposition, tissue protrusion); and (6) understanding causes of late stent failure (in-stent restenosis [ISR] hyperplasia, thrombosis, stent under expansion or fracture, or neoatherosclerosis).

IVUS/OCT Guided PCI

IVUS or OCT should be used as an adjunctive technology to improve long-term clinical outcomes after PCI. There have been algorithms used in the clinical trials that better define how to use intravascular imaging to improve outcomes and, at this time, operators should strive to adopt these best practices. Fig. 5.34 depicts the utility of IVUS and OCT across different clinical situations. Fig. 5.35 outlines the general algorithm for best stent sizing and optimization according to present data.

Multicenter Ultrasound Stenting in Coronaries Study

Originally published in 1998, the Multicenter Ultrasound Stenting in Coronaries Study (MUSIC) represents the first guide to optimal

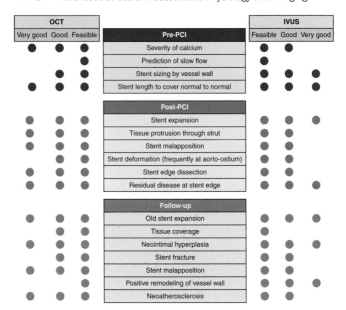

OCT				IVUS		
Very good	Good	Feasible	**Pre-PCI**	Feasible	Good	Very good
●	●	●	Severity of calcium	●	●	
		●	Prediction of slow flow	●		
	●	●	Stent sizing by vessel wall	●	●	●
●	●	●	Stent length to cover normal to normal	●	●	●
			Post-PCI			
●	●	●	Stent expansion	●	●	●
●	●	●	Tissue protrusion through strut	●	●	
●	●	●	Stent malapposition	●	●	
	●	●	Stent deformation (frequently at aorto-ostium)	●	●	
●	●	●	Stent edge dissection	●	●	
●	●	●	Residual disease at stent edge	●	●	●
			Follow-up			
●	●	●	Old stent expansion	●	●	●
	●	●	Tissue coverage	●		
●	●	●	Neointimal hyperplasia	●	●	●
	●	●	Stent fracture	●	●	
●	●	●	Stent malapposition	●	●	
		●	Positive remodeling of vessel wall	●	●	●
●	●	●	Neoatherosclerosis	●	●	

Figure 5.34 Intravascular ultrasound (IVUS) and optical coherence tomography (OCT): Usefulness in percutaneous coronary intervention (PCI). The ability of morphologic evaluation is shown as (very good), (good), or (feasible). In preintervention evaluation, OCT is better for evaluating the thickness of calcium, and IVUS can detect only the presence of calcium. Although IVUS can visualize the entire vessel wall, OCT cannot visualize the vessel wall when the wall thickness is beyond the penetration depth. In postintervention, both OCT and IVUS are good for evaluating stent expansion. A stent complication such as edge dissection is better visualized by OCT than IVUS. During follow-up, stent under expansion can be visualized by OCT. IVUS is sometimes difficult when neointimal calcification is present. Neoatherosclerosis is better visualized by OCT than IVUS. IVUS ¼ intravascular ultrasound; OCT ¼ optical coherence tomography; PCI ¼ percutaneous coronary intervention. (From Maehara A, Matsumura M, Ali ZA, Mintz GS, Stone GW. IVUS-guided versus OCT-guided coronary stent implantation: A critical appraisal. *JACC Cardiovasc Imaging.* 2017;10:1487–1503.)

stent implantation. Although done with an older generation of bare-metal stents (Palmaz-Shatz), the study did show that in the 81% of patients that met the IVUS optimization criteria, the target lesion revascularization rate was 4.5% at 6 months. The criteria described as "optimal" included:

- Minimum stent area (MSA) 90% of the average lumen area or at least 100% of the smaller reference area

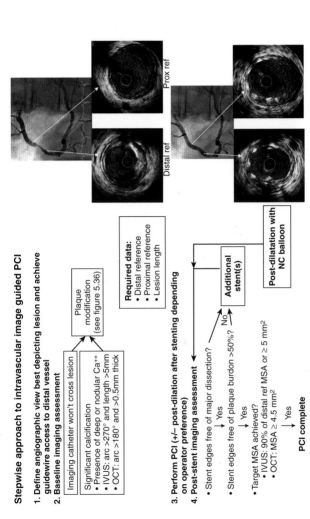

Stepwise approach to intravascular image guided PCI

1. Define angiographic view best depicting lesion and achieve guidewire access to distal vessel

2. Baseline imaging assessment

Imaging catheter won't cross lesion

Significant calcification
• Presence of deep or nodular Ca++
• IVUS: arc >270° and length >5mm
• OCT: arc >180° and >0.5mm thick

→ Plaque modification (see figure 5.36)

Required data:
• Distal reference
• Proximal reference
• Lesion length

3. Perform PCI (+/- post-dilation after stenting depending on operator preference)

4. Post-stent imaging assessment

• Stent edges free of major dissection?
 → Yes
• Stent edges free of plaque burden >50%?
 → Yes
• Target MSA achieved?
 • IVUS: 90% of distal ref MSA or ≥ 5 mm²
 • OCT: MSA ≥ 4.5 mm²
 → Yes

PCI complete

No → Additional stent(s)

Post-dilatation with NC balloon

Distal ref
Prox ref

Figure 5.35 Proposed intravascular imaging guided PCI algorithm steps to be followed that details the data supporting best long-term clinical results. *IVUS,* Intravascular ultrasound, *OCT,* Optical coherence tomography.

Or

• If the MSA was greater than 9 mm², then MSA of at least 80% of the average lumen area or at least 90% of the smaller reference lumen

Fig. 5.36 shows a proposed treatment algorithm for use in calcified vessels undergoing PCI/stenting.

ADAPT DES Study

This prospective, multicenter registry involved patients treated with at least one DES. Representing a more "modern" era of PCI, this trial incorporated the MUSIC criteria and further expanded the use of IVUS to guide stent implantation. Comparing IVUS-guided stent implantation with angiographic stent implantation, there were marked reductions in MACE.

Subsequently, multiple meta-analyses have been performed confirming similar findings, and operators should strive to embrace the algorithm for IVUS guidance. Table 5.11 provides a summary of effects of IVUS on outcomes. Table 5.12 provides key imaging criteria to assess optimal stent results.

Ilumien III and iSight: OCT-Guided Percutaneous Coronary Intervention

Because OCT images offer greater near-field resolution, investigators quickly attempted to mimic the use of IVUS measurements for OCT-guided PCI. The early results were that smaller luminal diameters were achieved after stenting. A novel OCT-specific strategy was then developed to use stenting to the EEL as seen on OCT and evaluated against IVUS and angiographically guided stenting. Both studies showed the superiority of intravascular image-guided stenting to angiographic guidance and similar stent areas achievable with IVUS and OCT. Table 5.13 lists the protocols for intravascular imaging that have been most studied to date.

Calcification

If one is evaluating the aforementioned algorithms for OCT or IVUS-guided PCI, it becomes clear that much of the benefit in clinical events is derived from maximizing the area of the stent. One of the principal barriers to achieving optimal stent area is calcium because it prevents expansion even with high atmosphere inflations and noncompliant balloons. Because intravascular imaging is particularly sensitive to determining the presence of calcium, it is easy to use these modalities to determine the need

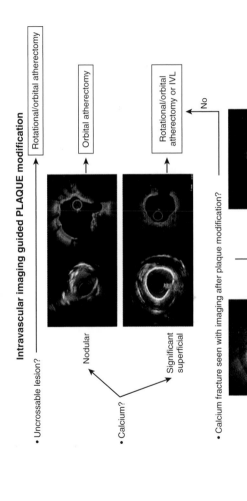

Figure 5.36 Proposed questions and options that facilitate best outcomes when treating calcified lesions. *IVL,* Intravascular lithotripsy.

Table 5.11

Impact of IVUS on Outcomes

	Steinvil (62)	Elgendy (61)	IVUS-XPL (60)	De la Torre Hernandez (64)	ADAPT-DES (4)
Uniqueness of study	Largest meta-analysis	Meta-analysis of randomized controlled trials	Largest randomized controlled trial, stent length ≥ 28 mm	Largest propensity matched pooled analysis of unprotected left main lesions	Largest all-comers registry
Percent IVUS guidance (N)	46.9 (31,283)	50 (3,192)	50 (1,400)	50 (1,010)	39 (8,582)
No. of studies included	25	7	1	4	1
Follow-up time, yrs	1 (in 56%)	1 (in 73%)	1	3	2
Unadjusted OR or HR					
	OR (95% CI)	OR (95% CI)	HR (95% CI)	Prevalence	HR (95% CI)
Major adverse cardiac event	0.76 (0.70–0.82)	0.60 (0.46–0.77)	0.48 (0.28–0.83)	11.7%/16%[a]	0.65 (0.54–0.78)
Death	0.62 (0.54–0.72)	0.46 (0.21–1.00)	3/5[a]	3.3%/6.0%[a]	.70 (0.51–0.96)
Myocardial infarction	0.67 (0.56–0.80)	0.52 (0.26–1.02)	0/1[a]	4.5%/6.5%[a]	0.62 (0.49–0.77)
Stent thrombosis	0.58 (0.47–0.73)	0.49 (0.24–0.99)	2/2[a]	0.6%/2.2%[a]	0.47 (0.28–0.80)
Target lesion revascularization	0.77 (0.67–0.89)	0.60 (0.43–0.84)	0.51 (0.28–0.91)	7.7%/6.0%	0.79 (0.85–0.95)

[a]IVUS guidance/angiography guidance.

CI, Confidence interval; HR, hazard ratio; IVUS, intravascular ultrasound; IVUS-XPL, Impact of Intravascular Ultrasound Guidance on Outcomes of Xience Prime Stents in Lesions; OR, odds ratio.
(From Mehran A. ivus v oct critical appraisal).

Table 5.12

Imaging Criteria to Assess Optimal Stent Result

- Stent expansion of > 80% (calculated as minimal stent area [MSA] divided by average reference lumen area)
- MSA > 5.5 mm^2 by intravascular ultrasound (IVUS) and > 4.5 mm^2 by optical coherence tomography (OCT) should be for nonleft main lesions.
- Extensive malapposition (> 0.5 mm) after stent implantation should be avoided and corrected if feasible. Acute malapposition of < 0.4 mm with longitudinal extension < 1 mm or malapposition should not be corrected because spontaneous neointimal integration is anticipated. Late acquired malapposition represents an established cause of late and very late stent thrombosis.
- Tissue prolapse in acute coronary syndrome (ACS) compared with stable coronary artery disease (CAD) is related to adverse outcomes, likely related to differences in the composition of the protruding tissue.
- Large dissections (by IVUS or OCT) are independent predictors of major adverse cardiac events (MACE). Extensive lateral (> 60 degrees) and longitudinal extension (> 2 mm), involvement of deeper layers (medial or adventitia), and localization distal to the stent increase the risk for adverse events.
- IVUS or OCT can clarify the appearance of a residual stent edge stenosis.

(Modified from Räber L, Mintz GS, Koskinas KC, et al. Clinical use of intracoronary imaging. *EuroIntervention*. 2018;14[6]:656–677.)

for lesion preparation with atherectomy or other specialized devices before stent deployment as seen in Fig. 5.35.

Ultra-Low Contrast Percutaneous Coronary Intervention

In patients with significant renal dysfunction, the most effective strategy to avoid postprocedure acute kidney injury is to limit the total contrast administered. Although this is sometimes easily achievable when performing PCI on simple single lesions, it becomes increasingly difficult when multiple lesions or lesion complexity increases. Ziad Ali and colleagues developed a strategy to use IVUS guidance and physiologic indexes and separate the diagnostic and PCI procedures by at least 1 week, which was shown to successfully avoid postprocedure renal dysfunction and MACE. For patients presenting with Stage 3 or higher chronic kidney disease, this type of approach should be strongly considered (Fig. 5.37).

Table 5.13

Protocols of OCT Used to Guide PCI in Randomized Trials of OCT vs. IVUS and/or Angiography

	Habara et al.	OPINION	ILUMIEN III	iSIGHT
Comparison	OCT vs. IVUS	OCT vs. IVUS	OCT vs. IVUS vs. angio	OCT vs. IVUS vs. angio
No. of Patients	70 (OCT: 35; IVUS: 35)	829 (OCT: 414; IVUS: 415)	450 (OCT: 158; IVUS: 146; Angio: 146)	150 (OCT: 50; IVUS: 51; Angio: 49)
Primary endpoint	Postprocedure stent expansion measured by IVUS	TLF (noninferiority of OCT vs. IVUS)	Postprocedure MSA measured by OCT (no-inferiority of OCT vs. IVUS)	Postprocedure stent expansion measured by OCT (noninferiority of OCT vs. IVUS)
Reference site selection	N/R	Most normal looking; no lipidic plaque	Regions with at least 180 degrees of the EEM visible; use of lumen profile	Most normal looking regions with largest lumen areas proximal and distal to the stenosis; lipid-free; use of lumen profile
Determination of stent diameter	• EEM and lumen border at both references quantifiable: use of largest lumen diameter either proximal or distal to the stenosis and with plaque burden < 50% • EEM not quantifiable: stent diameter and length determined by angio	Lumen diameter at proximal and distal references	• EEM ≥ 180 degrees: proximal and distal mean reference EEM diameter. Stent chosen by the smaller EEM diameter rounded down 0.25 mm • EEM < 180 degrees: proximal and distal reference lumen diameter	• EEM ≥ 180 degrees: reference sized by the mean EEM diameter • EEM ≥ 180 degrees: reference sized by the largest lumen diameter • Discrepancy between proximal and distal reference > 0.5 mm: smaller reference size used • Discrepancy between proximal and distal reference < 0.5mm: larger reference size used
Determination of stent length	Distance from distal to proximal reference	Distance from distal to proximal references	Distance from distal to proximal reference	Distance from distal to proximal reference

	In-stent MSA > 90% of the distal reference lumen area	In-stent MLA ≥ 90% of the average reference lumen area	Stent divided in 2 halves. MSA of each half should be ≥ 90% of the relative reference lumen area	In-stent MSA ≥ 90% of the average reference lumen area
Expansion criterion and goal				
Main results	• Pre-PCI EEM visible in 63% of distal and proximal references by OCT, and in 100% by IVUS • OCT-guided PCI resulted in significantly smaller MSA, mean stent area, and stent expansion than IVUS-guided PCI	• Smaller stents (2.92 ± 0.39, p = .005) and in-stent lumen gain (1.63 ± 0.47 mm vs. 1.72 ± 0.50 mm, p = .019) achieved in the OCT arm • Similar 8-month LLL (0.19 ± 0.29 mm vs. 0.17 ± 0.25, p = .58) • Similar 12-month TLF (5.2% vs. 4.9%, $p_{non-inferiority}$ .042)	• MSAs were 5.79 mm^2 (OCT) vs. 5.89 mm^2 (IVUS) vs. 5.49 mm^2 (angio). OCT noninferior to IVUS ($p_{non-inferiority}$ .01), and not superior to angio (p = .12) • Untreated major dissections (14% vs. 26%; p = .009) and major ISA (11% vs. 21%) were less frequent in OCT vs. IVUS • Stent chosen by EEM in 70% of cases by IVUS and OCT	• Stent expansions were 98.01% (OCT) vs. 91.69% (IVUS) vs. 90.53% (angio). OCT noninferior to IVUS ($p_{non-inferiority}$; < .001), and superior to angio (p = .041) • MSAs not significantly different in OCT (7.18 mm^2), IVUS (6.97 mm^2), and angio (7.26 mm^2) • Untreated ISA less frequent with OCT • Distal references more frequently sized by EEM in OCT (92% vs. 64.7%) and similar to IVUS in the proximal reference (80% vs. 70%)

Angio, Angiography; *EEM,* external elastic membrane; *ISA,* incomplete stent apposition; *IVUS,* intravascular ultrasound; *MLA,* minimum lumen area; *MSA,* minimum stent area; *N/R,* not reported; *OCT,* optical coherence tomography; *PCI,* percutaneous coronary intervention; *TLF,* target lesion failure.
(From Chamie D, Costa JR, Damiani LP, et al. Optical coherence tomography versus intravascular ultrasound and angiography to guide percutaneous coronary interventions – The iSIGHT trial. *Circ Cardiovasc Interv.* 2021;14:326–335 [Supp. Materials Table 6].)

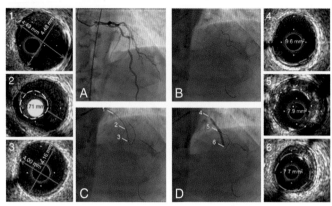

Figure 5.37 Case example of an ultralow contrast percutaneous coronary intervention (PCI). (A) Cineangiogram from diagnostic catheterization pulled up on the monitor in the lab to facilitate guiding catheter engagement and wiring of the lesion. (B) Noncontrast cineframe showing wire in the distal left anterior descending (LAD) with performance of intravascular ultrasound (IVUS). (1) IVUS measured proximal reference diameter (~4.5 mm). (2) IVUS measured minimal luminal area (3.71 mm^2). (3) IVUS measured distal reference diameter (~4.0 mm). (C) Coregistered cineframes are taken to "mark" the lesion and guide stent position. (D) 3.5 x 38 mm drug-eluting stent delivered with subsequent imaging of the proximal (4), mid (5), and distal (6) portions of the lesion used to determine criteria for optimal stent deployment. (From Ali Z, Galougahi KK, Nazif T, et al. Imaging- and physiology-guided percutaneous coronary intervention without contrast administration in advanced renal failure: a feasibility, safety, and outcome study. *European Heart J.* 2016; 37:3090-3095. Fig. 1.)

Key References

Ali Z, Galoughi KK, Nazif T, et al. Imaging- and physiology-guided percutaneous coronary intervention without contrast administration in advanced renal failure: a feasibility, safety, and outcome study. *Eur Heart J.* 2016;37:3090-3095.

Fearon W. Invasive coronary physiology for assessing intermediate lesions in advances in interventional cardiology. *Circ Cardiovasc Interv.* 2015;8:e001942.

Kogame N, Ono M, Kawashima H, et al. The impact of coronary physiology on contemporary clinical decision making. *JACC Cardiovasc Interv.* 2020;13:1617-1638.

Lofti A, Jeremias A, Fearon WF, et al. Expert consensus statement on the use of fractional flow reserve, intravascular ultrasound, and optical coherence tomography: a consensus statement of the society of cardiovascular angiography and interventions. *Catheter Cardiovasc Interv.* 2014;83:509-518.

Räber L, Mintz GS, Koskinas KC, et al. Clinical use of intracoronary imaging. Part 1: guidance and optimization of coronary interventions. An expert consensus document of the European Association of Percutaneous Cardiovascular Interventions. *EuroIntervention.* 2018;14:656-677.

References

Adjedj J, Toth GG, Johnson NP, et al. Intracoronary adenosine: dose-response relationship with hyperemia. *JACC Cardiovasc Interv*. 2015;8:1422-1430.

Ali ZA, Maehara A, Genereux P, et al. Optical coherence tomography compared with intravascular ultrasound and with angiography to guide coronary stent implantation (ILIUMIEN III:OPTIMIZE PCI): a randomized controlled trial. *Lancet*. 2016;388:2618-2628.

Chamie D, Costa JR, Damiani LP, et al. Optical coherence tomography versus intravascular ultrasound and angiography to guide percutaneous coronary interventions – the iSIGHT trial. *Circ Cardiovasc Interv*. 2021:14:326-335.

Fahrni G, Wolfrum M, De Maria GL, et al. Index of microcirculatory resistance at the time of primary percutaneous coronary intervention predicts early cardiac complications: insights from the OxAMI (Oxford Study in Acute Myocardial Infarction) Cohort. J Am Heart Assoc. 2017;6:e005409.

Fearon WF, Yong AS, Lenders G, et al. The impact of downstream coronary stenosis on fractional flow reserve assessment of intermediate left main coronary artery disease: human validation. *JACC Cardiovasc Interv*. 2015;8(3):398-403.

Johnson NP, Jeremias A, Zimmermann FM, et al. Continuum of vasodilator stress from rest to contrast medium to adenosine hyperemia for fractional flow reserve assessment. *JACC Cardiovasc Interv*. 2016;9:757-767.

Johnson NP, Johnson DT, Kirkeeide RL, et al. Repeatability of fractional flow reserve (FFR) despite variations in systemic and coronary hemodynamics. *JACC Cardiovasc Interv*. 2015;8(8):1018-1027.

Johnson NP, Li W, Chen X, et al. Diastolic pressure ratio: new approach and validation vs. the instantaneous wave-free ratio. *Eur Heart J*. 2019;40(31):2585-2594.

Leone AM, Martin-Reyes R, Baptista SB, et al. The multi-center evaluation of the accuracy of the contrast medium INduced Pd/Pa RaTiO in predicting FFR (MEMENTO-FFR) study. *EuroIntervention*. 2016;12:708-715.

Maehara A, Matsumura M, Ali ZA, Mintz GS, Stone GW. IVUS-Guided versus OCT-guided coronary stent implantation: a critical appraisal. *JACC Cardiovasc Imaging*. 2017;10:1487-1503.

Mintz GS, Ali Z, Maehara A. Use of intracoronary imaging to guide optimal percutaneous coronary intervention procedures and outcomes. *Heart*. 2021;107:755-764.

Taqueti VR, Di Carli MF. Coronary microvascular disease pathogenic mechanisms and therapeutic options: JACC state-of-the-art review. *J Am Coll Cardiol*. 2018;72:2625-2641.

Tonino PAL, Fearon WF, De Bruyne B, et al. Angiographic versus functional severity of coronary artery stenoses in the FAME study, fractional flow reserve versus angiography in multivessel evaluation. *J Am Coll Cardiol*. 2010;55:2816-2821.

Zimmermann FM, Ferrara A, Johnson NP, et al. Deferral vs. performance of percutaneous coronary intervention of functionally non-significant coronary stenosis: 15-year follow-up of the DEFER trial. *Eur Heart J*. 2015;36(45):3182-3188.

Adjunctive Tools: Atherectomy Devices, Laser, Thrombectomy

ABDUL AHAD KHAN • TAREK HELMY

KEY POINTS

- Intracoronary calcification creates significant challenges for interventional procedures due to suboptimal stent expansion and associated poor long-term clinical outcomes.

- Atherectomy tools are designed for modification of intracoronary calcification to allow balloon and stent expansion. Coronary thrombus presents a separate challenge and selective use of thrombectomy may improve outcomes.

- Other "niche" devices, including thrombectomy catheters and embolic protection filters are infrequently used but have benefit in carefully selected patients.

Introduction

Atherectomy devices were originally developed as a tool to decrease restenosis rates after PTCA. The use of atherectomy has changed considerably over the previous three decades. Rotational atherectomy (RA, introduced in 1988), helium laser angioplasty (ELCA, introduced in 1990), cutting balloon angioplasty (CBA, introduced in 1991), and orbital atherectomy (OA, introduced in 2008) have all been brought into routine use. Although the long-term results of these devices did not fulfill the promise of lowering the rates of target vessel revascularization with PTCA, the current era uses them to debulk heavily calcified vessels to facilitate delivery of stents and improve procedural results.

Rotational Atherectomy

Mechanism of Action

The principal mechanism for RA is differential cutting in which the diamond-tipped burr drills through rigid atherosclerotic plaque and calcium but spares the underlying elastic arterial structure. The resultant particulate matter is generally less than 10 μm in diameter, which passes through the microcirculation and is picked up by the reticuloendothelial system (without hindering the coronary microcirculation).

Indications and Contraindications

Although studies have shown that routine use of RA may not render a clinical benefit, there are several scenarios in which RA improves immediate angiographic results. Most commonly it is used to prepare vessels with severe fibrocalcific disease where in balloons or stents could not be passed. Additionally, attempts to pass stents through such ridgid, calcific lesions may result in inappropriate positioning, stent dislodgement, or erosion of the polymer–drug coating and inadequate drug delivery to the vessel wall.

Another scenario involving highly calcified nonyielding lesions is the need for high-pressure balloon expansion because of increased vessel stiffness, risking balloon rupture and vessel dissection or perforation. Delivering a stent in an incompletely dilated lesion inhibits its full expansion, which is a clear risk for stent thrombosis.

RA is also used to debulk bifurcation lesions to reduce plaque shift or the "snow-plowing" effect. Nevertheless, caution is advised in these scenarios because of the increased risk of dissection or perforation. Angulation of more than 60 degrees (between the main vessel and side branch) is a relative contraindication for RA, and bends of more than 90 degrees have a strong contraindication. Other contraindications are summarized in Table 6.1. A lesion that is more than 25 mm in length has a relative contraindication for RA. Smaller (<1.5mm) sized burrs should be used in these lesions should the operator so choose. A reduced ejection fraction (<30%) was previously a contraindication to RA, but the advent of mechanical support devices such as the Impella catheter has allowed physicians to consider RA for some of these patients (see Chapter 10 for more details).

Table 6.1

Indications and Contraindications to Rotational Atherectomy		
Indicated	**High-Risk**	**Contraindicated**
Single-vessel atherosclerotic coronary artery disease with a calcified plaque that *can* be passed with a guidewire	Severe, diffuse multivessel coronary artery disease	Occlusions where a guidewire cannot be passed
	Unprotected left main PCI	Saphenous vein graft PCI
Low-risk, multivessel coronary artery disease	Patients with compromised LV function (LVEF < 30%)	Angiographic evidence of significant dissection Type C or greater at the treatment site
De novo lesion < 25 mm in length	De novo lesion > 25 mm in length	
	Severely angulated (>45 degrees) lesions	
	Last remaining conduit with compromised LV function	
	Angiographic evidence of thrombus	

LV, Left ventricular; *LVEF*, left ventricular ejection fraction; *PCI*, percutaneous coronary intervention.

Device

The Rotablator system (Boston Scientific, Natick, MA) consists of a nickel-coated brass burr (Fig. 6.1A and 6.1B) that is coated with 2000 to 3000 microscopic diamond crystals that are 20 μm in size (with only 5 μm protruding from the nickel coating on its leading face). The burr is available in 1.25- to 2.50-mm sizes (0.25-mm increments) and is attached to a long, flexible drive shaft that is covered in a 4.3F Teflon sheath. The drive shaft can be inserted through various coronary guide catheters based on size (Table 6.2) over a RotaWire, which is 0.009 inch in diameter and 330 cm in length. The drive shaft is connected to an advancing console (Fig. 6.2) that houses a turbine driven by compressed nitrogen gas and that can rotate at speeds ranging from 140,000 to 220,000 rpm (Table 6.3). An emulsifier solution (Rotaglide) made of egg yolk, EDTA, and olive oil is infused along with saline via a pressurized system through the driveshaft to reduce friction and improve heat dissipation. The traditional Rotablator RA system involved the use of a foot pedal, console, and advancer. This has been largely replaced by the newer RotaPro RA system, which has added a digital console, eliminated the foot pedal,

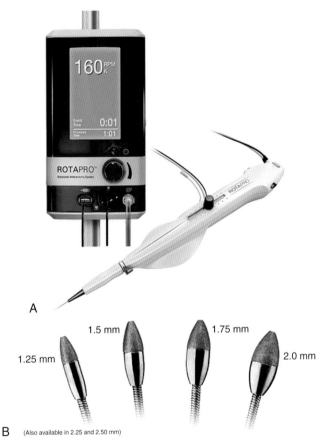

A

1.5 mm

1.75 mm

1.25 mm

2.0 mm

B (Also available in 2.25 and 2.50 mm)

Figure 6.1 (A) The RotaPro atherectomy system replaces the foot pedal with an advancer. A digital console has also been added. (B) Diagram of the rotational atherectomy burrs available between 1.25 to 2.5 mm. (Image provided courtesy of Boston Scientific. © 2022 Boston Scientific Corporation or its affiliates. All rights reserved.)

added buttons to the advancer that control device activation, and added a switch to turn to Dynaglide mode for easy burr retrieval.

Technical Tips

Once the decision to use RA is made based on the indications and contraindications discussed earlier, the next step is to determine

Table 6.2

Recommended Guide Catheter Sizes for Use With the Coronary Rotablator		
Rotablator Burr Size (mm)	Reference Vessel Diameter (mm)	Minimum Guide Size (French)[a]
1.25	2.5	5
1.50	3.0	6
1.75	3.5	6
2.00	4	7
2.15	4.3	7
2.25	4.5	8
2.50	5	9

[a]For a given size of catheter, the inside diameter varies from manufacturer to manufacturer. French sizes assume thin-wall (high-volume flow) catheters with side holes.

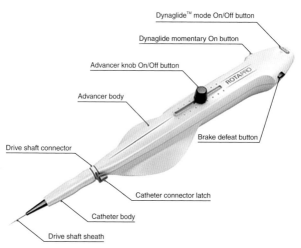

Figure 6.2 Rotablator advancer unit: The latest version incorporates all the controls on to the advancer. Ergonomic dynaglide design allows easy system removal. All individual cables have been added onto a hybrid harness. (Image provided courtesy of Boston Scientific. © 2022 Boston Scientific Corporation or its affiliates. All rights reserved.)

the burr size. For patent but stenotic vessels, a burr-to-artery ratio of less than 0.6 is appropriate. Although a larger ratio (>0.6) can aggressively debulk the lesion, it can increase the risk of dissections and perforations. For vessels with subtotal occlusions where the arterial size is difficult to ascertain, it is prudent to start with a

Table 6.3

Recommended Rotablator Advancer Turbine Speed			
Burr Size (mm)	Burr Size (French)	Design Rotational Speed Range (rpm)[a]	Optimum Rotational Speed Range (rpm; No Tissue Contact)
1.25	3.75	140,000–160,000	160,000
1.50	4.50	140,000–160,000	160,000
1.75	5.25	140,000–160,000	160,000
2.00	6.00	140,000–160,000	160,000
2.15	6.45	130,000–140,000	140,000
2.25	6.75	130,000–140,000	140,000
2.50	7.50	130,000–140,000	140,000

Rotablator Catheter Sheath Outer Diameter		
Size (mm)	Size (French)	Size (inch)
1.35	4.0	0.058

[a]Preset speed outside of the body at the higher rotational speed—for example, for a 1.25 mm Rotablator advancer, set speed outside body at 190,000 rpm.

small burr size (1.25 or 1.5 mm) to create a pilot channel and then upsize to a ratio of less than 0.6. Additionally, a smaller burr-to-artery ratio should also be used for vessels with lesions that are longer than 25 mm or if the vessel has mild tortuosity.

The next step is preparing the patient for RA. The patients usually already have aspirin on board; some operators use verapamil preemptively to prevent spasm. Heparin or bivalirudin can be given next to fully anticoagulate the patients. Traditionally, operators have chosen heparin because of its reversibility in case of vessel perforation, but studies have shown safety with bivalirudin as well. RA is associated with rotational speed-dependent platelet activation, and glycoprotein (GP) IIb/IIIA receptor antagonists can be used to counteract this effect. Standard use of temporary pacemakers before intervening on calcified lesions in the RCA left main is no longer needed. Smaller burrs at lower speeds have led to lower incidence of transient heart block. Many operators opt to use atropine, aminophylline, or vagolytic maneuvers as part of initial management of bradyarrhythmias, avoiding any complications of temporary pacemaker placement on a routine basis. Alternatively, a test run can be performed before RA of the RCA or dominant left circumflex to make sure bradycardia is not being induced.

A guide catheter with a gentle curve should be sized depending on the burr size (see Table 6.2). It is important to make sure that the guide catheter is coaxial to the vessel to prevent dissection of the vessel or retraction of the wire during RA. The RotaFloppy wire should be used for lesions that are more proximal and easily crossable to prevent guidewire bias in which a burr would differentially debride more on the lesser curvature of the vessel, which is straightened by a stiffer wire. The extrasupport RotaWire can be used for difficult-to-cross, heavily calcified or distal lesions. If a lesion cannot be crossed by the RotaWire, a 0.014-inch guidewire can be used to cross the lesion and then be exchanged for the RotaWire using a low-profile over-the-wire balloon or microcatheter.

Once the RA manifold is assembled, the burr speed is tested outside the body (140,000–160,000 rpm). Either saline or the Rotaflush solution (mix 4 mg of nitroglycerin and 5 mg of verapamil in 500 mL of saline to decrease spasm) is used to flush and lubricate the system. The Rotaglide solution is added to reduce friction. Before inserting the burr into the Y-adapter, one must also check for free movement of the burr with the advancer and test that the braking system holds the wire in place during rotation. The advance knob should be locked 2 cm from the distal end of its slidder slot.

After this, the burr is inserted via a Y-adapter and advanced over the wire through the guide catheter into the vessel to about 1 to 2 cm proximal to the lesion. The operator should hold the back end of the wire and apply gentle traction on the guidewire and catheter to limit acquired tension and thereby prevent the burr from leaping forward during the initial pass. This acquired tension is alleviated further by transiently activating the system proximal to the lesion. The system is then activated and the burr is brought into contact with the lesion in a "pecking" fashion in which 1 to 3 seconds of contact with the plaque is followed by pulling back the burr from the plaque surface for 3 to 5 seconds. This decreases the risk of sudden deceleration of the burr and allows the debris to clear from the distal circulation. It is important to prevent deceleration over 5000 rpm because such decelerations can lead to plaque heating, torsional dissection of the vessel, and formation of larger particles, which can lead to slow reflow or no reflow. Another important consideration during RA is that the operator should hold gentle forward pressure on the guide catheter and the wire to maintain wire position in the distal vessel. The total time taken for each pass should not exceed 30 seconds. There should be a 30- to 60-second interval wait between each atherectomy run to avoid no reflow phenomenon. Fig. 6.3 and Videos 6.1A–G demonstrate the use of RA in a severe left main stenosis. The slow pecking technique is important to prevent device entrapment beyond the target lesion, which is a rare but serious complication requiring expertise to extract the device or emergent surgery if other measures fail.

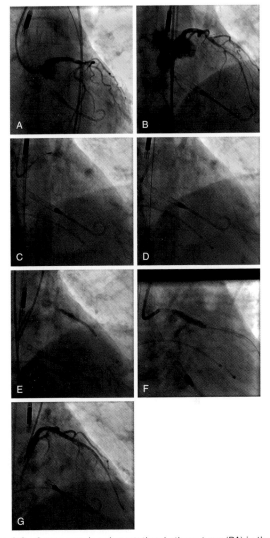

Figure 6.3 Case example using rotational atherectomy (RA) in the treatment of fibrocalcific left main (LM) and left anterior descending (LAD) disease. (A–B) Baseline angiography demonstrating calcified plaque of the LM and LAD in caudal and cranial projections. (C) RA using a 1.5-mm burr. (D) Post-RA angiography. (E) Stent deployment into the LAD. (F) Stenting of the LM into the LAD. (G) Angiography of the LM and LAD post stenting. *PTCA,* Percutaneous transluminal coronary angioplasty.

Box 6.1   Technical Notes and Tips on Performing Rotational Atherectomy

- A nitrogen compressed-gas cylinder with pressure regulator capable of delivering a minimum 140 L/min at 90 to 100 psi is required.
- The compressed-gas cylinder valve must be open to supply compressed gas to the console. The regulator should be adjusted so that the pressure does not exceed 100 psi.
- Angulated lesions and branch ostial lesions have a higher incidence of dissection and/or perforation; downsize initial burrs and stepwise increase burr size to achieve the final result.
- Rotational atherectomy (RA) can be performed on chronic total occlusions only if the guidewire is confirmed to be in true lumen distally.
- Perforations are uncommon. Covered stents should be available in all cardiac catheterization laboratories performing RA.

The most important factor in successfully using RA is to avoid complications such as dissection, perforation, and preventing no reflow or slow reflow (reduction in blood flow by 1 thrombolysis in myocardial infarction [TIMI] grade). Technical tips to prevent these adverse effects are listed in Box 6.1. When performed by an experienced operator with the appropriate precaution, RA proves to be an excellent method to debulk and modify plaque in preparation for stenting – with recent data suggesting that operator experience (i.e., number of cases performed every year) significantly reduces the occurrence of complications.

Orbital Atherectomy (OA)

The Diamondback 360-degree OA system (Cardiovascular Systems, St. Paul, MN) uses a diamond-coated crown (available in sizes 1.25–2.00 mm at 0.25-mm increments; Fig. 6.4) that orbits eccentrically over a coil made of three spiral wires. The elliptical motion of the crown is different from the burr used for RA such that the diameter and the depth of the OA depend on the velocity of crown rotation (80,000–200,000 rpm). Theoretically this elliptical motion of the crown makes deeper cuts and can ablate plaque in both antegrade and retrograde fashion and, at the same time, allows for greater blood flow and heat dissipation during atherectomy. The additional advantages of OA over RA are that the risk of entrapment of the device on the plaque is theoretically lower and the sanding motion results in smaller particulate matter.

The procedural technique for OA is similar to that of RA (PTRA) except that, when selecting lesions, the operator should

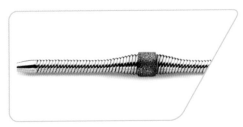

Figure 6.4 A diamond-coated crown for orbital atherectomy system. (Courtesy Cardiovascular Systems, St. Paul, MN.)

ensure the presence of calcium on both sides of the arterial wall using fluoroscopy or a 270-degree arc of calcium within the plaque via intravenous ultrasound (IVUS). A ViperWire (0.012-inch) can be used to cross the lesion instead of the RotaWire. Care should be taken not to advance the crown within 5 mm of the distal end of the ViperWire. The ViperSlide (composed of soybean oil, egg yolk phospholipids, glycerin, and water) solution is used for flush in place of the RotaFlush, and, unlike the RA system where the adequacy of flushing is determined by the operator, the OA system requires continuous flow of flush and automatically disables if the flow is interrupted. Finally, the preferred motion for the OA crown is slow continuous advancement as opposed to the pecking motion preferred for RA. The potential complications of OA are similar to RA and were discussed earlier.

To date, no randomized controlled trials have compared OA versus RA during PCI. A recent meta-analysis of retrospective studies comparing OA with RA by Khan et al. revealed no difference in overall major adverse cardiac events. OA had a lower fluoroscopy time but higher odds of causing coronary dissection and perforation. Table 6.4 describes the practical aspects associated with each atherectomy modality before its use.

Optimal Clinical Scenarios for Rotational Versus Orbital Atherectomy

With both technologies now readily accessible, operators have been faced with trying to find the best use for each of these tools. In general, there seems to be great equipoise between these devices and one should be used when treating heavily calcified vessels before stent deployment.

Table 6.4

Practical Considerations for Choice of Atherectomy Device

Choice Considerations	Rotational Atherectomy[a]	Orbital Atherectomy[b]
Guide Size	Usually 6-French (F) or larger	Usually 6F
Arterial Access	Radial or femoral	Radial or femoral
Ostial lesions	Offers more control and the preferred choice for severe aorto-ostial lesions	Ostial ablation is possible provided crown can be advanced through the lesion. Ablation has to be backward (i.e., distal to proximal)
Presence of a stent	Technically challenging but feasible and reported	Contraindicated
Wire	Flimsy and hard to manipulate	User friendly and comparable to workhorse wires
Insertion/ removal	Dynaglide mode helps make delivery/removal of the burr much less cumbersome. Single-operator technique being adopted at some centers	Glide assist feature facilitates crown delivery often using just a single operator
Vessel size	Similar to orbital atherectomy in lesions with smaller lumens. Larger vessels need gradual burr upsizing.	Preferred for larger vessels because of superior debulking.
Tortuosity	Tighter turns easier to navigate	Better suited for straighter segments
Cutting Direction	Forward	Forward and backward
Foot Pedal	Replaced by an advancer knob in the newer generation (Rota-Pro)	No foot pedal

[a]Rotational atherectomy: Boston Scientific, Natick, MA, USA
[b]Orbital atherectomy: Cardiovascular Systems, Inc., St. Paul, MN, USA

RA is primarily indicated for plaque modification of severely calcified de novo coronary lesions followed by subsequent angioplasty and stenting, particularly when intravascular imaging shows most of this calcification to be superficial. RA can either be performed as an upfront strategy or as a secondary approach after an initial unsuccessful attempt to dilate a lesion. OA has been advocated for preparing larger vessels before stenting or when intravascular imaging finds that the calcium is more deeply imbedded into the vessel wall. Safety appears to be comparable with the two approaches, although the upfront approach is associated with lower procedure time, fluoroscopy time, contrast volume, and decreased likelihood of stent loss.

RA should not be done in occlusions through which a guide-wire will not pass, although it may be the preferred strategy for balloon-uncrossable lesions and aorto-ostial lesions because of its forward ablation (in contrast to OA, which uses side ablation). Degenerative saphenous vein grafts have an increased risk of perforation, and atherectomy (RA and OA) should generally be avoided. RA can generally be done safely in old stents and has also been performed within recently placed stents that fail to expand. RA in recently placed stents carries an increased risk for burr entrapment, distal embolization, and stent distortion. Higher burr speeds should be used to avoid burr entrapment in such cases. Stent reimplantation is often warranted in such cases because of disruption of the previously placed stents.

Cutting Balloon Angioplasty (CBA)

Mechanism of Action

CBA involves three to four 0.1- to 0.4-mm-thick atherotomes (long stainless steel blades) mounted on a noncompliant balloon designed to make microincisions on plaque during inflation. CBA requires lower inflation pressures compared with PTCA and thus theoretically renders the advantage of lower barotrauma and thereby reduces neointimal proliferation. The atherotomes make controlled incisions that do not exceed the entire radius of the plaque and thereby reduce the incidence of plaque fracture. Because the incisions are limited within the plaque, theoretically there is a lower chance of vessel dissection.

Equipment

The Wolverine Cutting Balloon (Boston Scientific, Marlborough, MA) is available in monorail and over-the-wire configurations and contains three or four atherotomes (microsurgical blades) that protrude 0.005 inches from the surface of the balloon in a longitudinal fashion and modify the target lesion by creating initiation sites for crack propagation. This process, also known as atherotomy, allows for dilatation of the target lesion at lower pressures. The device is available in 6-mm, 100-mm, and 15-mm lengths (Fig. 6.5). In contrast to the AngioSculpt and Chocolate

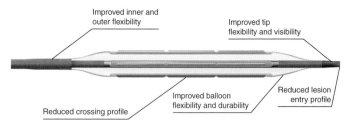

Figure 6.5 Wolverine cutting balloon in its inflated state. Microtomes can be seen extending outward from the balloon. (©2022 Boston Scientific Corporation or its affiliates. All rights reserved.)

balloons (see later), cutting balloons have a high crossing profile and require very slow inflations to avoid vessel injury (typically 1 atm every 5 seconds).

Technique and Technical Tips

The atherotomes make cutting balloons less flexible than conventional balloons and hence more difficult to deliver. One can predilate the lesion with a conventional 1.5- or 2-mm balloon to allow the cutting balloon to pass. Inflation should be performed slowly to allow for appropriate deployment of the atherotomes in a perpendicular fashion to the atheroma in the vessel wall. Another technique is to partially inflate the cutting balloon as it enters the lesion and then advance the balloon through the lesion as it deflates. For difficulty in crossing lesions, operators can consider using a (buddy) 0.014-inch wire in addition to the guidewire to support the guide catheter while advancing the cutting balloon through a lesion within a stent or in a tortuous segment. In addition, for tortuous vessels, there is a potential for guidewire bias. This can be reduced using a Wiggle wire (Abbott Vascular, Abbott Park, IL).

The potential complications of CBA are atherotome fracture or retention, vessel perforation, and inappropriate folding of the device on deflation (device "winging") making it difficult to retrieve. These can be mitigated by ensuring that the ratio of balloon to vessel size is 1:1, not exceeding the recommended inflation pressures for given balloon and desired vessel size, and slowly inflating the balloon during angioplasty, followed by slow deflation of the balloon before pulling negative before retrieval. Multiple slow inflations maintained over 60 to 90 seconds allow for smooth, flat incisions and provide good angiographic results.

Scoring Balloon Angioplasty

The AngioSculpt Scoring Balloon (AngioScore, Freemont, CA) has a nitinol spiral element with three spiral struts that wrap around a semicompliant balloon. This provides a more flexible alternative to the CBA catheter, which has three or four linear struts on a noncompliant balloon (Fig. 6.6). The increased flexibility provides better crossing capability compared with CBA, but the data for clinical use are limited. One nonrandomized study showed greater stent expansion compared with direct stenting or conventional PTCA before stenting. Currently there are no randomized trials to evaluate the use of scoring balloon angioplasty in coronary intervention.

Chocolate (Telescope)

The Chocolate balloon has a mounted nitinol constraining structure that creates "pillows" and "grooves" as the semicompliant balloon expands. The pillows apply force to allow vessel dilatation without cutting or scoring, and the grooves allow for stress leave minimizing the risk of dissection. This is also known as "constrained semicompliant balloon angioplasty" (Fig. 6.7).

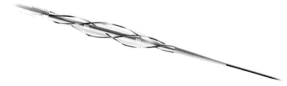

Figure 6.6 The AngioSculpt scoring balloon (AngioScore, Freemont, CA) has a nitinol spiral element with three spiral struts that wrap around a semicompliant balloon. (Courtesy of Philips, Amsterdam, the Netherlands (Image caption: The Philips Scoring Balloon Catheter RX – AngioSculpt Evo –has a ninitol spiral element with three spiral struts that wrap around a semicompliant balloon).)

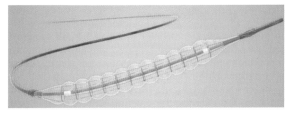

Figure 6.7 The Chocolate balloon has a mounted nitinol constraining structure that creates "pillows" and "grooves" as the semicompliant balloon expands. (Courtesy Teleflex, Wayne, PA.)

Optimal Clinical Scenarios for the Use of Plaque Modification Balloons

These devices have proven to be useful for bifurcation lesions, ostial lesions, and in-stent restenosis (ISR). For bifurcation lesions, the challenges for routine PTCA are plaque shift and high restenosis rates. The lower inflation pressure and microincisions of these balloons reduce plaque shift and neointimal proliferation, resulting in lower restenosis rates than PTCA. There is a lower incidence of balloon slippage (watermelon seeding) with these balloons compared with PTCA, thereby reducing trauma to the healthy vessel beyond the target lesion; this gives CBA an advantage in the treatment of ostial lesions and ISR.

Balloon angioplasty with plaque modification balloons is reasonable in deep wall calcification compared with superficial and nodular calcifications, which are best treated with atherectomy. Use of these balloons may also be useful for lesion preparation of relatively smaller-sized side branch ostia, where there is concern for watermelon seeding and consequent injury to the main vessel branch. Plaque modification balloons can decrease unwanted movement of the balloon and decrease the risk of dissecting the main vessel. Their larger crossing profile can sometimes make deliverability to the target lesion challenging.

Routine use of plaque modification balloons for standard lesions is not indicated and is particularly disadvantageous for vessels that are very tortuous or are less than 2 mm in size; lesions that are greater than 20 mm long; heavily calcified lesions; and chronic total occlusions (CTOs).

Shockwave Lithotripsy

Established on the principle of kidney stone treatment, the Shockwave coronary intravascular lithotripsy (IVL) system consists of a portable and rechargeable generator, a connector with push button activation, and a catheter that can be railed across any standard workhorse guidewire (Fig. 6.8). Miniaturized and arrayed lithotripsy emitters produce an electric spark that vaporizes the saline/contrast mixture contained within the integrated balloon. The resulting acoustic pressure wave radiates spherically outward, selectively modifying vascular calcium while leaving soft tissue undisturbed.

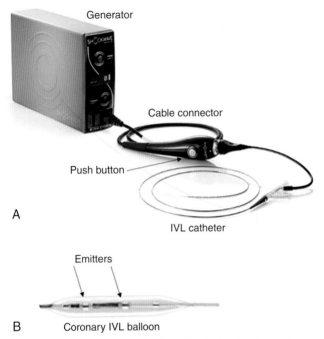

A

B

Figure 6.8 (A) Intravascular lithotripsy (IVL) device. (B) IVL emitters produce an electric spark that vaporizes the saline/contrast mixture contained within the integrated balloon. The resulting acoustic pressure wave radiates spherically outward. (Courtesy Shockwave Medical.)

The IVL balloon is sized with a 1:1 ratio to the reference vessel diameter. The IVL balloon is inflated to 4 atm at target lesion for 10 seconds with up to 80 pulses of energy delivered per balloon. Eccentric calcifications may sometimes need more shock pulses compared with concentric calcific lesions because of the circumferential nature of the sonic pressure wave forms. The presence of ventricular ectopy at the time of ultrasonic impulse generation is also a common phenomenon. Recent RCTs, such as the Disrupt Coronary Artery Disease (CAD) I and Disrupt CAD II, have shown excellent procedural success rates (98%–100% stent deployment), relatively low MACE (5.8%–8.5%), and no major intraprocedural complications, including perforation, embolization, slow flow, or no reflow.

IVL is currently very early in clinical use and specific lesion types, vessels, or patients in which it may be more advantageous compared with atherectomy or plaque modification balloons remain unknown.

Laser Angioplasty

The ELCA system emits ultraviolet (UV) laser light (300 nm wavelength) that ablates plaque using vaporization (photothermal effect), direct breakdown of chemicals (photochemical dissociation), and ejection of the debris from tissue (photoacoustic effect). The process is associated with the formation of a vapor bubble that can be mitigated by infusing saline at a rate of 2 to 3 mL/sec via the guide catheter during the ablation. Commonly seen complications may include dissection or perforation, which can be reduced by limiting the size of the laser catheter to less than two-thirds the size of the reference vessel. Infusing contrast during laser application delivers more energy to the vessel wall but is considered an off-label use and carries a higher risk of complications. The clinical experience in RCTs comparing ELCA with other modalities have failed to show benefit. In some trials, however, ELCA was successful in recanalizing CTO or subtotal occlusions that were not crossable with conventional guidewires. ELCA also has approval for saphenous vein graft (SVG) lesions and ostial lesions that are not amenable to RA and OA. An emerging lesion subset where laser is helpful is in treating ISR, especially in cases where the stent is underexpanded because of a calcified nonyielding lesion. Laser can provide lesion modification through the stent struts, allowing for effective dilation and full expansion of the stent.

Thrombectomy

Primary PCI has been shown to improve clinical outcomes compared with conservative medical therapy using fibrinolytic or thrombolytic agents; it has become the treatment of choice and is the standard of care for patients with acute ST-elevation myocardial infarction (STEMI).

One of the main concerns during primary PCI, or in lesions with large thrombus burden, is embolization of thrombotic or plaque debris and vasoactive substances into the distal coronary circulation resulting in no reflow or slow reflow. The frequency of this complication has been reported to be between 15% and 20% during primary PCI. Despite distal embolization, the reduction of distal coronary flow is usually transient; however, adverse outcomes have been associated even with transient minimal reductions in coronary microvascular flow during PCI.

Background

Angiographically, thrombus is visualized in 75.9% of patients with non-STEMI acute coronary syndrome (ACS) and almost 100% of patients with STEMI. Fig. 6.9 shows angiographic thrombus.

Thrombectomy should be considered when thrombus is present in a culprit artery of sufficient diameter such that it can allow safe passage of the thrombectomy catheters. Fiberoptic angioscopy is the gold standard for detection of intracoronary thrombus; however, most cardiac catheterization laboratories do not possess this technique. As a result, IVUS or optical coherence tomography (OCT) is an alternate method for detection of intracoronary

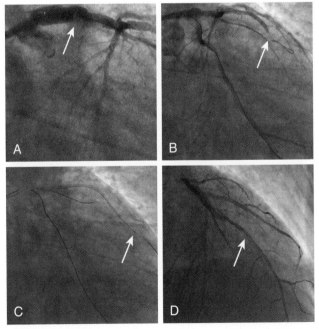

Figure 6.9 Angiographic appearance of intracoronary thrombus. (A) Contrast staining noted in distal right coronary artery (RCA) suggestive of intracoronary thrombus. (B) Complete occlusion of flow distal to the intracoronary thrombus.

thrombus. On coronary angiography, thrombus is recognized as a filling defect in the lumen of the coronary artery with or without persistent contrast staining. IVUS and OCT reveal the presence of thrombus as a low echogenic mass with a globular or layered appearance protruding from the attached vessel wall. It is challenging to definitively differentiate thrombus from soft plaque on IVUS imaging, and OCT is a better modality for thrombus imaging and diagnosis.

Aspiration of the intracoronary thrombus can be performed manually using any one of the several available manual aspiration catheters or a high-pressure rheolytic thrombectomy system (AngioJet, Boston Scientific, Maple Grove, MN). Of these, the AngioJet catheter uses high-pressure water jets that are directed backward into the catheter to create a strong negative suction (Venturi current) at the space of the catheter tip (Fig. 6.10). This not only evacuates the thrombus effectively but also macerates the thrombus into very small particles.

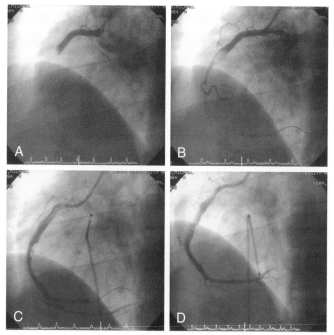

Figure 6.10 AngioJet rheolytic thrombectomy system cross-stream technology.

Mechanical Thrombectomy

Technical Tips

Mechanical aspiration thrombectomy devices are dual-lumen catheters that are passed across the culprit lesion over a standard 0.014-inch guidewire. Of the two lumens, the smaller lumen consists of the guidewire using a rapid exchange monorail system. The larger lumen connects the distal opening to the proximal port and serves as the aspiration lumen, using a large (30–50 mL) lockable aspiration syringe that is attached to the proximal port. Currently, the most frequently used aspiration thrombectomy catheters are the Export XT Aspiration Catheter (Medtronic, Inc., Minneapolis, MN, Fig. 6.11), the Pronto V3 Extraction Catheter (Vascular Solutions, Inc., Minneapolis, MN), and the Extract Catheter (Volcano Therapeutics, Rancho Mirage, CA). All these catheters are available in both 6-French (F) and 7F sizes. These catheters also vary in the degree of rigidity or support to cross difficult lesions. The Pronto LP has a stiletto, stiffening the catheter and allowing for more pushability and crossability.

Mechanical aspiration should be performed in an antegrade fashion (i.e., from proximal to distal) while crossing the lesion, and this should be continued while the aspiration catheter is being withdrawn into the guide catheter. This can be repeated multiple times as long as there is continuous collection of the thrombus into the lockable syringe. Continuous aspiration ensures that there is no premature release of the distal thrombus into the proximal part of the coronary artery, other coronary branches, or the aortic root. Operators should exercise caution because large thrombus particles may be attached to the tip of the aspiration catheter even if there is no flow into the syringe. At the end of aspiration, sufficient back-bleeding should be performed to ensure that both the guide catheter and the connector are clear of the entire thrombus burden.

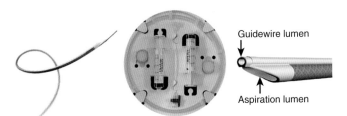

Guidewire lumen

Aspiration lumen

Figure 6.11 The Medtronic Export XT aspiration catheter. (Courtesy Medtronic, Inc., Minneapolis, MN.)

Aspiration Using the Penumbra System

Thrombectomy using the penumbra system (Fig. 6.12) is similar to aspiration thrombectomy, except the device is attached to a pump that allows for stronger and continuous suction for removal of thrombus.

Clinical Outcomes Data

Routine use of thrombectomy should not be performed in all cases for which intracoronary thrombus can be detected. This is because of the multiple trials performed using these catheters that failed to show a consistent beneficial effect and because of the finding of an increased risk of stroke associated with them. At present, use of selective and bailout aspiration thrombectomy remains recommended when vessels with a large thrombus burden are being treated.

Figs. 6.13 and 6.14 illustrate the use of thrombectomy for STEMI.

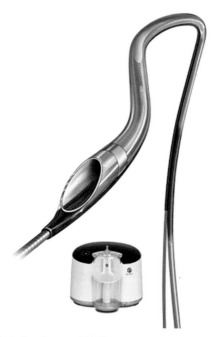

Figure 6.12 Indigo System CAT RX aspiration catheter and Penumbra ENGINE. The Penumbra system is indicated for the removal of fresh soft emboli and thrombi from vessels in the coronary and peripheral vasculature. (Courtesy Penumbra, Inc., Alameda, CA.)

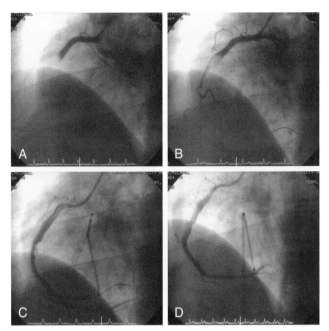

Figure 6.13 Case example using mechanical thrombectomy. (A) Heavy thrombus burden in the left main coronary artery (*arrow*). (B) Embolization of thrombus to the mid left anterior descending (LAD) artery occluding distal flow (*arrow*). (C) Aspiration thrombectomy (*arrow*). (D) Restoration of flow to the distal LAD.

Embolic Protection Devices

SVGs develop atherosclerotic luminal disease much more commonly than arterial grafts do. In fact, within 10 years, approximately half of these vein grafts develop complete or significant occlusion. In the majority of these cases, PCI is preferred over redo CABG surgery because of the inherent risks associated with repeat surgical revascularization. PCI of the SVGs is associated with multiple technical challenges, the most concerning being the high risk of no reflow phenomenon because of embolization of thrombotic debris into the distal vessel. Epicardial vasodilators such as nitroglycerin are of little value in restoring distal flow, but microvascular vasodilators such as adenosine or nicardipine may have a beneficial role in treating the no reflow phenomenon. This has led to the development of embolic protection devices to prevent or

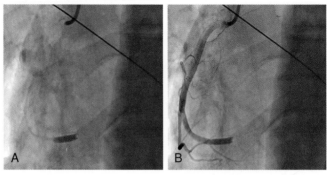

Figure 6.14 Example of AngioJet thrombectomy in a 37-year-old man 8 hours after the onset of chest pain for acute inferior wall myocardial infarction. (A) Right coronary artery with thrombus in proximal portion. (B) Angioplasty guidewire traversing lesion with large amount of clot in the proximal portion of the artery. (C) Right coronary artery after 4-French (F) AngioJet. A temporary pacemaker was also inserted. (D) The thrombus was almost completely extracted from the vessel. The final angiogram demonstrates residual distal embolic occlusions but good patency, with thrombolysis in myocardial infarction (TIMI) grade 3 flow.

minimize distal embolization and, in turn, improve both procedural and clinical outcomes.

Embolic protection devices are developed to decrease embolization of thrombotic or friable plaque material into the distal vessel during PCI. Although the data do not support the use of embolic protection devices during primary PCI in STEMI patients, these devices have been shown to improve outcomes in patients undergoing PCI on SVGs.

Distal Filter Device Technique

The Filterwire EZ embolic protection system (Boston Scientific Corporation, Natick, MA; Fig. 6.15) is the most commonly used device for this technique. This device consists of a symmetric 110-micron pore basket filter fixed to a guidewire. When this filter is released, it expands up to 5.5 mm. This technique requires crossing the lesion and placing the Filterwire EZ system distal to the lesion before deploying the filter. After completing the PCI, the filter is collapsed into a retrieval catheter, thus trapping the thrombotic debris and preventing distal embolization. In practice, the major limitation is the need for an adequate "landing zone" approximately 25 to 30 mm distal to the edge of the lesion to deploy the device.

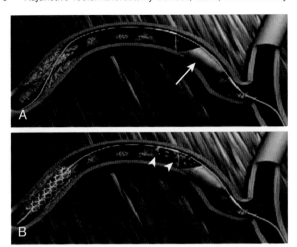

Figure 6.15 The Boston Scientific Filterwire EZ embolic protection system. (A) The filter (*arrow*) is deployed distal to the lesion. (B) Embolic material (*arrowheads*) is captured during intervention. (Courtesy Boston Scientific Corp., Natick, MA.)

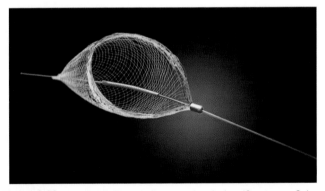

Figure 6.16 The SpiderFX embolic protection device. (Courtesy ev3, Inc., Plymouth, MN.)

The SpiderFX embolic protection device (ev3, Inc., Plymouth, MN; Fig. 6.16) is another device that uses the distal filter technique and can be used during PCI of SVGs. This device is heparin-coated and comes in a range of sizes from 3.0 mm to 7.0 mm. This device has an advantage over the Filterwire EZ embolic protection system in that it does not have a fixed guidewire and allows for use of any standard 0.014-inch interventional guidewire. The filter is delivered distal to the lesion using a 3.2F catheter by means of a rapid exchange system (SpideRX); at the end of the procedure, it is retrieved using a separate 4.2F or 4.6F SpideRX retrieval catheter.

Key References

Chambers JW, Feldman RL, Himmelstein SI, et al. Pivotal trial to evaluate the safety and efficacy of the orbital atherectomy system in treating de novo, severely calcified coronary lesions (ORBIT II). *JACC Cardiovasc Interv*. 2014;7:510-518.

Khan AA, Murtaza G, Khalid MF, et al. Outcomes of rotational atherectomy versus orbital atherectomy for the treatment of heavily calcified coronary stenosis: a systematic review and meta-analysis. *Catheter Cardiovasc Interv*. 2021;98(5): 884-892.

Latif F, Vidovich MI. *Rotational vs. Orbital Atherectomy: How to Choose?*. https://scai. org/rotational-vs-orb ital-atherectomy-how-choose, 2020. Available at:Accessed August 03, 2021.

Levine GN, Bates ER, Blankenship JC, et al. 2011 ACCF/AHA/SCAI guideline for percutaneous coronary intervention. A report of the American College of Cardiology Foundation/American Heart Association Task Force on Practice Guidelines and the Society for Cardiovascular Angiography and Interventions. *J Am Coll Cardiol*. 2011;58:e44-e122.

Parikh K, Chandra P, Choksi N, et al. Safety and feasibility of orbital atherectomy for the treatment of calcified coronary lesions: the ORBIT I trial. *Catheter Cardiovasc Interv*. 2013;81:1134-1139.

Takebayashi H, Haruta S, Kohno H, et al. Immediate and 3-month follow-up outcome after cutting balloon angioplasty for bifurcation lesions. *J Interv Cardiol*. 2004;17:1-7.

Tian W, Lhermusier T, Minha S, et al. Rational use of rotational atherectomy in calcified lesions in the drug-eluting stent era: review of the evidence and current practice. *Cardiovasc Revasc Med*. 2015;16:78-83.

Shah M, Najam O, Bhindi R, De Silva K. Calcium modification techniques in complex percutaneous coronary intervention. *Circ Cardiovasc Interv*. 2021;14(5):e009870.

Sharma SK, Tomey MI, Teirstein PS, et al. North American expert review of rotational atherectomy. *Circ Cardiovasc Interv*. 2019;12(5):e007448.

Bifurcation PCI

EMMANOUIL S. BRILAKIS • YIANNIS CHATZIZISIS •
ALLISON BARBARA HALL • SUBHASH BANERJEE •
YVES R. LOUVARD

KEY POINTS

- Percutaneous coronary intervention (PCI) of bifurcation lesions can be complex requiring several equipment types and intraprocedural decision making.

- Various classification systems exist for bifurcations to guide treatment decisions, but the Medina classification is most commonly used.

- There are a variety of well-known "two-stent" bifurcation strategies available which have specific technical steps to achieve procedural success.

- Intravascular imaging assists operators to guide and plan bifurcation PCI.

Disclosures

Dr. Brilakis has received consulting/speaker honoraria from Abbott Vascular, American Heart Association (Associate Editor Circulation), Amgen, Biotronik, Boston Scientific, Cardiovascular Innovations Foundation (Board of Directors), ControlRad, CSI, Ebix, Elsevier, GE Healthcare, InfraRedx, Medtronic, Siemens, and Teleflex; research support from Regeneron and Siemens; owner, Hippocrates LLC; shareholder, MHI Ventures.
Dr. Chatzizisis has received consulting/speaker honoraria and research support from Boston Scientific and research support from Medtronic; holds patent.
Dr. Hall has received speaker honoraria from Medtronic, OpSens Medical and Cardiovascular Innovations Foundation.
Dr. Banerjee has received honoraria from Medtronic, Cordis, Livmor, AngioSafe.
Dr. Louvard: none.

Definition and Classification

The European Bifurcation Club (EBC) has defined bifurcation lesions as lesions occurring at or adjacent to a significant division of a major epicardial coronary artery. What is "significant" remains subjective and is determined by the treating physician as branches that, if compromised during percutaneous coronary intervention (PCI), can cause symptoms or periprocedural myocardial infarction (MI). A recent computed tomography (CT) analysis by Kim et al. showed that only 20% of non-left main bifurcations supply at least 10% of the myocardium.

There are multiple classifications of bifurcation lesions, but one of the simplest and most commonly used currently is the Medina classification (Fig. 7.1), which records any narrowing of 50% or more in each of the three arterial segments of the bifurcation in the following order: proximal main vessel (MV), distal main vessel, and proximal side branch (SB). The presence of

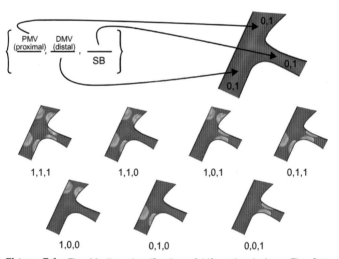

Figure 7.1 The Medina classification of bifurcation lesions. The first number describes the PMV, the second number the DMV, and the third number the SB. Each segment is described as "1" if the segment has a diameter stenosis of at least 50% by visual estimation; otherwise, it is described as "0." *DMV,* Distal main vessel; *PMV,* proximal main vessel; *SB,* side branch. (Reprinted from Brilakis ES. *Manual of Percutaneous Coronary Intervention: A Step-By-Step Approach.* Elsevier; 2020.)

significant stenosis is marked as "1" and the absence as "0." A limitation of the Medina classification is that it does not account for other lesion characteristics, such as angulation, plaque location, length, and calcification.

Basics of Bifurcation Lesion Percutaneous Coronary Intervention

PCI of bifurcation lesions can result in both acute (such as SB occlusion and periprocedural MI) and long-term (such as restenosis and/or stent thrombosis) complications. Several strategies for bifurcation PCI are summarized in the Main, Across, Distal, Side (MADS) classification based on how the first stent is implanted (Fig. 7.2).

Large (such as 7 French [F] or 8F) guide catheters may facilitate bifurcation PCI because they allow more treatment options, especially for two-stent strategies or if a complication occurs. Nevertheless, 6F guides (with or without radial access) are adequate for most bifurcation PCIs and are used by most operators. Wiring both the MV and SB should be done for all bifurcations with important SBs. Keeping the wires organized (e.g., by using a towel to separate them and by using guidewires with different shaft color) can facilitate performance of the procedure. The most challenging branch to wire should be wired first, and the wires should be kept in the same position on the table as on the working projection to prevent twisting. Drug-eluting stents (DES) significantly reduce the risk of in-stent restenosis (ISR) and are preferred for bifurcation lesions. The minimum number of stents should be used, and intracoronary imaging should be used in most cases to optimize stent expansion and stent strut apposition and help detect tissue protrusion and stent edge dissections.

A practical approach for selecting a treatment strategy for bifurcation lesion PCI follows.

Algorithmic Approach to Bifurcation Percutaneous Coronary Intervention

See Video 7.1.

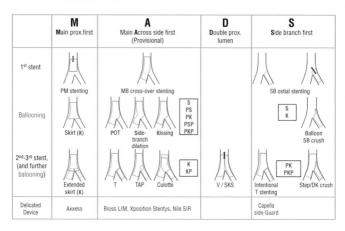

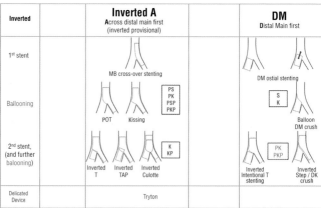

Figure 7.2 The MADS (Main-Across-Distal-Side)-2 Classification of Bifurcation Lesion Stenting. The figure includes two panels. The upper panel shows the standard techniques, and the lower panel shows the "inverted" techniques. Blue capital letters describe ballooning techniques, as follows:

1. P: Postdilation of the proximal main vessel (usually reported as proximal optimization technique [POT])
2. S: balloon dilation of the side branch (SB) ostium
3. K: balloon inflation in the main vessel (MV) and SB (usually reported as kissing balloon inflation technique).

Common combinations of ballooning techniques are described as the sequential blue capital letters. (Reprinted from Burzotta F, Lassen JF, Louvard Y, et al. European Bifurcation Club white paper on stenting techniques for patients with bifurcated coronary artery lesions. *Catheter Cardiovasc Interv.* 2020;96:1067–1079.)

Determine Whether a Side Branch Needs to Be Preserved

Bifurcation lesions with SBs that supply a small amount of myocardium and are unlikely to cause symptoms if they become occluded or highly stenotic are approached with MV stenting without attempts to maintain the side branch patency (Fig. 7.3).

Determine the Likelihood of Side Branch Occlusion During Bifurcation PCI

The likelihood of SB occlusion is estimated based on vessel size, angulation, and proximal disease. A study of 1601 consecutive bifurcation PCIs demonstrated SB occlusion in 7.37%. SB occlusion was associated with the following six parameters (RESOLVE [Risk Prediction of Side Branch Occlusion in Coronary Bifurcation Intervention] score):

1. Plaque distribution at the same side as the SB
2. Lower MV thrombolysis in MI (TIMI) flow grade before stenting

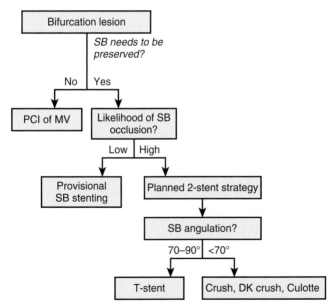

Figure 7.3 Algorithmic approach to bifurcation percutaneous coronary intervention. *DK crush,* Double kissing crush; *MV,* main vessel; *SB,* side branch; *TAP,* T and protrusion.

3. Higher preprocedure diameter stenosis of the bifurcation core (central part of the bifurcation, which begins where the common vessel starts to split into two branches and ends at the carinal point)

4. Higher bifurcation angle

5. Higher diameter ratio between MV/SB

6. Higher diameter stenosis of SB before MV stenting

In the DEFINITION II trial, complex bifurcations at high risk for SB occlusion were defined as those fulfilling one major criterion (SB lesion length $\geq$ 10 mm with diameter stenosis of SB $\geq$ 70% for distal LM bifurcation lesions or diameter stenosis of SB $\geq$ 90% for non-LM bifurcation lesions) plus any two minor criteria (moderate-to-severe calcification, multiple lesions, bifurcation angle < 45 degrees or > 70 degrees, MV reference vessel diameter < 2.5 mm, thrombus-containing lesions, or MV lesion length $\geq$ 25 mm) by visual estimation.

SBs at high risk for compromise are best treated with an upfront two-stent strategy.

Significant Side Branch at Low Risk for Occlusion

The preferred strategy for such lesions is *provisional SB stenting*. Both branches are wired and the MV is stented first, followed by ballooning and/or stenting of the SB only if the SB develops a severe stenosis (often patients develop electrocardiographic changes or angina) or its flow is compromised (Figs. 7.4–7.6 and Videos 7.2 and 7.3). Predilation of the MV is usually performed to ensure subsequent expansion of the stent, whereas predilation of the SB is not needed for most cases unless there is significant ostial SB disease (or severe calcification or angulation that could hinder access to the SB after MV stenting) or reduced flow after wiring. DES are preferred, sized to the diameter of the distal MV, but allowing expansion to the reference diameter of the proximal MV. According to Finet's formula, the diameter of the proximal MV is equal to (distal main vessel diameter + SB diameter) × 0.678. Hence the chosen stent has to accommodate two diameters: the one of the distal MV (no oversizing to avoid carina shift and compromise of the SB) and the one of the proximal MV (to prevent stent underexpansion and malapposition). Expansion of the proximal MV portion of the stent is achieved using the proximal optimization technique (POT; i.e., inflation with a short noncompliant balloon adequately sized for the proximal MV with the distal radiopaque marker positioned at the carina and inflated at high pressures). POT facilitates rewiring of the SB (if needed), minimizes the risk of substent wire crossing, and

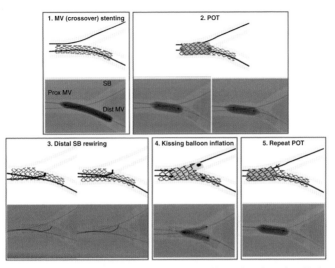

Figure 7.4 Illustration of the Provisional Bifurcation Stenting Technique. Panel 1: The main vessel (MV) and side branch (SB) are both wired. Consider predilation of the SB (if it has significant disease; most times predilation is not needed because it may cause dissection that can lead to implantation of a SB stent). The MV is stented across the SB take-off with a drug-eluting stent (DES) sized 1:1 according to the distal MV diameter. Panel 2: Proximal optimization technique with balloon sized 1:1 to proximal MV. Note that, because of long stented area in the proximal MV, two inflations were needed to appropriately postdilate the entire proximal MV stent segment. If the SB does not become compromised (significant angiographic stenosis or decrease in antegrade flow) after MV stenting, no further treatment is required. Otherwise, SB rewiring, kissing balloon inflation and repeat proximal optimization technique [POT] is performed as shown in panels 3 to 5. Panel 3: Rewire the SB through a distal stent strut. Note the double bended guidewire tip shape that may facilitate entering the distal part of the SB ostium. Panel 4: Kissing balloon inflation with MV balloon sized 1:1 according to distal MV and SB balloon sized 1:1 according to SB diameter. Panel 5: Repeat POT with a balloon sized 1:1 with the proximal MV. (Reprinted from Burzotta F, Lassen JF, Louvard Y, et al. European Bifurcation Club white paper on stenting techniques for patients with bifurcated coronary artery lesions. *Catheter Cardiovasc Interv.* 2020;96:1067–1079.)

facilitates equipment advancement through the proximal portion of the MV stent.

Several studies have shown better outcomes with provisional SB stenting compared with a routine two-stent strategy, although these studies have been criticized for including nontrue bifurcation

Provisional Technique

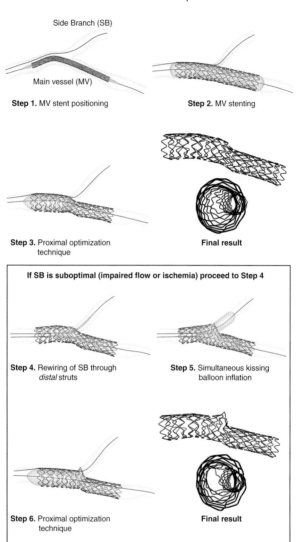

Step 1. MV stent positioning

Step 2. MV stenting

Step 3. Proximal optimization technique

Final result

If SB is suboptimal (impaired flow or ischemia) proceed to Step 4

Step 4. Rewiring of SB through *distal* struts

Step 5. Simultaneous kissing balloon inflation

Step 6. Proximal optimization technique

Final result

Figure 7.5 Illustration of the provisional bifurcation stenting technique. (Courtesy Dr. Yiannis Chatzizisis.)

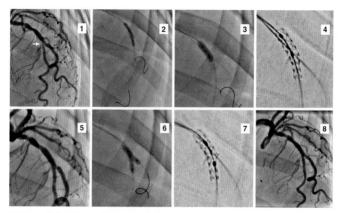

Figure 7.6 Illustrative case of bifurcation stenting using the provisional side branch stenting technique. A bifurcation of the left anterior descending artery and the diagonal branch (panel 1) was treated with crossover stenting after wiring both branches (panel 2). After proximal optimization technique (panel 3), the side branch (diagonal) was rewired (panel 4) and given a proximal side branch lesion (panel 5), and kissing balloon inflation was performed (panel 6) with an excellent final result (panel 7 and 8). (Courtesy Dr. Yves Louvard.)

lesions, stenting small SBs, and not performing a two-step final kissing balloon inflation. In the DK CRUSH V trial, provisional stenting was associated with worse outcomes compared with the double kissing crush (DK crush) technique in left main bifurcation lesions. In the DEFINITION II trial, a two-stent strategy was associated with better outcomes compared with provisional stenting in complex bifurcation lesions. In general, two-stent techniques are easier to perform when the SB is stented first, but a provisional SB technique may obviate the need for SB stenting in the majority of treated bifurcations.

Routine SB ballooning after MV stenting is generally *not* recommended except when the SB ostium is compromised by significant diameter stenosis, dissection, and/or reduced flow. Kissing balloon inflation can cause SB dissection requiring SB stenting and should be done with short noncompliant balloons inflated at low pressure (10–12 atm). Fractional flow reserve (FFR) of jailed SBs can be useful because many lesions that appear severe by angiography may not be hemodynamically significant (FFR was <0.75 in only 27% of 73 jailed SBs with ≥ 75% angiographic stenosis in a study by Koo et al.) and may not require stenting. Advancing the pressure wire through the jailed SB can be challenging.

Rewiring a jailed SB can be challenging (although POT can significantly facilitate rewiring) and should be performed through a distal stent strut because wiring through a proximal stent strut can result in suboptimal SB ostium coverage and metal overhang into the MV. Optical coherence tomography (OCT) could be used to confirm rewiring through a distal stent strut. As discussed earlier, the POT technique should be performed before rewiring attempts if there is a mismatch between the proximal and distal MV diameter. Rewiring through a jailed side branch may be facilitated by (Fig. 7.7):

- Having a jailed wire in the SB that marks the SB origin and changes the access angle
- Use of polymer-jacketed guidewires
- Use of a microcatheter, especially an angulated microcatheter such as the Supercross and the Venture (Vascular Solutions, Minneapolis, MN; see Fig. 7.7D), or a dual-lumen microcatheter, such as the Twin-Pass (Vascular Solutions) and Sasuke (Asahi Intecc; see Fig. 7.7E), that can prevent crossing through proximal stent struts
- Use of the reversed guidewire technique (see Fig. 7.7F–H)
- Use of the guidewire exchange technique (i.e., pulling back the MV wire to advance it into the SB through a distal stent cell [using the jailed SB wire as marker] and removing the jailed wire from the SB [under fluoroscopy to prevent deep intubation of the guide catheter] and advancing it into the distal MV [preferably after creating a loop at the tip to prevent crossing under the proximal MV struts])

If the SB cannot be rewired after stenting and flow is compromised, a small balloon can be advanced over the jailed guidewire to restore flow into the SB before continued rewiring attempts.

After SB rewiring, balloon advancement through the stent struts can be challenging and can be facilitated by:

- Use of a small balloon (1.0–1.5 mm, such as the Sapphire II Pro [OrbusNeich] balloon, which is the smallest diameter balloon currently available in the US, the Threader [Boston Scientific, Natick, MA], or the Glider balloon [Teleflex, Morrisville, NC])
- If even a small balloon will not pass, sometimes a microcatheter will, which can facilitate exchange to a more supportive wire and also create a tract for subsequent balloon passage.
- If everything else fails, rewiring with another wire through another strut can be attempted.

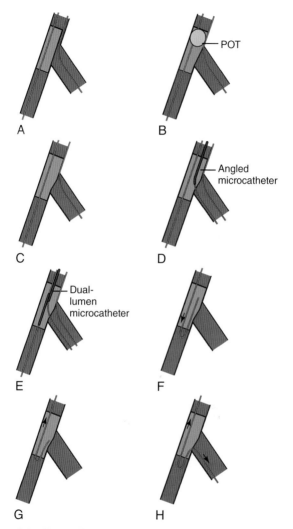

Figure 7.7   How to Rewire a Jailed Side Branch. 1, Before rewiring, the proximal optimization technique (POT) is performed if the proximal main vessel is larger than the distal main vessel to optimize proximal stent strut apposition and prevent substent guidewire advancement (A–C). 2, An angled microcatheter (D), a dual-lumen microcatheter (E), or a knuckled guidewire (F–H) can be used to prevent inadvertent substent guidewire entry. Alternatively, the side branch (SB) could be rewired by withdrawing the main vessel guidewire.

If SB stenting is needed in provisional SB technique after MV stenting, the following techniques can be used depending on SB angulation (Fig. 7.8):

- 70–90 degrees: Use the T-stenting (if the bifurcation angle is nearly 90 degrees, which can allow stent coverage of the SB ostium without stent protrusion into the MV) or more commonly the T and protrusion (TAP) technique (Figs. 7.9 and 7.10 and Video 7.4). In the TAP technique, the SB stent is deployed with minimal protrusion into the MV while an uninflated balloon is kept in the MV, followed by slight withdrawal of the SB balloon, kissing balloon inflation (without rewiring the SB), and final POT.
- Less than 70 degrees: Use the reverse crush (also called "internal crush") or culotte technique.
- In the reverse crush technique (Fig. 7.11, Video 7.5), the SB stent is deployed with protrusion in the MV stent, followed by crush and POT, rewiring of the SB stent, kissing balloon inflation, and final POT.
- In the culotte technique (described in more detail later), the SB stent is deployed into the MV stent, followed by POT, rewiring of the MV stent through a distal strut, high-pressure balloon inflation into the MV, kissing balloon inflation, and final POT. The culotte technique may be preferred when the MV diameter is similar to the SB diameter, but both techniques require rewiring and final kissing balloon inflation, followed by final POT. The culotte technique was originally designed as a bailout for SB compromise during the provisional approach but can also be performed by implanting the first stent into the SB, a sequence that is called "inverted" culotte.

Significant Side Branch at High Risk for Occlusion

Such bifurcation lesions are best treated with an upfront two-stent strategy (MV and SB). Lesion preparation (with balloon angioplasty and/or cutting balloon inflation or atherectomy) is important for both MV and SB before stenting to facilitate stent delivery and expansion. The most commonly used two-stent strategies are the T-stent and TAP technique (for 70- to 90-degree angulation) and the DK crush or culotte (for <70-degree angulation):

- 70 to 90 degrees: Use T-stenting if angulation is nearly 90 degrees and TAP for lesser angulation
- Less than 70 degrees: Use the DK crush or culotte technique
  - DK crush (Figs. 7.12 and 7.13, Videos 7.6–7.8) is currently the preferred two-stent bifurcation technique by many operators

Text continued on page 285

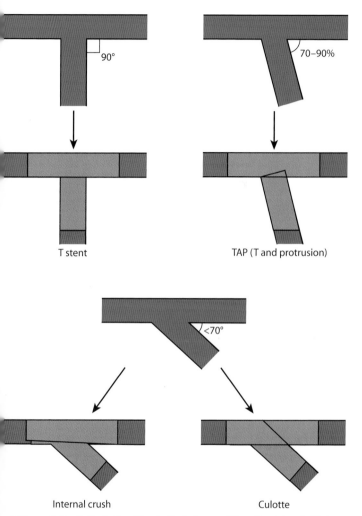

Figure 7.8 Bailout Two-Stent Techniques After Provisional Main Vessel (MV) Stenting. Technique selection depends on side branch (SB) angulation.

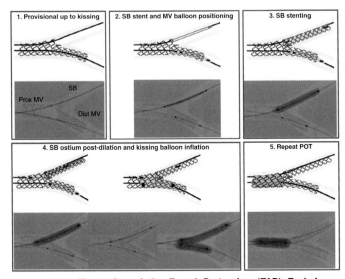

Figure 7.9 Illustration of the T and Protrusion (TAP) Technique.
Panel 1: The recommended steps of provisional have been followed up to kissing balloon inflation. Panel 2: Side branch (SB) stent and main vessel (MV) balloon positioning: An appropriately sized SB stent is placed in the SB and a balloon sized 1:1 according to the distal MV is advanced in the distal MV. Panel 3: SB stenting: When the best position (to allow cover the SB ostium and minimally protruding inside the MV) for SB stent has been selected, the SB stent is deployed with the MV balloon left uninflated. Panel 4: SB ostium postdilation and kissing balloon inflation: After SB stent deployment, the balloon of the stent is slightly pulled back and repeat infla-tion at high pressure is performed to warrant optimal stent expansion at the level of SB ostium (the balloon inside the MV is still kept uninflated during this phase). Then, after alignment of the MV balloon and SB stent's balloon, kissing balloon inflation is performed by inflating simultaneously the two balloons. Panel 5: Repeat proximal optimization technique (POT). This step is not mandatory. If this step is adopted, the POT balloon is inflated in the proximal MV in a position that is far from the metallic neocarina. (Reprinted from Burzotta F, Lassen JF, Louvard Y, et al. European Bifurcation Club white paper on stenting techniques for patients with bifurcated coronary artery lesions. *Catheter Cardiovasc Interv.* 2020;96:1067–1079.)

T and Protrusion (TAP) Technique

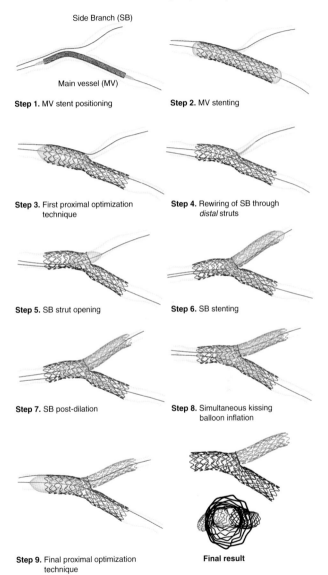

Figure 7.10 Illustration of the T and protrusion (TAP) technique. (Courtesy Dr. Yiannis Chatzizisis.)

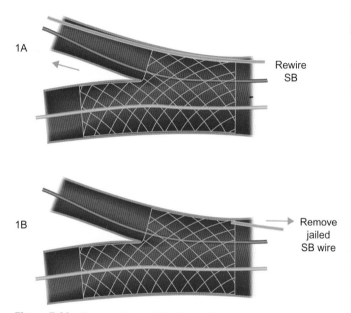

1A

Rewire
SB

1B

Remove
jailed
SB wire

Figure 7.11   Reverse Crush (Also Called "Internal Crush") Technique After Main Vessel (MV) Stenting.
Step 1: Rewire SB (side branch) and remove jailed guidewire. A balloon can be advanced into the MV at this time (instead of advancing it in step 3) because after SB ballooning some struts may protrude, making it challenging to advance the MV balloon.

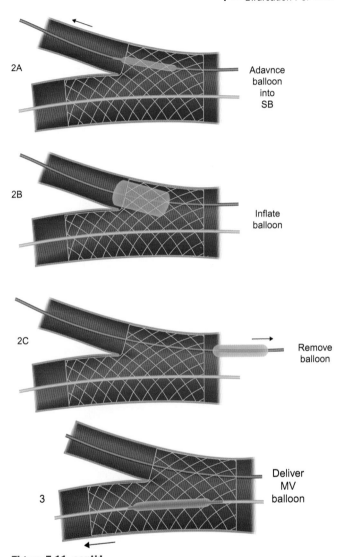

Figure 7.11, cont'd
Step 2. Dilate SB.
Step 3. Deliver MV balloon.

Continued

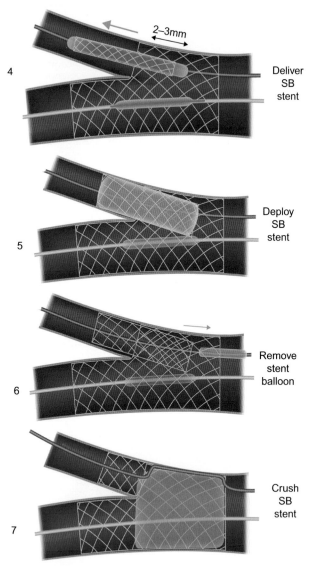

Figure 7.11, cont'd
Step 4. Deliver SB stent.
Step 5. Deploy SB stent.
Step 6. Remove stent balloon.
Step 7. Crush SB stent.

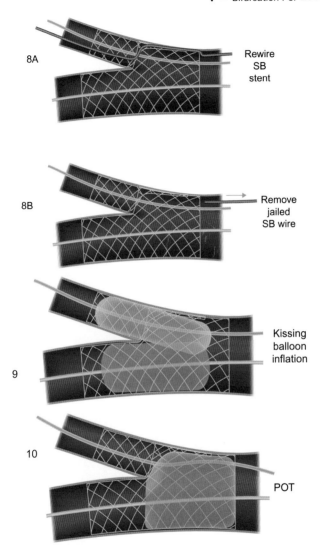

Figure 7.11, cont'd

Step 8. Rewire SB stent and remove jailed guidewire. Proximal optimization technique (POT) is needed if there is discrepancy in the size of the distal versus proximal MV.

Step 9. Kissing balloon inflation.

Step 10. POT.

Continued

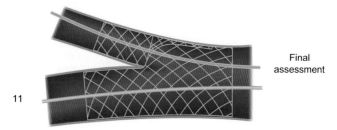

11

Figure 7.11, cont'd
Step 11. Final assessment. (Reprinted from Brilakis ES. *Manual of Percutaneous Coronary Intervention: A Step-By-Step Approach*. Elsevier; 2020.)

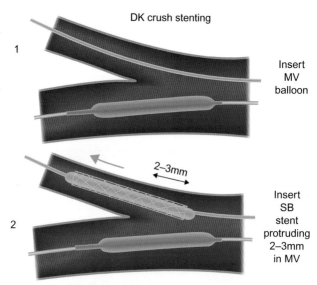

Figure 7.12 Illustration of the Double-Kissing Crush (DK Crush) Technique.
Step 1: Insert main vessel (MV) balloon (sized 1:1 with the distal MV) in the MV at or distal to the side branch (SB) origin.
Step 2. Deliver SB stent protruding 2–3 mm in the MV.

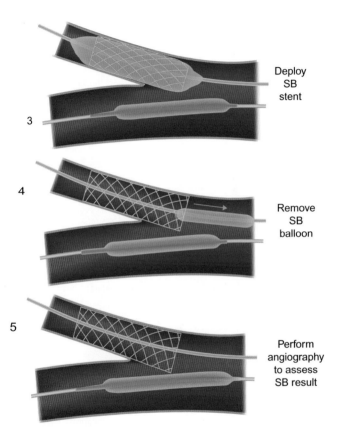

3 — Deploy SB stent

4 — Remove SB balloon

5 — Perform angiography to assess SB result

Figure 7.12, cont'd

Step 3. Deploy SB stent.
Step 4. Remove SB balloon.
Step 5. Perform angiography to assess SB result. Additional percutaneous coronary intervention (PCI) of the SB may be needed (in case of stent underexpansion or distal dissection); failure to optimize the SB result may hinder rewiring.

Continued

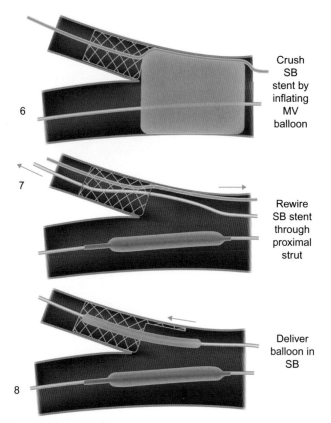

6   Crush SB stent by inflating MV balloon

7   Rewire SB stent through proximal strut

8   Deliver balloon in SB

Figure 7.12, cont'd

Step 6. Crush SB stent by inflating MV balloon (could jail the SB guidewire, although most operators remove the SB guidewire before crushing the stent). If the MV balloon is sized according to the proximal main branch (same size for doing a proximal optimization technique [POT]), it should not be advanced past the carina to minimize the risk of distal MV dissection. Alternatively, the MV balloon is sized according to the distal MV diameter, followed by POT.

Step 7. Rewire SB through crushed stent (through proximal strut), then remove jailed SB wire.

Step 8. Deliver balloon in SB.

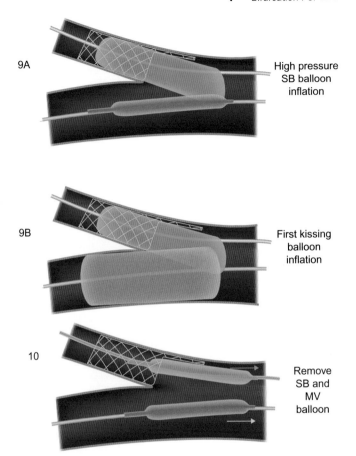

9A — High pressure SB balloon inflation

9B — First kissing balloon inflation

10 — Remove SB and MV balloon

Figure 7.12, cont'd
Step 9. First kissing balloon inflation.
Step 10. Remove SB and MV balloon (may or may not leave SB wire in).

Continued

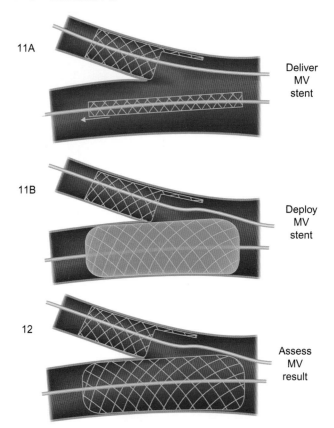

11A

Deliver
MV
stent

11B

Deploy
MV
stent

12

Assess
MV
result

Figure 7.12, cont'd
Step 11. Deliver and deploy MV stent.
Step 12. Assess MV stent result—Additional PCI of the MV distally may be
needed.

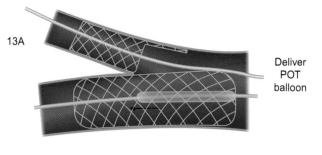

13A

Deliver
POT
balloon

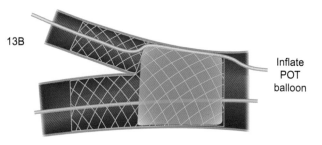

13B

Inflate
POT
balloon

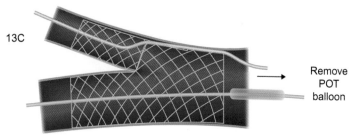

13C

Remove
POT
balloon

Figure 7.12, cont'd

Step 13. POT (if proximal MV has significant size mismatch from distal MV).
1. Place POT balloon (sized 1:1 to proximal MV) with its distal edge at the bifurcation carina.
2. Inflate POT balloon.
3. Remove POT balloon.

Continued

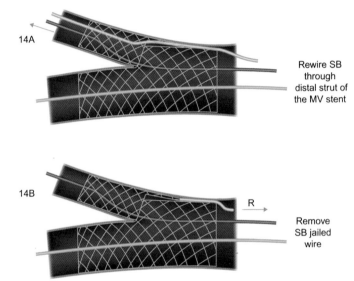

14A

Rewire SB
through
distal strut of
the MV stent

14B

R →

Remove
SB jailed
wire

Figure 7.12, cont'd
Step 14. Rewire SB through MV stent (then remove the jailed SB wire if it had been left in).
  1. Rewire SB though MV stent (through distal strut, in contrast to the first rewiring).
  2. Remove jailed SB wire.

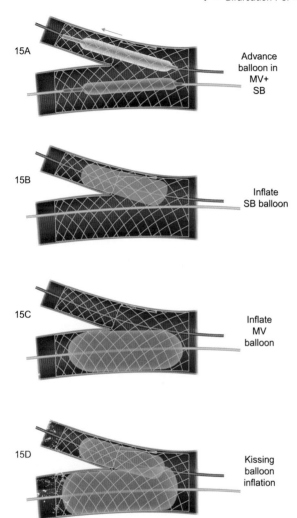

Figure 7.12, cont'd

Step 15. Second kissing balloon inflation (two-step kiss):
1. Advance SB balloon and MV balloon (it does not matter which one goes first).
2. Inflate SB (or MV) balloon at high pressure.
3. Inflate MV (or SB) balloon at high pressure.
4. Inflate both MV and SB balloon at 12–14 atm.

Continued

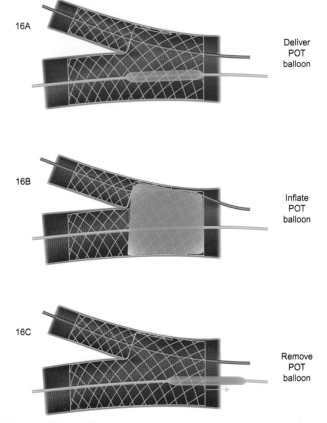

16A

Deliver
POT
balloon

16B

Inflate
POT
balloon

16C

Remove
POT
balloon

Figure 7.12, cont'd

Step 16. Final POT.
  1. Place POT balloon (sized 1:1 to proximal MV) with its distal edge at the carina of the bifurcation.
  2. Inflate POT balloon.
  3. Remove POT balloon.

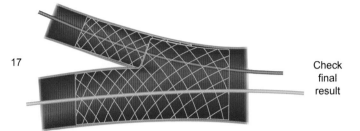

17

Check final result

Figure 7.12, cont'd
Step 17. Final angiography (and intravascular imaging) to assess final result. (Reprinted from Brilakis ES. *Manual of Percutaneous Coronary Intervention: A Step-By-Step Approach.* Elsevier; 2020.)

because it has the strongest clinical data. In DK crush, kissing balloon inflation is performed twice: after crushing the first stent with a balloon before deploying the second stent, and after deploying the second stent after rewiring of the SB. DK crush facilitates access to the SB, which is a limitation of the standard crush technique but can be technically challenging (Video 7.9). The steps of the DK crush technique are shown in Fig. 7.12.

- Culotte is performed as illustrated in Figs. 7.14 and 7.15 and Videos 7.10 and 7.11. Culotte is preferred when the MV and SB have similar diameters; however, the DK CRUSH III trial demonstrated higher rates of restenosis and target vessel revascularization in unprotected left main bifurcation lesions treated with the culotte versus DK crush technique.

There are several other two-stent techniques, such as the simultaneous kissing stent (SKS) technique, in which two stents are positioned in both the MV and SB with their proximal portions being parallel to each other and deployed. Although SKS allows continuous wire access to both MV and SB, it is not currently recommended except in emergency salvage cases because it creates a long new metal carina and recrossing may be challenging to achieve.

Double Kissing (OK) Crush Technique

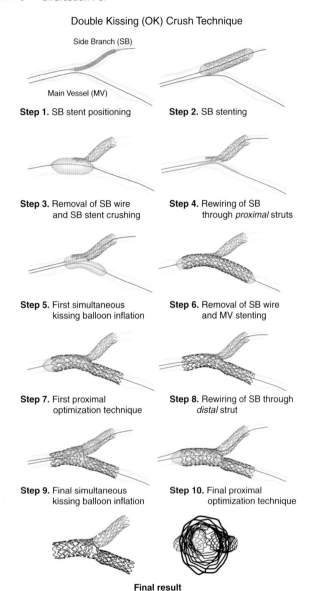

Step 1. SB stent positioning

Step 2. SB stenting

Step 3. Removal of SB wire and SB stent crushing

Step 4. Rewiring of SB through *proximal* struts

Step 5. First simultaneous kissing balloon inflation

Step 6. Removal of SB wire and MV stenting

Step 7. First proximal optimization technique

Step 8. Rewiring of SB through *distal* strut

Step 9. Final simultaneous kissing balloon inflation

Step 10. Final proximal optimization technique

Final result

Figure 7.13 Illustration of the DK crush technique. (Courtesy Dr. Yiannis Chatzizisis.)

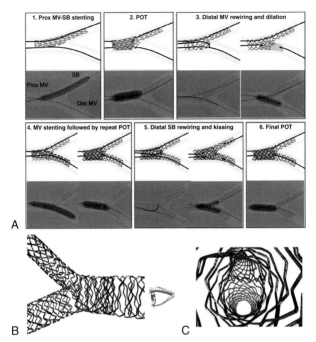

Figure 7.14 The Culotte Technique. (A) Recommended steps for culotte stenting (in the case of elective double stenting):

Step 1. Stent implantation from proximal main vessel (MV) into the side branch (SB) across distal MV with drug-eluting stent (DES) sized 1:1 according to SB. When culotte is used for elective double stenting, usually a short proximal MV coverage may be selected to limit the area with overlapping stents.

Step 2. Proximal optimization technique (POT) with balloon sized 1:1 to proximal MV.

Step 3. Distal MV rewiring and dilation. Distal MV rewiring is performed according to the pullback technique. Distal MV dilation may be performed either using kissing balloon inflation (see inverted provisional) or by simple balloon dilation with balloon selected 1:1 according to distal MV size.

Step 4. MV stenting followed by repeat POT: After SB guidewire removal, stent implantation across the SB with DES diameter selected 1:1 according to the distal MV size is performed. Thereafter, repeat POT with balloon sized 1:1 to proximal MV is done.

Step 5. Distal SB rewiring and kissing: Distal SB rewiring is performed according to the pullback technique. Simultaneous kissing balloon inflation (usually with noncompliant balloons at high pressure) is performed selecting MV balloon sized 1:1 according to distal MV and SB balloon sized 1:1 according to SB diameter.

Step 6. Final POT performed with balloon sized 1:1 to proximal MV. (B–C) Micro-computed tomography (CT) image of stent conformation obtained by culotte. (Reprinted from Burzotta F, Lassen JF, Louvard Y, et al. European Bifurcation Club white paper on stenting techniques for patients with bifurcated coronary artery lesions. *Catheter Cardiovasc Interv.* 2020;96:1067–1079.)

Culotte Technique

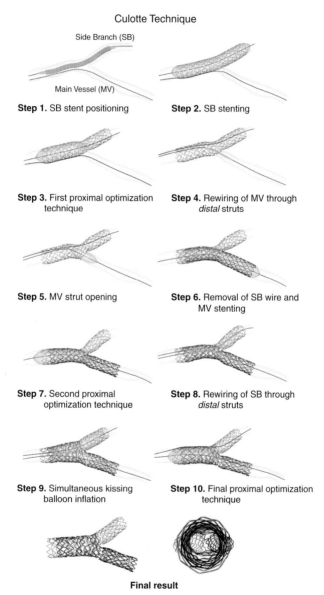

Step 1. SB stent positioning

Step 2. SB stenting

Step 3. First proximal optimization technique

Step 4. Rewiring of MV through *distal* struts

Step 5. MV strut opening

Step 6. Removal of SB wire and MV stenting

Step 7. Second proximal optimization technique

Step 8. Rewiring of SB through *distal* struts

Step 9. Simultaneous kissing balloon inflation

Step 10. Final proximal optimization technique

Final result

Figure 7.15 Illustration of the culotte technique. (Courtesy Dr. Yiannis Chatzizisis.)

Intravascular Imaging and Functional Assessment for Bifurcation Stenting

Intravascular imaging (intravascular ultrasound [IVUS] and OCT) is highly recommended for bifurcation PCI, both before stenting (to assess lesion composition and the need for pretreatment and to select the optimal stent sizes) and after stenting (to confirm adequate stent expansion, stent-strut apposition and lack of tissue protrusion, edge dissection, and stent distortion).

The following minimum stent areas should be achieved at various locations during left main stenting:

- Left main proximal to the point of confluence: 8 mm^2
- Point of confluence: 7 mm^2
- Left anterior descending (LAD) artery ostium: 6 mm^2
- Circumflex ostium: 5 mm^2
- Particular attention should be paid to the circumflex ostium that is the most common site of ISR during left main stenting.

Imaging of a jailed SB during provisional stenting should be avoided to prevent stent deformation, but imaging of both branches is highly recommended for two-stent bifurcation PCI techniques. Physiologic assessment of the SB after provisional stenting can help determine whether additional treatment of the SB is needed, as previously described.

Antiplatelet Therapy After Bifurcation Stenting

Patients undergoing bifurcation stenting may be at increased risk for stent thrombosis. As a result, more intensive (e.g., aspirin + ticagrelor or aspirin + prasugrel) or prolonged (>12 months) dual antiplatelet therapy may be considered after bifurcation stenting, especially for two-stent bifurcation PCI techniques.

SUMMARY

Several treatment techniques are available for treating bifurcation lesions. A provisional SB stenting strategy is preferred for lesions with insignificant SB or SB at low risk for occlusion. For bifurcations requiring an upfront two-stent strategy, the T-stenting and TAP technique is preferred when the bifurcation angle

Continued

SUMMARY—cont'd

is 70 degrees or greater and the DK crush or culotte technique when the bifurcation angle is less than 70 degrees. The two-step kissing balloon inflation technique (for two-stent bifurcation stenting) followed by final proximal optimization technique (for all bifurcations) can help optimize the bifurcation stenting results.

Acknowledgment

We would like to acknowledge the invaluable help of Saurabhi Samant, MBBS, Behram Khan, MBBS, Shijia Zhao, PhD, and Muhammad Fayaz, MBBS who created the video animations.

Key References

Burzotta F, Lassen JF, Lefevre T, et al. Percutaneous coronary intervention for bifurcation coronary lesions. The 15th consensus document from the European Bifurcation Club. *EuroIntervention*. 2021;16(16):1307–1317.

Burzotta F, Lassen JF, Louvard Y, et al. European Bifurcation Club white paper on stenting techniques for patients with bifurcated coronary artery lesions. *Catheter Cardiovasc Interv*. 2020;96:1067-1079.

Brilakis ES. *Manual of Percutaneous Coronary Intervention: A Step-By-Step Approach*. Elsevier; 2020.

References

Chen SL, Xu B, Han YL, et al. Comparison of double kissing crush versus culotte stenting for unprotected distal left main bifurcation lesions: results from a multicenter, randomized, prospective DKCRUSH-III study. *J Am Coll Cardiol*. 2013;61:1482–1488.

Chen SL, Zhang JJ, Han Y, et al. Double kissing crush versus provisional stenting for left main distal bifurcation lesions: DK CRUSH-V randomized trial. *J Am Coll Cardiol*. 2017;70:2605–2617.

Di Gioia G, Sonck J, Ferenc M, et al. Clinical outcomes following coronary bifurcation PCI techniques: a systematic review and network meta-analysis comprising 5,711 patients. *JACC Cardiovasc Interv*. 2020;13:1432–1444.

Hall AB, Chavez I, Garcia S, et al. Double-kiss-crush bifurcation stenting: Step-by-step troubleshooting. *EuroIntervention*. 2021;17(4):e317–e325. doi: 10.4244/EIJ-D-19-00721.

Zhang JJ, Ye F, Xu K, et al. Multicentre, randomized comparison of two-stent and provisional stenting techniques in patients with complex coronary bifurcation lesions: The DEFINITION II trial. *Eur Heart J*. 2020;41:2523–2536.

Zimarino M, Angiolillo DJ, Dangas G, et al. Antithrombotic therapy after percutaneous coronary intervention of bifurcation lesions. *EuroIntervention*. 2021;17(1):59–66. doi: 10.4244/EIJ-D-20-00885.

Chronic Total Occlusion Interventions

EMMANOUIL S. BRILAKIS • ALLISON BARBARA HALL • M. NICHOLAS BURKE

KEY POINTS

- Percutaneous coronary intervention (PCI) of chronic total occlusions (CTOs) has become safer and more successful with the advent of improved, dedicated equipment and an algorithmic approach.

- The principal indication for CTO PCI is to improve angina and quality of life.

- Terminology, equipment, and techniques specific to CTO PCI have been developed.

- Objective scores have been developed to give the operator insights into the likelihood of success and into potential complications during the planning phase of the procedure.

- Preparedness for treating complications requires specialized equipment; it is essential that the Cath lab staff can quickly locate complication management equipment and that operators are familiar with its use to minimize the impact of a complication.

Disclosures

Dr. Brilakis has received consulting/speaker honoraria from Abbott Vascular, American Heart Association (Associate Editor Circulation), Amgen, Biotronik, Boston Scientific, Cardiovascular Innovations Foundation (Board of Directors), ControlRad, CSI, Ebix, Elsevier, GE Healthcare, InfraRedx, Medtronic, Siemens, and Teleflex; research support from Regeneron and Siemens; owner, Hippocrates LLC; shareholder: MHI Ventures. Dr. Hall has received speaker honoraria from Medtronic, OpSens Medical, and Cardiovascular Innovations Foundation. Dr. Burke has received speaker honoraria from Opsens and is a shareholder of Egg Medical and MHI Ventures.

Chronic total occlusions (CTOs) are completely occluded coronary arteries with thrombolysis in myocardial infarction (TIMI) 0 flow with an estimated duration of at least 3 months. CTO percutaneous coronary intervention (PCI) can be challenging; however, 85% to 90% success rates can currently be achieved at experienced centers around the world. A global consensus was recently reached on the key principles underlying CTO PCI (Table 8.1).

Indications

CTO PCI should be performed when the anticipated benefit is greater than the potential risk (Fig. 8.1). The main benefit of CTO PCI is symptom improvement (i.e., angina and dyspnea in most patients). The more symptomatic the patient, the higher the potential benefit of CTO PCI. CTO PCI can improve exercise capacity, increase anaerobic threshold, and alleviate depression. It continues to be debated whether CTO PCI can improve left ventricular systolic function and reduce the risk of arrhythmias or death.

The risks of CTO PCI can be acute during the perioperative period (such as acute myocardial infarction, perforation, need for

Table 8.1

Key Principles on the Indications and Technique of Chronic Total Occlusion Percutaneous Coronary Intervention

1	The principal indication for CTO PCI is to improve symptoms.
2	Dual coronary angiography and thorough, structured angiographic review should be performed in every case.
3	Use of a microcatheter is essential for guidewire support.
4	There are four CTO crossing strategies: antegrade wire escalation, antegrade dissection/reentry, retrograde wire escalation, and retrograde dissection/reentry.
5	Change of equipment and technique increases the likelihood of success and improves the efficiency of the procedure.
6	Centers and physicians performing CTO PCI should have the necessary equipment, expertise, and experience to optimize success and minimize and manage complications.
7	Every effort should be made to optimize stent deployment in CTO PCI, including the frequent use of intravascular imaging.

CTO, Chronic total occlusion; *PCI*, percutaneous coronary intervention.
Reproduced with permission from Brilakis ES, Mashayekhi K, Tsuchikane E, et al. Guiding principles for chronic total occlusion percutaneous coronary intervention. *Circulation.* 2019;140:420–433.

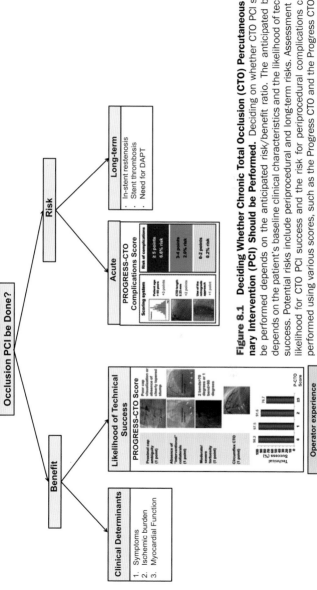

Figure 8.1 Deciding Whether Chronic Total Occlusion (CTO) Percutaneous Coronary Intervention (PCI) Should be Performed. Deciding on whether CTO PCI should be performed depends on the anticipated risk/benefit ratio. The anticipated benefit depends on the patient's baseline clinical characteristics and the likelihood of technical success. Potential risks include periprocedural and long-term risks. Assessment of the likelihood for CTO PCI success and the risk for periprocedural complications can be performed using various scores, such as the Progress CTO and the Progress CTO Complications score. (Reproduced with permission from Brilakis ES. *Manual of Coronary Chronic Total Occlusion Interventions. A Step-By-Step Approach.* 2nd ed. Elsevier; 2017.)

emergency coronary artery bypass graft [CABG] surgery, or death) or chronic (such as restenosis and stent thrombosis).

The optimal coronary revascularization modality in patients with coronary CTOs depends on coronary anatomy and comorbidities, with "best practice" currently involving individualizing patient treatment decisions with discussion between cardiac surgery, cardiology, and interventional cardiology in a Heart Team approach. Some patients with coronary CTOs may be better served with CABG surgery, especially if they have multivessel complex coronary artery disease and they are diabetic. Other patients may be better served by CTO PCI, especially if they have had prior CABG, if they are poor surgical candidates, or if they have single vessel coronary artery disease (Fig. 8.2).

In the 2021 American College of Cardiology (ACC)/American Heart Association (AHA) PCI guidelines, CTO PCI carries a class IIB/level of evidence B recommendation: "In patients with suitable anatomy who have refractory angina on medical therapy, after treatment of non-CTO lesions, the benefit of PCI of a CTO to improve symptoms is uncertain." In the 2018 European Society of Cardiology (ESC)/European Association of Cardiothoracic Surgery (EACS) guidelines on myocardial revascularization, CTO PCI carries a class IIA/level of evidence B recommendation: "Percutaneous recanalization of CTOs should be considered in patients with angina resistant to medical therapy or with large area of documented ischemia in the territory of the occluded vessel.

In summary, at present the main goal of CTO PCI is to improve patient symptoms that are caused by myocardial ischemia (angina, exertional dyspnea, and sometimes fatigue) despite optimal medical therapy. A detailed conversation with patients who are candidates for CTO PCI is critical to ensure full understanding of the potential risks and benefits of the procedure.

Planning for CTO PCI: Dual Angiography Performance and Interpretation

Dual angiography is critical for the success and safety of CTO PCI. It should be done in nearly all cases, except when the collateral circulation is originating exclusively from the CTO vessel. The donor vessel is injected first, followed by injection of the CTO vessel 2 to 3 seconds later using low magnification and avoiding panning that can result in degradation of the image quality. Coronary computed tomography angiography (CCTA) is another imaging technique that can help assess the anatomy of the CTO vessel.

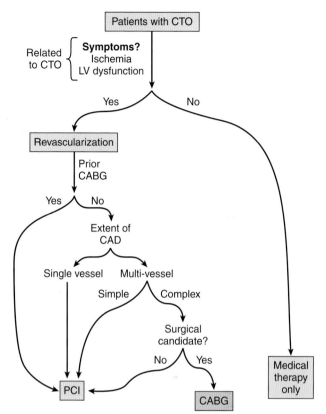

Figure 8.2 Revascularization Options for Patients With Coronary Chronic Total Occlusions (CTOs). Algorithm for determining the need for coronary revascularization in patients with coronary chronic total occlusions. Revascularization is indicated in patients with symptoms, significant ischemia, and left ventricular dysfunction attributable to the CTO(s). Patients with prior coronary bypass graft surgery (CABG) are almost always treated with percutaneous coronary intervention (PCI) given the increased risk of redo CABG. In patients without prior CABG, CTO PCI and CABG surgery are both treatment options, with CABG preferred for patients with multivessel complex disease and PCI (including CTO PCI) preferred for patients with simple multivessel or single vessel disease or patients who are poor candidates for CABG. (Reproduced with permission from Brilakis ES. *Manual of Coronary Chronic Total Occlusion Interventions. A Step-By-Step Approach.* 2nd ed. Elsevier; 2017.)

Angiographic review of the CTO anatomy focuses on the following four characteristics (Fig. 8.3): (1) proximal cap morphology; (2) occlusion length, course, and composition (e.g., calcium); (3) quality of the distal vessel; and (4) collateral circulation. Moreover, non-CTO lesions are reviewed because the presence of additional lesions can help determine the optimal coronary revascularization strategy (PCI vs. CABG), and if PCI is selected, decisions must be made about the sequence in which CTO and non-CTO lesions will be revascularized.

Proximal Cap Morphology

Proximal cap ambiguity is very important for selecting the initial and subsequent CTO crossing strategies because attempting to cross an ambiguous proximal cap could cause a perforation. Additional angiographic projections using dual injection, selective contrast injection through a microcatheter located near the proximal cap, use of intravascular ultrasound (IVUS), and preprocedural or real-time CCTA may help identify the location of the proximal cap. If the location of the proximal cap remains unclear despite additional imaging, a retrograde approach or "move the cap" dissection/reentry techniques can be used as the initial crossing strategy.

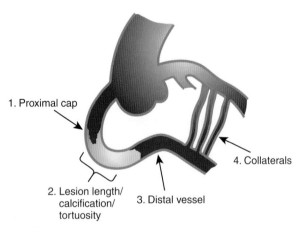

1. Proximal cap
4. Collaterals
2. Lesion length/ calcification/ tortuosity
3. Distal vessel

Figure 8.3 The four key angiographic parameters that need to be assessed to plan chronic total occlusion percutaneous coronary intervention. (Reproduced with permission from Brilakis ES. *Manual of Coronary Chronic Total Occlusion Interventions. A Step-By-Step Approach.* 2nd ed. Elsevier; 2017.)

Lesion Length, Course, and Composition

Antegrade-only injections of the CTO vessel often lead to overestimation of the lesion length because of underfilling and poor opacification of the distal vessel, from competing antegrade and retrograde coronary flow, leaving uncertainty about the location and morphology of the distal cap. Crossing the CTO can be very challenging in the presence of severe calcification and tortuosity of the occluded segment. Using a knuckled (J-shaped) guidewire or using the retrograde approach is often preferred when the vessel course is unclear or highly tortuous because a knuckled guidewire allows advancement within the vessel architecture with low risk of perforation.

Distal Vessel

CTO vessels with small and diffusely diseased distal segments are more challenging to recanalize, especially after subintimal guidewire entry. Sometimes, however, distal vessels may appear small because of hypoperfusion and increase in size after recanalization. Distal vessel calcification may hinder wire reentry into the true lumen in the case of subintimal guidewire position.

Collateral Circulation

Assessing the collateral circulation is critical for determining the feasibility of the retrograde approach. High-quality dual angiography (ideally obtained during breath hold and without panning) with complete opacification of collateral vessels and obtained in optimal angiographic projections can help determine the presence and characteristics of the collateral circulation. Retrograde crossing can be attempted through septal collaterals, epicardial collaterals, or (patent or occluded) bypass grafts. The ability to cross a collateral vessel with a guidewire depends on its size, tortuosity, bifurcations, angle of entry to and exit from the collateral, and distance from the collateral exit to the distal cap. The size of the collaterals is often assessed using the Werner classification (CC0: no continuous connection; CC1: threadlike connection; CC2: side branch-like connection). Sometimes invisible septal collaterals can be crossed with the surfing technique (advancement of a guidewire with simultaneous rotation without angiographic guidance). Previous angiograms should be reviewed for multiple potential collateral pathways because the predominant collateral may change before or during the procedure ("shifting collaterals"). Previously visualized collaterals that disappear at the time of the procedure may still be crossable. Selective contrast tip injections through a microcatheter can help visualize the collateral anatomy. Aortocoronary bypass grafts (both patent and occluded) are often favorable retrograde conduits because of the absence of side branches, predictable course, and large caliber. Septal collaterals are preferred over epicardial collaterals because of lower risk of perforation causing tamponade.

Septal collaterals are typically safer and easier to navigate using very soft tip and polymer-jacketed guidewires compared with epicardial collaterals. In contrast to epicardial collaterals, septal collaterals can be safely dilated with small balloons to facilitate microcatheter or device crossing.

CTO Scores

Several scores that include angiographic and clinical characteristics have been developed to estimate the difficulty of CTO PCI and the likelihood of success and complications. The oldest and most commonly used score is the J-CTO (Multicenter CTO Registry of Japan) score, developed to estimate the likelihood of successful antegrade guidewire crossing within 30 minutes based on 5 criteria (at least 1 bend of > 45 degrees in the CTO entry or CTO body, occlusion length > 20 mm, calcification, blunt proximal stump, and previously failed attempt; Fig. 8.4). Other scores include the PROGRESS-CTO score (Fig. 8.5), the RECHARGE (REgistry of Crossboss and Hybrid Procedures in FrAnce, the NetheRlands, BelGium and UnitEd Kingdom) registry score, the CL-score (Clinical and Lesion-related score), and the CASTLE (CABG history, Age ≥ 70 yrs, Stump anatomy [blunt or invisible], Tortuosity degree [severe or unseen], Length of occlusion ≥ 20 mm, and Extent of calcification [severe]) score. There are also CCTA-based scores, such as the CT-RECTOR multicenter registry (Computed Tomography Registry of Chronic Total Occlusion Revascularization) score and the Korean Multicenter CTO CT Registry Score.

The risk of CTO PCI complications can be assessed using the Progress-CTO complications score, which uses three variables (age ≥ 65 years, lesion length > 23 mm, and use of the retrograde approach) to stratify patients according to periprocedural complication risk (Fig. 8.6).

An online calculator for multiple scores is located at: https://www.ctomanual.org/cto-scores. CTO score calculation requires detailed review of the angiogram and can facilitate decision making. For example, medical therapy may be preferred over CTO PCI in mildly symptomatic patients with highly complex occlusions. Complex CTOs (e.g., those with J-CTO score ≥ 2) are more likely to require dissection reentry and retrograde-crossing techniques and should be performed by experienced operators.

J-CTO Score

494 native CTO lesions Crossing within 30 minutes

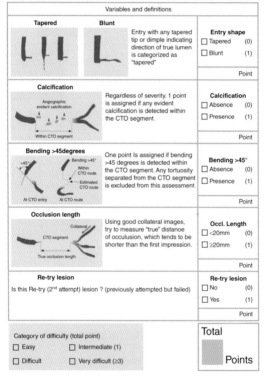

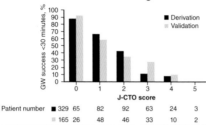

Figure 8.4 The J-CTO (Multicenter Chronic Total Occlusion Registry in Japan) Score. Description of the components of the J-CTO score, which was developed to predict the likelihood of successful guidewire crossing of the occlusion within 30 minutes. (Reproduced with permission from Morino Y, Abe M, Morimoto T, et al. Predicting successful guidewire crossing through chronic total occlusion of native coronary lesions within 30 minutes: the J-CTO score as a difficulty grading and time assessment tool. *JACC Cardiovasc Interv.* 2011;4:213–221.)

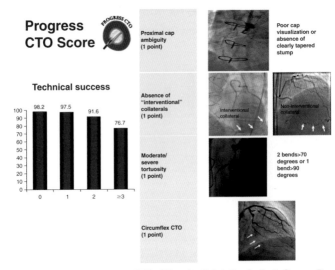

Figure 8.5 The Progress-CTO (Chronic Total Occlusion) Score. Description of the components of the Progress-CTO score, which was developed to predict technical success of CTO percutaneous coronary intervention (PCI). (Reproduced with permission from Christopoulos G, Kandzari DE, Yeh RW, et al. Development and validation of a novel scoring system for predicting technical success of chronic total occlusion percutaneous coronary interventions: The PROGRESS CTO [Prospective Global Registry for the Study of Chronic Total Occlusion Intervention] Score. *JACC Cardiovasc Interv.* 2016; 9:1–9.)

CTO Crossing

Advancing a guidewire through the occlusion is often the most challenging step of CTO PCI. A microcatheter should be routinely used for supporting the guidewire and facilitating guidewire exchanges and tip reshaping. Microcatheters improve the precision of guidewire advancement and can alter the penetration force of the wire (guidewires become more penetrating when a microcatheter is advanced close to the guidewire tip). Microcatheters can help cross retrograde collateral channels and also protect them from wire-induced trauma. Similar to guidewires, microcatheter selection depends on the CTO characteristics, availability, and expertise. Strong guide catheter support (e.g., by using large guide catheters or guide catheter extensions) can also facilitate CTO crossing.

There are four CTO crossing techniques, classified according to wiring direction (antegrade and retrograde) and whether or not the subintimal space is used (wiring vs. dissection and reentry; Fig. 8.7).

Progress CTO complications score

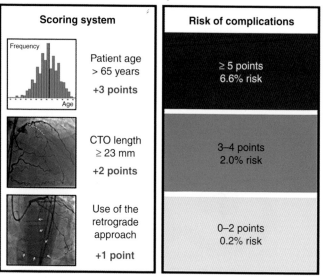

Scoring system		Risk of complications
Frequency / *Age*	Patient age > 65 years +3 points	≥ 5 points 6.6% risk
	CTO length ≥ 23 mm +2 points	3–4 points 2.0% risk
	Use of the retrograde approach +1 point	0–2 points 0.2% risk

Figure 8.6 The Progress-CTO (Chronic Total Occlusion) Complications Score. Description of the components of the Progress-CTO Complications score, which was developed to predict periprocedural complications during CTO percutaneous coronary intervention (PCI). Periprocedural complications included any of the following adverse events before hospital discharge: death, myocardial infarction, recurrent symptoms requiring urgent repeat target vessel revascularization with PCI or coronary artery bypass graft (CABG), tamponade requiring either pericardiocentesis or surgery, and stroke. (Reproduced with permission from Danek BA, Karatasakis A, Karmpaliotis D, et al. Development and validation of a scoring system for predicting periprocedural complications during percutaneous coronary interventions of chronic total occlusions: The Prospective Global Registry for the Study of Chronic Total Occlusion Intervention (PROGRESS CTO) Complications Score. *J Am Heart Assoc.* 2016;5.)

Antegrade Wiring

Antegrade wiring (guidewire advancement in the original direction of blood flow) is the most commonly used CTO crossing technique. The initial and subsequent guidewire selection depends on CTO lesion characteristics. Polymer-jacketed, low-penetration-force, tapered guidewires are usually used initially for CTOs with a tapered proximal cap, with subsequent escalation to intermediate and high-penetration-force guidewires as required. Intermediate-penetration-force polymer-jacketed guidewire, or composite core guidewires are

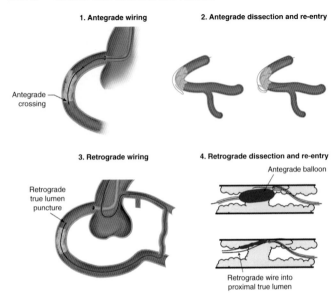

1. Antegrade wiring

Antegrade crossing

2. Antegrade dissection and re-entry

3. Retrograde wiring

Retrograde true lumen puncture

4. Retrograde dissection and re-entry

Antegrade balloon

Retrograde wire into proximal true lumen

Figure 8.7 Illustration of the chronic total occlusion crossing techniques. (Reproduced with permission from Brilakis ES. *Manual of Coronary Chronic Total Occlusion Interventions. A Step-By-Step Approach.* 2nd ed. Elsevier; 2017.)

often used in CTOs with a blunt proximal cap. Stiff, high-penetration-force guidewires are often needed in highly resistant proximal caps or to cross areas of resistance within the occlusion. After crossing the areas of resistance, these guidewires should be changed to less penetrating guidewires (de-escalation) to navigate through the CTO segment.

Contralateral injection and orthogonal angiographic projections help determine guidewire position during crossing attempts. If the guidewire enters into the distal true lumen, the microcatheter is advanced into the distal true lumen and the CTO crossing guidewire is exchanged for a workhorse guidewire through the microcatheter to minimize the risk of distal vessel injury and perforation during balloon angioplasty and stenting. If the guidewire exits the vessel architecture, it should be withdrawn and redirected without advancing other equipment over it. If the guidewire enters the subintimal space, it can be redirected or left in place to serve as a marker guiding advancement of a second guidewire

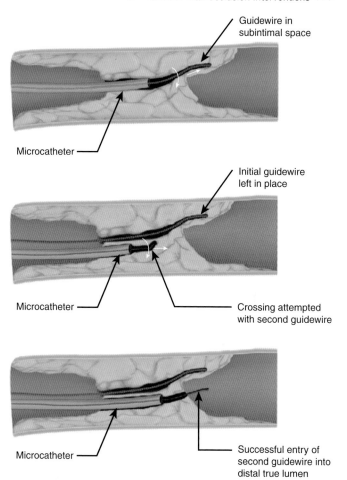

Figure 8.8 Illustration of the parallel wire technique. (Reproduced with permission from Brilakis ES. *Manual of Coronary Chronic Total Occlusion Interventions. A Step-By-Step Approach.* 2nd ed. Elsevier; 2017.)

into the distal true lumen (parallel wire technique; Fig. 8.8). Another option is to use antegrade dissection/reentry techniques to reenter into the distal true lumen. Subintimal guidewires should not be advanced distal to the distal cap to prevent hematoma formation that can cause luminal compression and hinder guide-wire crossing.

Antegrade Dissection and Reentry

As the name implies, in antegrade dissection and reentry, a guidewire is advanced in the subintimal space, followed by subintimal crossing of the CTO and reentry into the distal true lumen. Antegrade dissection and reentry can be performed intentionally or after subintimal guidewire entry during antegrade wiring attempts.

The STAR (Subintimal Tracking And Reentry) technique was the first dissection/reentry technique; it uses nontargeted reentry into the distal lumen by pushing a knuckled wire distally through the occluded segment until it spontaneously reenters the true lumen at any location, sometimes quite distally. This often requires stenting long coronary segments and is associated with high rates of in-stent restenosis (ISR) and reocclusion. The STAR technique is currently only used for bailout without stent implantation in preparation for a repeat CTO PCI attempt (subintimal plaque modification or "investment" procedure).

Limited dissection/reentry techniques are preferred because they minimize the extent of dissection by facilitating reentry immediately distal to the distal cap, usually using a dedicated reentry device, such as the Stingray balloon. Limited antegrade dissection/reentry techniques minimize vascular injury, limit the length of dissection and subsequent stent length, and increase the likelihood of side branch preservation with favorable clinical outcomes.

The Retrograde Approach

In the retrograde approach, the guidewire is advanced against the original direction of blood flow. A guidewire is advanced into the artery distal to the occlusion through a collateral channel or a bypass graft, followed by placement of a microcatheter at the distal CTO cap. Retrograde CTO crossing is then attempted either with retrograde wiring (usually for short occlusions, especially when the distal cap is tapered) or with retrograde dissection/reentry techniques. The 10 steps of the retrograde approach are shown in Fig. 8.9.

The most commonly used retrograde crossing technique is reverse controlled antegrade and retrograde tracking (reverse CART), in which a balloon is inflated over the antegrade guidewire, followed by retrograde guidewire advancement into the space created by the antegrade balloon (see Fig. 8.7). In challenging reverse CART cases, use of intravascular ultrasound or guide catheter extensions can facilitate guidewire crossing.

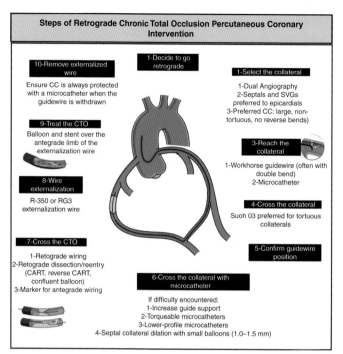

Steps of Retrograde Chronic Total Occlusion Percutaneous Coronary Intervention

10-Remove externalized wire
Ensure CC is always protected with a microcatheter when the guidewire is withdrawn

9-Treat the CTO
Balloon and stent over the antegrade limb of the externalization wire

8-Wire externalization
R-350 or RG3 externalization wire

7-Cross the CTO
1-Retrograde wiring
2-Retrograde dissection/reentry (CART, reverse CART, confluent balloon)
3-Marker for antegrade wiring

1-Decide to go retrograde

1-Select the collateral
1-Dual Angiography
2-Septals and SVGs preferred to epicardials
3-Preferred CC: large, non-tortuous, no reverse bends)

3-Reach the collateral
1-Workhorse guidewire (often with double bend)
2-Microcatheter

4-Cross the collateral
Suoh 03 preferred for tortuous collaterals

5-Confirm guidewire position

6-Cross the collateral with microcatheter
If difficulty encountered:
1-Increase guide support
2-Torqueable microcatheters
3-Lower-profile microcatheters
4-Septal collateral dilation with small balloons (1.0–1.5 mm)

Figure 8.9 The 10 Steps of Retrograde Chronic Total Occlusion (CTO) Percutaneous Coronary Intervention. *CART,* Controlled antegrade and retrograde tracking; *CC,* collateral channel; *SVG,* saphenous vein graft. (Reproduced with permission from Megaly M, Xenogiannis I, Abi Rafeh N, et al. Retrograde approach to chronic total occlusion percutaneous coronary intervention. *Circ Cardiovasc Interv.* 2020;13:e008900.)

Crossing Strategy Selection

Selecting the initial and subsequent crossing strategies depends on the CTO lesion characteristics and local equipment availability and expertise.

Several algorithms have been developed to facilitate crossing strategy selection, such as the hybrid (Fig. 8.10), Asia Pacific, and Euro-CTO algorithms. Antegrade crossing is preferred over retrograde crossing as the initial crossing strategy in all algorithms because the retrograde approach carries a higher risk of complications and antegrade lesion preparation is needed even when the retrograde approach is eventually required. Some retrograde CTO

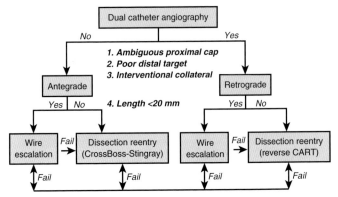

Figure 8.10 The "hybrid" chronic total occlusion (CTO) crossing algorithm. (Reproduced with permission from Brilakis ES, Grantham JA, Rinfret S, et al. A percutaneous treatment algorithm for crossing coronary chronic total occlusions. *JACC Cardiovasc Interv.* 2012;5:367–379.)

PCI complications are caused by antegrade crossing attempts. The retrograde approach has significantly increased the success rates of CTO PCI, especially in more complex CTOs, but needs to be performed by experienced operators to minimize the occurrence of complications and to facilitate their treatment should they occur.

A primary retrograde approach is sometimes needed (e.g., in CTOs with proximal cap ambiguity that cannot be resolved using other techniques or in flush aorto-ostial CTOs).

Change of Crossing Strategy

In many cases, the initially selected crossing strategy fails to cross the CTO. Changes in procedural strategy, minor or significant, are constantly required to increase the likelihood of success. Examples of small changes are reshaping the guidewire tip or changing the guidewire or microcatheter. Example of bigger changes are changing from antegrade wiring to antegrade dissection/reentry or to retrograde crossing.

When and how to change crossing strategy depends on the operator's experience, preprocedural planning, the risk of the alternative strategies, and the progress of the procedure. More experienced operators are usually faster at implementing changes. Persisting with strategies that are failing to achieve progress increases contrast and radiation dose and reduces the likelihood of success.

When to Stop

CTO PCI should be stopped in most cases if there is a complication, a high radiation dose (usually >5 Gray air kerma dose in the absence of lesion crossing or substantial progress), high contrast volume (>3.7 times the estimated creatinine clearance or lower depending the patient's baseline renal function), exhaustion of crossing options, or patient or physician fatigue. Failing may be better than pursuing highly aggressive strategies that may lead to serious complications.

Optimization of Stent Deployment

Stent optimization is critical for optimizing the short-term (such as stent thrombosis) and long-term (such as ISR) outcomes of CTO PCI because implantation of multiple stents in heavily calcified, diffusely diseased, and negatively remodeled vessels is often needed. The CTO lesions should be fully expanded before stent implantation by predilation with properly sized balloons or with use of plaque modification strategies such as atherectomy. Intravascular imaging is critical for assessing vessel size and calcification before stenting and ensuring optimal stent expansion, apposition, and lesion coverage. CTO vessels often have diffuse disease and negative remodeling distal to the CTO: stenting the distal segments is usually avoided because it often enlarges over time after restoring vessel patency.

Preventing and Treating Complications

CTO PCI is associated with a higher risk of complications (Fig. 8.11) compared with PCI of non-CTO lesions. The average complication risk is approximately 3% but varies widely between studies and is higher in more complex lesions. Some complications are unique to CTO PCI, such as perforation of septal and epicardial collaterals or donor vessel dissection when dual injection is being used. Insertion of a "safety" guidewire in the CTO donor vessel can facilitate treatment if donor vessel injury occurs. To minimize the risk of donor vessel thrombosis, the goal activated clotting time (ACT) is at least 300 seconds for antegrade cases and at least 350 seconds for retrograde cases with frequent checks (at least every 30 minutes) during the procedure.

CTO PCI is associated with an increased risk of perforation: use of dual injection and orthogonal projections to assess equipment

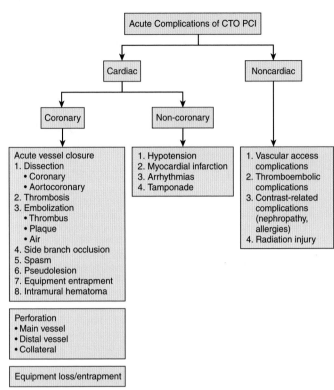

Figure 8.11 Complications of chronic total occlusion (CTO) percutaneous coronary intervention (PCI). (Reproduced with permission from Brilakis ES. *Manual of Percutaneous Coronary Intervention: a step-by-step approach.* Elsevier; 2020.)

position during all stages of the procedure can help reduce this risk. Large vessel perforations are usually treated with covered stents, whereas distal vessel and collateral vessel perforation usually require embolization (embolization should be performed from both directions in epicardial collateral perforations). Availability and experience in using covered stents and coils are essential for CTO PCI programs. Coronary perforation in prior CABG patients may carry an increased risk because it can lead to life-threatening and difficult to access loculated hematomas or bleeding in the mediastinum or pleural cavities.

CTO PCI may require a high radiation dose, potentially leading to radiation skin injury. Minimizing radiation dose can be achieved by low-frame-rate fluoroscopy and the "fluoroscopy store" function for documenting balloon and stent inflation instead of cine-angiography, using collimation, minimizing the distance of the image receptor from the patient, and changing the position of the image receptor during the procedure. Patients who receive high radiation dose (>5 Gray air kerma dose) should be followed up to evaluate for subacute skin injury. Contrast administration should also be minimized and carefully tracked during the procedure to reduce the risk for contrast nephropathy.

Key References

Brilakis ES. *Manual of Coronary Chronic Total Occlusion Interventions. A Step-By-Step Approach.* 2nd ed. Elsevier; 2017. www.ctomanual.org.

Brilakis ES. *Manual of Percutaneous Coronary Intervention: A Step-by-Step Approach.* Elsevier; 2020. www.pcimanual.org.

Brilakis ES, Mashayekhi K, Tsuchikane E, et al. Guiding principles for chronic total occlusion percutaneous coronary intervention. *Circulation.* 2019;140:420-433.

Jang Y. *Perctuaneous Coronary Intervention for Chronic Total Occlusion: A Guide to Success.* Spinger; 2019.

Rinfret S, ed. *Percutaneous Intervention for Coronary Chronic Occlusion: The Hybrid Approach.* Springer; 2016.

Spratt JC, ed. *A Guide to Mastering Antegrade CTO PCI.* Optima Education Ltd; 2019. Online: www.ctoibooks.com.

Spratt JC, ed. *A Guide to Mastering Retrograde CTO PCI.* Optima Education Ltd; 2015. Online: www.ctoibooks.com.

PCI in STEMI, NSTEMI, and Shock

MIR BABAR BASIR • ALEJANDRO LEMOR

KEY POINTS

- Acute myocardial infarction (AMI) is best treated with timely revascularization using percutaneous coronary intervention (PCI).

- ST-segment elevation myocardial infarction (STEMI) systems of care are crucial in allowing patients with AMI to have the opportunity for timely care at a PCI-capable center.

- A focused history and electrocardiogram (ECG) interpretation are of great importance to rapidly diagnose STEMI and initiate activation of the cardiac catheterization laboratory.

- Nonculprit PCI with the goal of providing complete revascularization should be the goal in the majority of patients. In STEMI without cardiogenic shock, this can occur carefully in the index procedure or in a staged fashion, taking into account patient hemodynamics. In cardiogenic shock, this should occur in a staged fashion.

- AMI complicated by cardiogenic shock is a deadly condition associated with significant morbidity and mortality.

- Technological advancements will lead to continued development of more mobile, smaller-caliber, and more

Disclosures

MBB is a consultant for Abbott Vascular, Abiomed, Cardiovascular Systems Inc, Chiesi and Zoll. AL reports no conflicts to disclose.

powerful mechanical circulatory support devices. Understanding the mechanism of action and physiologic effects of these devices is important.

- Mechanical circulatory support devices are increasingly used to support and prevent hemodynamic collapse. Intra-aortic balloon pumps (IABPs) have been found to have limited utility in AMI with cardiogenic shock (AMI-CS), whereas more robust support devices, including venoarterial extracorporeal membrane oxygenation (VA-ECMO) and Impella, are currently enrolling in large scale randomized control trials to elicit their use in AMI-CS.

- Although these large-scale studies are being conducted, the use of shock protocols and teams has been associated with improved outcomes in AMI-CS.

Incidence

Approximately 1 million Americans have an acute myocardial infarction (AMI) every year, corresponding to one AMI every 40 seconds. An ST-elevation myocardial infarction (STEMI) should be considered in patients who present with ischemic symptoms (angina, chest pressure/pain, heartburn, nausea, indigestion, diaphoresis, shortness of breath) and corresponding electrocardiographic (ECG) ST-elevation (Table 9.1). Prompt recognition of STEMI is crucial to activate the cardiac catheterization laboratory and provide percutaneous coronary intervention (PCI). ECGs also serve as an important tool to localize injury (Fig. 9.1).

Non-STEMI (NSTEMI) are typically diagnosed in the presence of ischemic symptoms and elevated biomarkers. Ischemic changes on ECG can still be present (Fig. 9.2). High-risk features that should prompt early consideration for revascularization in NSTEMI include ongoing ischemic symptoms despite medical therapy, cardiogenic shock, arrhythmia, or a Global Registry of Acute Coronary Events (GRACE) risk score greater than 140.

Hospital mortality after AMI has steadily decreased and is currently less than 5%, with most patients now being discharged home within 1 to 3 days. This is largely driven by the ability to provide rapid early revascularization through PCI using current STEMI systems of care.

Table 9.1

ECG Criteria for STEMI				
STEMI Anatomic Location	ECG Leads with ST Elevation	Males <40 years	Males ≥40 years	Females (all Ages)
Anterior	V2–V4	V2, V3 > 2.5 mm, V4 > 1 mm	V2, V3 > 2 mm V4 > 1 mm	V2, V3 > 1.5 mm, V4 > 1 mm
Septal	V1–V2	V1 > 1 mm V2 > 2.5 mm	V1 > 1 mm V2 > 2 mm	V1 > 1mm V2 > 1.5 mm
Inferior	II, III, aVF	> 1 mm	> 1 mm	> 1 mm
Lateral	I, aVL, V5–V6	> 1 mm	> 1 mm	> 1 mm

ECG, Electrocardiogram; *STEMI*, ST-segment elevation myocardial infarction.

Pathophysiology

The pathophysiology of an AMI is outlined in Fig. 9.3. Plaque deposition leads to progressive atherosclerosis. Plaque rupture can result in thrombosis and decreased blood flow, leading to myocardial ischemia and necrosis. This injury can be measured by biomarkers, such as troponin. AMI can result in diastolic dysfunction and an increase in left ventricular (LV) end-diastolic pressure. If not promptly treated, AMI can progress to systolic dysfunction and decreasing stroke volume, which can lead to cardiogenic shock (CS) and death.

Revascularization

Methods of revascularization in patients suffering from AMI have evolved from thrombolytic therapy to mechanical revascularization using coronary artery bypass grafting (CABG) or PCI. Thrombolytics can achieve infarct artery patency in approximately 50% to 70% of patients presenting with an AMI within 90 minutes. Primary percutaneous balloon angioplasty and stenting, however, restores TIMI (thrombolysis in myocardial infarction) grade 3 coronary blood flow in over 95% of patients. Thrombolytic therapy has also been associated with complications, such as bleeding and stroke. PCI is thus the standard mode of revascularization in patients presenting with AMI, with a goal of reducing infarct size, preserving LV function, and improving survival.

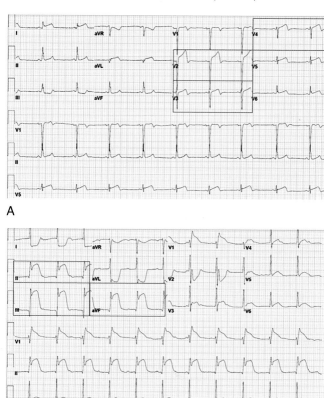

A

B

Figure 9.1 (A) Anterior ST-segment elevation myocardial infarction (STEMI) with ST elevation in leads V1 to V4. (B) Inferior STEMI with ST elevation in leads II, III, and aVF. *Continued*

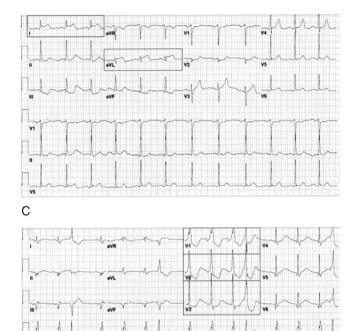

C

D

Figure 9.1, cont'd (C) Lateral STEMI with ST elevation in leads I, aVL, V5, and V6. (D) Posterior STEMI with ST depression in leads V1 to V3.

STEMI Systems of Care

To facilitate timely revascularization, an enormous infrastructure has been developed over the past three decades to provide rapid access to the cardiac catheterization laboratory for patients presenting with AMI. The creation of this STEMI system-of-care has allowed more than 80% of Americans access to the cardiac catheterization laboratory for PCI. For those patients who cannot be transferred to a PCI-capable center within 120 minutes, thrombolytics remain a therapeutic option (Fig. 9.4).

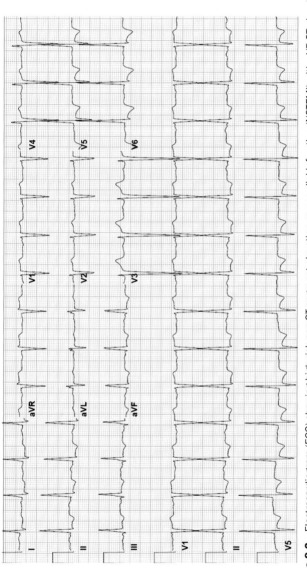

Figure 9.2 Electrocardiogram (ECG) showing high-risk non-ST segment elevation myocardial infarction (NSTEMI) with aVR ST elevation and diffuse ST depression and T-wave inversions.

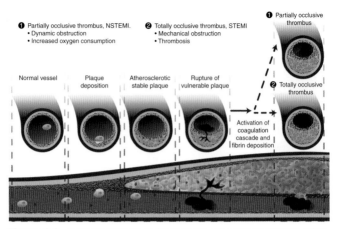

Figure 9.3 Pathophysiology of ST-segment elevation myocardial infarction (STEMI) and non-STEMI (NSTEMI).

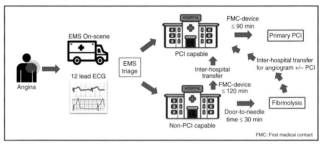

Figure 9.4 Emergency Medical Services (EMS) and ST-segment elevation myocardial infarction (STEMI) system of care.

The COVID-19 pandemic has highlighted vulnerabilities in providing such services at certain unforeseen times. Modified actions plans should be in place for the rare event in which either Emergency Medical Services (EMS) or cardiac catheterization laboratory personnel cannot provide such services.

STEMI Mimickers

The importance of a detailed history cannot be overemphasized because STEMI mimickers are frequently identified (Table 9.2).

These can include the presence of hyperkalemia or left bundle branch blocks and diseases such as LV aneurysm, Brugada syndrome, pericarditis, and pulmonary embolism.

Complications of Acute Myocardial Infarction

When timely reperfusion is not provided because of delays in presentation, unrecognized AMI, untimely revascularization, or complicated revascularization, mechanical complications of AMI can occur. Common complications of AMI are listed in Table 9.3. In the era of primary PCI, the incidence of mechanical complications is 0.3% in patients presenting with STEMI compared with 6.2% of patients in the thrombolytic era. Mechanical complications are more common in STEMI than NSTEMI and are seen more commonly in patients who are older, female, or presenting with their first AMI.

Pharmacotherapy

Dosing for antiplatelet therapy (Table 9.4A), anticoagulation (see Table 9.4B), and important post-PCI medications (Fig. 9.5) are listed. Potent oral antiplatelet therapies have been shown to be superior to clopidogrel in AMI. It is important to consider intravenous (IV) antiplatelet therapies, particularly when PCI is performed using a radial approach, because patients with AMI have significant risk factors for poor absorption of oral medications, including the use of opioids, the presence of nausea and vomiting, mechanical ventilation, and cardiac arrest. Interventional pharmacology is discussed in more detail in Chapter 3.

Reperfusion Injury

Primary PCI and the resumption of blood flow to a myocardial bed can induce myocardial injury and cell death in a process termed *ischemic reperfusion injury.* Reperfusion injury results in a neurohumoral cascade from oxidative free radicals, leading to myocardial injury. It is suspected that reperfusion injury is one of the main factors of post-AMI scar and can also result in arrhythmias and no-reflow.

No-Reflow

No-reflow, or lack of antegrade perfusion despite a patent artery, can occur commonly in patients who present with AMI. This

Table 9.2

Pathologies With Similar ECG as STEMI

Pathology	ECG Characteristics	ECG Example
Hyperkalemia	Symmetric, narrow, peaked T waves without ST elevation	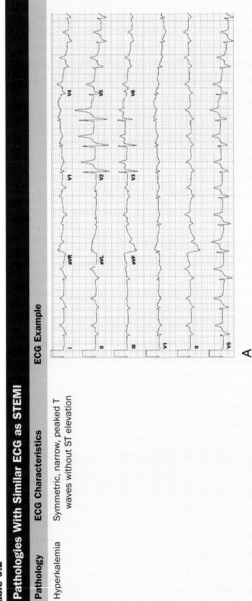

A

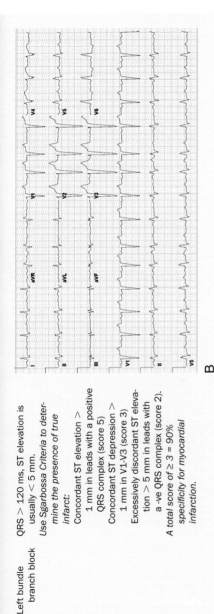

Left bundle branch block	QRS > 120 ms, ST elevation is usually < 5 mm. Use *Sgarbossa Criteria* to determine the presence of true infarct: Concordant ST elevation > 1 mm in leads with a positive QRS complex (score 5) Concordant ST depression > 1 mm in V1-V3 (score 3) Excessively discordant ST elevation > 5 mm in leads with a -ve QRS complex (score 2). A total score of ≥ 3 = 90% specificity for myocardial infarction.

B

Continued on following page

Table 9.2

Pathologies with Similar ECG as STEM (Continued)

Pathology	ECG Characteristics	ECG Example
Left ventricular aneurysm	Persistent ST elevations after a myocardial infarction, associated with Q waves in the location of the infarct	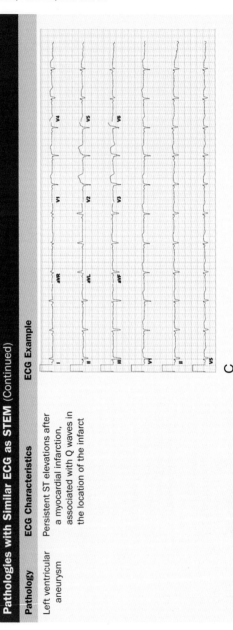

C

Brugada syndrome Na+ channel mutation. Type 1 and 2 will have ST elevation in V1–V3.

Continued on following page

Table 9.2

Pathologies with Similar ECG as STEM (Continued)

Pathology	ECG Characteristics	ECG Example
Acute pericarditis	Diffuse ST elevations along with PR depression. Reciprocal changes are not present.	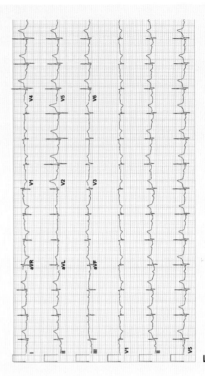

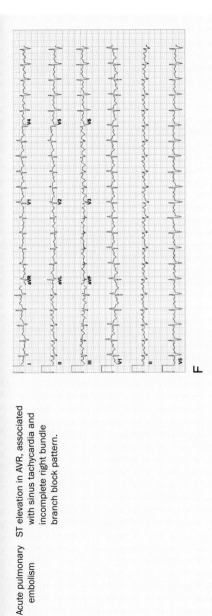

Acute pulmonary embolism ST elevation in AVR, associated with sinus tachycardia and incomplete right bundle branch block pattern.

ECG, Electrocardiogram; *STEMI,* ST-segment elevation myocardial infarction.

Table 9.3

Complications After a STEMI

	Time of onset	Presentation	Management	Mortality
Mechanical Complications				
Papillary muscle rupture and acute mitral regurgitation	Within 7 days post-MI	Acute pulmonary edema, cardiogenic shock	Urgent surgery, inotropes, ECMO, diuretics	10%–30%
Ventricular septal rupture	Within 7 days post-MI	Chest pain, acute heart failure	Urgent surgery, inotropes, ECMO, diuretics	50%–90%
Free wall rupture	Within 7 days post-MI	Cardiogenic shock, tamponade, cardiac arrest	Urgent surgery, pericardiocentesis, ECMO	50%–90%
Nonmechanical Complications				
Pericarditis (Dressler syndrome)	10–14 days	Chest pain, persistent ST elevation, fever, friction rub on exam	Aspirin 650 mg TID	Low
Ventricular arrhythmias	0–48 hours	Palpitations, syncope	Beta-blocker, ICD placement	Low
Cardiogenic shock	0–24 hours	Hypotension, altered mental status, acute respiratory failure	Right heart catheterization, mechanical circulatory support, inotropes	50%

ECMO, Extracorporeal membrane oxygenation; *ICD,* implantable cardioverter-defibrillator; *MI,* myocardial infarction; *STEMI,* ST-segment elevation myocardial infarction; *TID,* thrice daily.

Table 9.4A

Antiplatelets Therapies in Acute Coronary Syndrome

Antiplatelets	Target	Loading Dose	Maintenance Dose	Onset of action	Offset of action
Aspirin	COX-1	150–325 mg PO	81–100 mg daily	60 min	7–10 days
Clopidogrel	P2Y12 receptor (I)	600 mg PO	75 mg daily	2 hours	7–10 days
Ticagrelor	P2Y12 receptor (R)	180 mg PO	90 mg twice a day	30 min	3–5 days
Prasugrel	P2Y12 receptor (I)	60 mg PO	10 mg daily	30 min	7–10 days
Cangrelor	P2Y12 receptor (R)	30 mcg/kg IV	Infusion rate: 4 mcg/kg/min IV	2 min	1 hour
Abciximab	GP IIb/IIIa receptor (I)	0.25 mg/kg IV	0.125 µg/kg/min IV for 12 hours	10 min	48–72 hours
Eptifibatide	GP IIb/IIIa receptor (R)	180 µg/kg IV	2 µg/kg/min for 18–24 hours	5–60 min	4 hours
Tirofiban	GP IIb/IIIa receptor (R)	0.4 µg/kg IV bolus	0.1µg/kg/min for 18–24 hours	10 min	4 hours

(I), Irreversible blockade; IV, intravenous; PO, oral; (R), Reversible blockade.

Table 9.4B

Anticoagulation Therapies in Acute Coronary Syndrome

Anticoagulation	Target	Half-life	Monitoring	Use if GFR < 30
Unfractionated heparin	Factor Xa and IIa (thrombin)	1 hour	Anti Xa level, PTT	Yes
Low-molecular-weight heparin	Factor Xa and IIa (thrombin)	3–6 hours	Anti-Xa level 4 hrs post dose	Contraindicated
Bivalirudin	Direct thrombin inhibitor	25 minutes	PTT	Yes (needs dose reduction)
Fondaparinox	Factor Xa	17–21 hours	Anti-Xa level 4 hrs post dose	Contraindicated

GFR, Glomerular filtration rate.

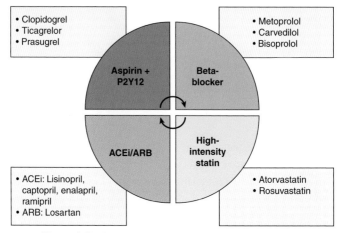

Figure 9.5 Routine therapies in acute coronary syndrome.

has been attributed to secondary distal embolization, endothelial injury, and microvascular obstruction after an AMI. High-risk features for the occurrence of no-reflow include those who present with delays to revascularization, those with organized and highly thrombotic lesions, and patients who do not achieve adequate anticoagulation and platelet inhibition. No-reflow also increases the risk for mechanical complications, larger myocardial infarct sizes, and mortality. Therapeutic options include the use of vasodilators or intracoronary epinephrine. These agents are ideally used before aggressive PCI to limit the risk of no reflow.

Nonculprit Percutaneous Coronary Intervention

Nonculprit lesions are commonly found when treating patients with AMI. In patients who present with AMI without cardiogenic shock, complete revascularization leads to decreased rates of cardiac death, myocardial infarction (MI), and ischemic driven revascularization. It is important to point out that revascularization can occur in the index procedure or in a staged manner after the index procedure.

In patients who present in cardiogenic shock, however, culprit-only PCI during the index procedure leads to better outcomes. The difference between those who present in shock and those who present without shock are important. In cardiogenic shock, the heart is failing and under tremendous physiologic stress. PCI results in temporary cessation of blood flow and microembolization, which can worsen myocardial function. In cardiogenic shock, therefore, every additional PCI may lead to worsening LV function and risk worsening hemodynamic collapse, particularly when performed without mechanical circulatory support (MCS). Careful consideration of nonculprit PCI in cardiogenic shock should therefore occur when considering such scenarios and may be better tolerated in patients with the use of MCS devices (Fig. 9.6).

NSTEMI

PCI is commonly performed in patients presenting with NSTEMI and accounts for a large percentage of the annual volume in most catheterization labs in the United States. These patients can suffer from plaque rupture and subsequent thrombus generation without complete occlusion of the culprit coronary vessel and are typically treated with anticoagulation before arrival to the lab. Anticoagulation should be driven by institutional protocols favoring the use of either IV unfractionated heparin or subcutaneous (SC) enoxaparin. Aspirin pretreatment also remains ubiquitous in all patients with NSTEMI, but there remains large variation in preloading a second antiplatelet agent before

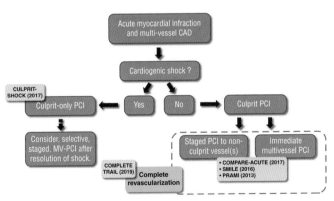

Figure 9.6 Nonculprit percutaneous coronary intervention (PCI) in ST-segment elevation myocardial infarction (STEMI) and in cardiogenic shock.

catheterization (i.e., defining the coronary anatomy). Table 9.5 highlights the critical considerations when performing PCI in a patient with NSTEMI compared with patients with stable ischemic heart disease.

Cardiogenic Shock

Definition

CS is a low-output state that frequently leads to significant end-organ hypoperfusion. CS has been classically defined as a systolic blood pressure less than or equal to 90 mm Hg for at least 30 minutes or the need for vasopressors or MCS to maintain a systolic blood pressure of at least 90 mm Hg. Definitions of CS typically include the presence of end-organ hypoperfusion, which can be variably defined as the presence of decreasing urine output, altered mental status, or an elevated serum lactate (>2.0 mmol/L). CS can also be defined using hemodynamic parameters, such as the presence of a cardiac index less than or equal to 2.2 L/min/m², cardiac power output of less than 0.6 W in the setting of a pulmonary capillary wedge pressure of at least 15 mm Hg. Although this definition does not fully address the spectrum of shock severity, nor does it take into account the etiology of shock, it does serve as a starting point for identifying these high-risk patients.

A consensus statement on the classification of CS was put forth by the Society for Coronary Angiography and Intervention (SCAI). These shock stages stratify patients according to biochemical markers, clinical findings, and hemodynamics into five categories: A "At Risk," B "Beginning," C "Classic," D "Deteriorating," or E "Extremis." Validation of the SCAI classification of CS has shown it to be a reproducible predictor of in-hospital mortality among similar CS phenotypes (Fig. 9.7).

Incidence, Mortality, and Pathophysiology

CS occurs in 5% to 10% of patients presenting with AMI. Patients presenting with AMI-CS who do not receive invasive therapies have less than 20% survival. With early revascularization, the risk of mortality in STEMI without shock in less than 2%; however, in those who present with shock, mortality is approximately 50% (Fig. 9.8). Independent predictors of mortality in AMI-CS include advanced age; Killip class IV symptoms on admission; low systolic blood pressure on admission; and presentation with STEMI, peripheral arterial disease, and/or stroke.

The most common etiology of AMI-CS is LV failure, although there is significant heterogeneity within this shock phenotype:

Table 9.5

Issues and Considerations for PCI in Patients With NSTEMI

Issue	Recommendations	Supportive Evidence
Timing of catheterization	An urgent/immediate invasive strategy (diagnostic angiography with intent to perform revascularization if appropriate based on coronary anatomy) is indicated in patients (men and women) with NSTE-ACS who have refractory angina or hemodynamic or electrical instability (without serious comorbidities or contraindications to such procedures).	ACC/AHA 2014 Guidelines, Class I (A)
	An early invasive strategy (diagnostic angiography with intent to perform revascularization if appropriate based on coronary anatomy) is indicated in initially stabilized patients with NSTE-ACS (without serious comorbidities or contraindications to such procedures) who have an elevated risk for clinical events.	ACC/AHA 2014 Guidelines, Class I (B)
	It is reasonable to choose an early invasive strategy (within 24 hours of admission) over a delayed invasive strategy (within 25–72 hours) for initially stabilized high-risk patients with NSTE-ACS. For those not at high/intermediate risk, a delayed invasive approach is reasonable.	ACC/AHA 2014 Guidelines, Class IIa (B)
Aspirin	Patients already taking daily aspirin before PCI should take 81 mg to 325 mg non–enteric-coated aspirin before PCI.	ACC/AHA 2014 Guidelines, Class I (B)
	Patients not on aspirin therapy should be given non–enteric-coated aspirin 325 mg as soon as possible before PCI.	
P2Y12 Inhibitors	A loading dose of a P2Y$_{12}$ receptor inhibitor should be given before the procedure in patients undergoing PCI with stenting. *(Level of Evidence: A)* Options include: Clopidogrel: 600 mg *(Level of Evidence: B)* or Prasugrel: 60 mg *(Level of Evidence: B)* or Ticagrelor: 180 mg *(Level of Evidence: B)*	ACC/AHA 2014 Guidelines, Class I

Continued on following page

Table 9.5

Issues and Considerations for PCI in Patients With NSTEMI (Continued)

Issue	Recommendations	Supportive Evidence
GP IIb/IIIa Inhibitors	In patients with NSTE-ACS and high-risk features (e.g., elevated troponin) not adequately pretreated with clopidogrel or ticagrelor, it is useful to administer a GP IIb/IIIa inhibitor (abciximab, double-bolus eptifibatide, or high-dose bolus tirofiban) at the time of PCI.	ACC/AHA 2014 Guidelines, Class I (A)
Anticoagulant Therapy	An anticoagulant should be administered to patients with NSTE-ACS undergoing PCI to reduce the risk of intracoronary and catheter thrombus formation.	ACC/AHA 2014 Guidelines, Class I (C)
	Intravenous UFH is useful in patients with NSTE-ACS undergoing PCI.	ACC/AHA 2014 Guidelines, Class I (C)
	Bivalirudin is useful as an anticoagulant with or without prior treatment with UFH in patients with NSTE-ACS undergoing PCI.	ACC/AHA 2014 Guidelines, Class I (B)
	An additional dose of 0.3 mg/kg IV enoxaparin should be administered at the time of PCI to patients with NSTE-ACS who have received fewer than two therapeutic subcutaneous doses (e.g., 1 mg/kg SC) or received the last subcutaneous enoxaparin dose 8–12 hours before PCI.	ACC/AHA 2014 Guidelines, Class I (B)
	If PCI is performed while the patient is on fondaparinux, an additional 85 IU/kg of UFH should be given IV immediately before PCI because of the risk for catheter thrombosis (60 IU/kg IV if a GP IIb/IIIa inhibitor used with UFH dosing based on the target-activated clotting time).	ACC/AHA 2014 Guidelines, Class I (B)
Complete Revascularization	A strategy of multivessel PCI, in contrast to culprit lesion-only PCI, may be reasonable in patients undergoing coronary revascularization as part of treatment for NSTE-ACS.	ACC/AHA 2014 Guidelines, Class IIb (B)

ACC, American College of Cardiology; AHA, American Heart Association; IU, international units; IV, intravenous; NSTE-ACS, non-ST segment elevation acute coronary syndrome; PCI, percutaneous coronary intervention; UFH, unfractionated heparin.

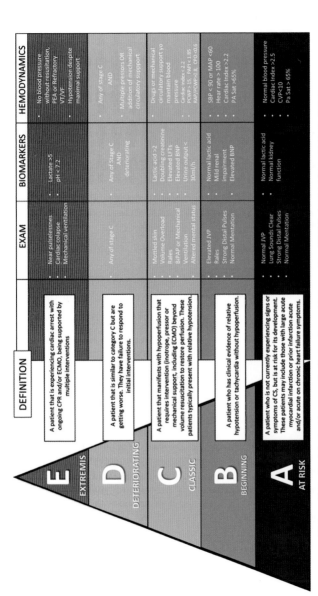

Figure 9.7 Society for Coronary Angiography and Intervention (SCAI) stages of cardiogenic shock.

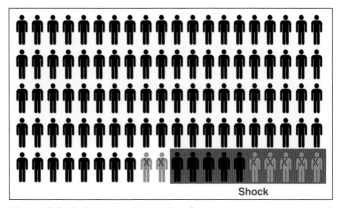

Figure 9.8 Incidence and mortality of acute coronary syndrome and cardiogenic shock.

- Patients can present with a large MI, resulting in significant stunning, ischemia, and infarction, to a large area of myocardium, resulting in acute pump dysfunction, hypotension, and hemodynamic compromise.

- Patients can present with multivessel coronary artery disease, with an AMI in a small or moderate territory, which may result in a large ischemic insult because of underlying disease in a noninfarct artery. For example, a patient with a chronically occluded left anterior descending (LAD) artery and an inferior MI can present with hemodynamic collapse because the right coronary artery frequently supplies collaterals to the LAD territory. Patients with multivessel disease similarly may develop global ischemia because of poor coronary perfusion in the setting of systemic hypotension and preexisting stenosis in noninfarct-related arteries.

- Patients with underlying cardiomyopathy can present with an ischemic insult, which may result in hemodynamic compromise because of baseline cardiac dysfunction with poor myocardial reserve and tenuous hemodynamics.

- Lastly, patients with AMI and prolonged cardiac arrest can develop rapid global end-organ hypoperfusion, often resulting in advanced stages of metabolic shock.

In all of these pathophysiologic subtypes, the final common pathway occurs via the ischemic cascade in which reduced compliance of the LV is associated with increased LV end diastolic pressure, LV dilation, and reduced systolic function. Compensatory tachycardia and peripheral vasoconstriction lead to further myocardial ischemia by increasing myocardial oxygen demand. Reduction in systolic function leads to further systemic hypotension, activation of the inflammatory cascade via inflammatory mediators, and ultimately multisystem organ failure.

Right Ventricular Failure

Isolated right ventricular (RV) infarction leading to CS is relatively rare, making up 3% to 5% of cases. RV infarction most commonly accompanies a posterior or inferior AMI. RV failure does not occur with every posterior/inferior AMI because the myocardial oxygen demand of the RV is lower compared with the LV. Also the RV is typically supplied by left-sided collaterals, which can limit infarction.

When RV infarction does occur, it results in decreased RV compliance and contractile function. With acute dysfunction of the RV, the RV cannot adequately fill the LV, causing an acute reduction in cardiac output. As the failing RV dilates, the interventricular septum shifts leftward and the interdependence between the two ventricles is altered. This adversely affects the LV contractility, leading to further reductions in cardiac output and LV compliance. RV infarctions are also frequently associated with sinus bradycardia and atrioventricular block, which can further worsen hemodynamics.

Hemodynamic Markers of Right Ventricular Failure

Several echocardiographic and hemodynamic parameters have been studied to characterize RV dysfunction in the setting of CS (Table 9.6). Hemodynamic parameters, including the right atrial to pulmonary capillary wedge pressure (RA:PCWP) ratio, RV stroke work index, and the pulmonary artery pulsatility index (PAPi), correlate to echocardiographic findings of RV dysfunction and clinical outcomes. Of the parameters studied, PAPi in the setting of a high RA pressure was identified as having the highest sensitivity and specificity for identifying patients with RV dysfunction.

Systemic Inflammatory Response Syndrome

Hypoperfusion initiates a cascade of neurohormonal responses that trigger the hemodynamic and metabolic effects seen in CS. The release of catecholamines, vasopressin, and angiotensin II leads to peripheral vasoconstriction and sodium retention, which transiently improves coronary and peripheral perfusion; however, it also results

Table 9.6

Parameters to Identify Right Ventricular Failure		
Parameter	**Definition**	**Right Ventricular Failure**
CVP	Mean right atrial pressure	> 12–15 mm Hg
CVP/PCWP	Ratio of mean right atrial pressure by the pulmonary capillary wedge pressure	> 0.8
PAPI	(Systolic PA pressure – diastolic PA pressure) / CVP	< 1.0
RVSWI	(Mean PA pressure − CVP) × SVI	< 300 g·m/m^2

CVP, Central venous pressure; *PA*, pulmonary artery; *PAPI*, pulmonary artery pressure index; *PCWP*, pulmonary capillary wedge pressure; *RVSWI*, right ventricular stroke work index; *SVI*, stroke volume index.

in increased afterload and volume, resulting in pulmonary edema and further exacerbation of cardiac dysfunction. In the 24 to 72 hours after an AMI, cytokine levels have been shown to be elevated in patients with cardiogenic shock. Patients in the late stages of CS go on to develop a systemic inflammatory response characterized by low systemic vascular resistance progressing to vasodilatory shock. This physiology is seen in one-fifth of patients with AMI-CS and is associated with a twofold increase in the risk of death.

Inotropes and Vasopressors

The most commonly used vasoactive medications and their mechanisms of action are listed in Table 9.7. The dose of vasopressor or inotrope required to establish hemodynamic stability is variable. These medications also typically increase myocardial oxygen consumption and can negatively impact myocardial recovery and salvage. Knowing patient level hemodynamics and the mechanism of action of vasoactive medications allows for a tailored patient-specific treatment strategy to optimize hemodynamic performance and restore tissue perfusion.

In patients presenting with normotensive CS because of a low stroke volume, decreased cardiac output, and elevated systemic vascular resistance, use of inodilators, such as dobutamine and milrinone, should be considered first line. In states of hypotensive CS, inoconstrictors (i.e., norepinephrine, epinephrine, and dopamine) should be considered first line to augment cardiac output and hypotension. In general, norepinephrine is regarded as the

Table 9.7

Vasopressors and Inotropes Used in Shock					
				Effect	
Drug	Usual Dose Range	Target	Cardiac Output	Systemic Vascular Resistance	Pulmonary Vascular Resistance
Milrinone	0.125–0.750 mcg/kg/min	cAMP	↑↑↑	↓↓	↓↓
Dobutamine	2.5–10 mcg/kg/min	α β1 β2	↑↑↑	↓	↓
Dopamine	1–4 mcg/kg/min	D	↑	↓	
	5–10 mcg/kg/min	α β1 D	↑↑	↔	
	10–20 mcg/kg/min	α β1 D	↑	↑↑	↑
Epinephrine	1–20 mcg/min	α β1 β2	↑↑	↑	
Norepinephrine	1–40 mcg/min	α β1	↑	↑↑	
Phenylephrine	40–180 mcg/min	α	↔	↑↑↑	↑↑
Vasopressin	0.01–0.06 U/min	v1, v2	↔	↑↑↑	↓

preferred inoconstrictor over dopamine or epinephrine. The final vasoactive agents used in the management of CS are vasoconstrictors, such as phenylephrine and vasopressin. These medications have limited use in the management of AMI-CS and are generally reserved for low afterload states or when inotropy is harmful, such as with tachyarrhythmia or LV outflow tract obstruction.

Mechanical Circulatory Support

Given the high mortality associated with AMI-CS, MCS devices have been increasingly used to provide hemodynamic support. Use of

MCS is supported in the US and European guidelines; however, data from well-powered randomized control trials (RCTs) have been lacking, given the difficulties in conducting trials in critically ill patients and because use of MCS has been historically limited to large tertiary care centers. Technological advancements, however, have led to the development of mobile, percutaneous, MCS devices with growing adoption from interventional and heart failure cardiologists. MCS differ in their mechanism of action, implantation, size, flow, and complication risk (Fig. 9.9 and Table 9.8).

Intra-Aortic Balloon Pumps

The most commonly used MCS has been intra-aortic balloon pumps (IABPs). IABPs deflate during systole, reducing afterload,

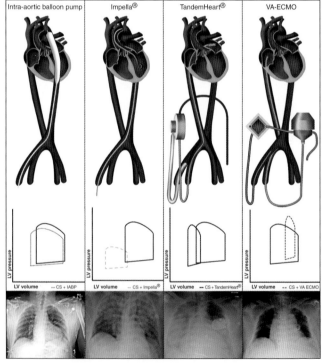

Figure 9.9 Left ventricular mechanical support devices.

Table 9.8

Types and Characteristics of Left Ventricular Mechanical Circulatory Support Devices

	IABP	Impella	Tandem	VA-ECMO
Flow (L/min)	0.5–1	2.5 3.5 5.0 5.5	3.5–4.5	3–6
Mechanism of action	Counterpulsation	Transvalvular micro-axial pump	Centrifugal cardiac bypass	Centrifugal cardiopulmonary bypass
Access site	Femoral or axillary artery	Femoral or axillary artery	Femoral artery Femoral vein	Femoral artery Femoral vein
Sheath size	7–8F	2.5F–13F CP–14 F 5.0F–33F 5.5F–19F (cut down)	Inflow – 17F Outflow – 15F–19F	Inflow – 21F–29F Outflow – 15F–19F
Effect on cardiac output	↑	↑↑	↑↑	↑↑
Effect on afterload	↓	↓	↑	↑↑
Effect on LVEDP	↓	↓↓	↓↓	↑↓
Effect on coronary perfusion	↑	↑	↑	↑
Advantages	Simple cannulation, low hemolysis profile, easy to transport patient	Simple cannulation, unloading of the LV, antegrade flow	Unloading of the LV	Biventricular support, oxygenation, simple cannulation
Disadvantages	Requires intrinsic heart function, modest hemodynamic support	Large-bore access, risk of hemolysis	Large-bore access, retrograde blood flow, requires atrial septostomy	Large-bore access, retrograde blood flow

IABP, Intra-aortic balloon pump; *LV,* left ventricle; *LVEDP,* left ventricular end diastolic pressure; *VA-ECMO,* venoarterial extracorporeal membrane oxygenation.

and inflate during diastole, increasing coronary perfusion. IABPs require a 7 to 8 French (F) access and can be placed percutaneously in the femoral, axillary, and brachial arteries. IABPs are easy for clinical staff to use, portable, and can be removed at bedside. IABPs are frequently used for patients with cardiogenic shock, with decompensated heart failure, and as a bridge to definitive therapies such as CABG, PCI, or advanced heart failure therapies. In appropriately selected patients, early use of an IABP can restore hemodynamics and preserve end-organ function until definitive therapies can be administered. In patients with cardiogenic shock from decompensated heart failure, there can be up to a fivefold greater cardiac output augmentation with IABP compared with patients with AMI and cardiogenic shock. This is because IABPs rely on intrinsic heart function, which needs to be maintained. IABP provides a modest hemodynamic support (typically around 0.5 L/min) and therefore in cardiogenic shock may not provide enough support to preserve end-organ function. Multiple RCTs and large meta-analyses have demonstrated that routine use of IABP in AMI-CS does not improve survival.

Axial-Flow Transvalvular Pumps

Impella (Abiomed, Danvers, MA) is an axial-flow, transvalvular MCS device. Currently there are five commercially available devices with incremental levels of hemodynamic support. LV support devices include the percutaneous Impella 2.5 and CP (3.5L), which use a 13F and 14F arterial access and the surgically delivered 5.0 and 5.5. The RV support device, called the Impella RP, uses a similar motor as the 5.0 L device and is percutaneously implanted using a 22F venous access.

Impellas provide continuous flow, reducing LV end diastolic pressure, decreasing pressure-volume area and myocardial oxygen consumption, and increasing coronary perfusion pressures. The Impella platforms decrease LV wall stress, thereby facilitating LV unloading and myocardial recovery. Impella devices are large-bore MCS devices that require careful implantation and are associated with bleeding and vascular access complications.

Extracorporeal Membrane Oxygenation

Venoarterial extracorporeal membrane oxygenation (VA-ECMO) functions as a cardiopulmonary bypass circuit typically requiring a 21F to 27F venous cannula and a 15F to 19F arterial cannula. Blood is taken out of the right atrium through a centrifugal pump, oxygenated, and returned to the femoral artery using a typical peripheral cannulation strategy. VA-ECMO circuits can be constructed using numerous configurations, including central cannulation, which require surgical implantation.

VA-ECMO is the only MCS currently available that supports both the RV and LV using a single circuit. It also provides robust support based on the size of the cannula used and can achieve 3 to 6 L/min of cardiac output. VA-ECMO is used in cases of refractory cardiogenic shock and for assisted cardiopulmonary resuscitation (eCPR). ECMO typically requires dedicated nurses or perfusionists to manage the circuit. Given the added level of expertise, widespread adoption of VA-ECMO has been limited to select tertiary care hospitals. As technological advancements have led to smaller, more mobile pumps and with dissemination of shock management from surgical to cardiology led teams, there has been increasing utilization.

Physiologically, VA-ECMO, unlike IABP and axial flow devices, may increase afterload. In these scenarios, modes to allow for LV venting are preferred to facilitate myocardial recovery. Importantly, given the large-bore cannulas and retrograde delivery of blood in typical peripheral ECMO circuits, there are high rates of bleeding, vascular injury, and stroke in current practice, highlighting the importance of patient selection.

Left Atrium-to-Femoral Artery Bypass

TandemHeart is a centrifugal flow left atrium-to-femoral artery bypass circuit, which diverts blood from the left atrium to the iliofemoral system. It indirectly unloads the LV and reduces LV wall stress. It similarly improves coronary perfusion pressure by decreasing the LV end diastolic pressure and increasing the diastolic mean arterial pressure. A TandemHeart requires the expertise of a transseptal puncture and is associated with similar complication profiles as VA-ECMO and Impella.

Shock Protocols and Teams

Greater familiarity with MCS devices, including large-bore access and closure, has led to increasing use of MCS in the cardiac catheterization laboratory (Figs. 9.10 and 9.11). This includes community programs without LV assist device (LVAD) and transplant programs. Given the variability in experience with MCS devices, many centers have adopted multidisciplinary cardiogenic shock teams to formalize care for patients requiring MCS devices.

Shock protocols allow for a uniform treatment strategy in an effort to provide patients, nurses, and clinicians with a systematic pathway of care (Fig. 9.12). They allow clinicians to cater to the individual based on operator and institutional expertise. Despite the need for ongoing study, the use of such protocols and teams has been associated with improving outcomes (Fig. 9.13).

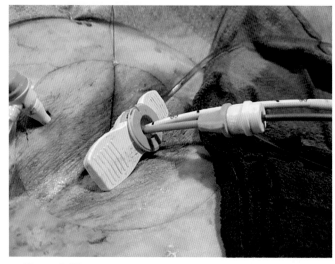

Figure 9.10 Single access through 14 French (F) Impella sheath.

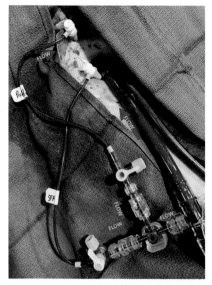

Figure 9.11 Right femoral artery and vein extracorporeal membrane oxygenation (ECMO) cannulation with reperfusion sheaths to profunda femoris and superficial femoral artery.

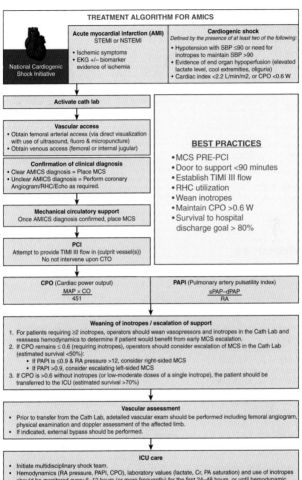

TREATMENT ALGORITHM FOR AMICS

Acute myocardial infarction (AMI) STEMI or NSTEMI	Cardiogenic shock *Defined by the presence of at least two of the following:*
• Ischemic symptoms • EKG +/– biomarker evidence of ischemia	• Hypotension with SBP ≤90 or need for inotropes to maintain SBP >90 • Evidence of end organ hypoperfusion (elevated lactate level, cool extremities, oliguria) • Cardiac index <2.2 L/min/m2, or CPO <0.6 W

National Cardiogenic Shock Initiative

Activate cath lab

Vascular access
• Obtain femoral arterial access (via direct visualization with use of ultrasound, fluoro & micropuncture)
• Obtain venous access (femoral or internal jugular)

Confirmation of clinical diagnosis
• Clear AMICS diagnosis = Place MCS
• Unclear AMICS diagnosis = Perform coronary Angiogram/RHC/Echo as required.

Mechanical circulatory support
Once AMICS diagnosis confirmed, place MCS

PCI
Attempt to provide TIMI III flow in (culprit vessel(s))
No not intervene upon CTO

BEST PRACTICES
• MCS PRE-PCI
• Door to support <90 minutes
• Establish TIMI III flow
• RHC utilization
• Wean inotropes
• Maintain CPO >0.6 W
• Survival to hospital discharge goal > 80%

CPO (Cardiac power output) $$\frac{MAP \times CO}{451}$$	PAPI (Pulmonary artery pulsatility index) $$\frac{sPAP-dPAP}{RA}$$

Weaning of inotropes / escalation of support
1. For patients requiring ≥2 inotropes, operators should wean vasopressors and inotropes in the Cath Lab and reassess hemodynamics to determine if patient would benefit from early MCS escalation.
2. If CPO remains ≤ 0.6 (requiring inotropes), operators should consider escalation of MCS in the Cath Lab (estimated survival <50%):
   • If PAPI is ≤0.9 & RA pressure >12, consider right-sided MCS
   • If PAPI >0.9, consider escalating left-sided MCS
3. If CPO is >0.6 without inotropes (or low-moderate doses of a single inotrope), the patient should be transferred to the ICU (estimated survival >70%)

Vascular assessment
• Prior to transfer from the Cath Lab, adetailed vascular exam should be performed including femoral angiogram, physical examination and doppler assessment of the affected limb.
• If indicated, external bypass should be performed.

ICU care
• Initiate multidisciplinary shock team.
• Hemodynamics (RA pressure, PAPI, CPO), laboratory values (lactate, Cr, PA saturation) and use of inotropes should be monitored every 6–12 hours (or more frequently) for the first 24–48 hours, or until hemodynamic stabilization.
• Patient requiring escalating doses of inotropes, rising lactate levels, worsening hemodynamics (CPO≤0.6W), and/or the development of RV failure (PAPI≤0.9, RA pressure >12, or frequent suction alarms despite proper MCS positioning) should be considered for escalation of MCS in suitable candidates.
• Daily vascular assessment.
• Monitor for signs of hemolysis and adjust MCS position as indicated.

Device weaning
• If CPO is >0.6 (ideally >0.8) without inotropes (or low doses of a single inotrope), MCS should weaned.

Bridge to decision
• Patients who do not regain myocardial recovery within 24–72 hours, should be considered for transfer to a LVAD/transplant center.
• Patients who are not candidates for advanced therapies and cannot be weaned off MCS should have discussions with palliative care as clinically appropriate.

Figure 9.12 The National Cardiogenic Shock treatment algorithm for acute myocardial infarction and cardiogenic shock.

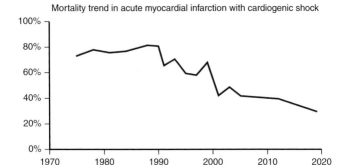

Figure 9.13 Mortality trend in acute myocardial infarction with cardiogenic shock.

References

Amsterdam EA, Wenger NK, Brindis RG, et al. 2014 AHA/ACC guideline for the management of patients with Non-ST-Elevation Acute Coronary Syndromes: a report of the American College of Cardiology/American Heart Association Task Force on Practice Guidelines. *J Am Coll Cardiol.* 2014;64(24):e139-e228. Erratum in: *J Am Coll Cardiol.* 2014;64(24):2713-2714. Dosage error in article text.

Anderson ML, Peterson ED, Peng SA, et al. Differences in the profile, treatment, and prognosis of patients with cardiogenic shock by myocardial infarction classification: a report from NCDR. *Circ Cardiovasc Qual Outcomes.* 2013;6(6):708-715.

Basir MB, Kapur NK, Patel K, et al. Improved outcomes associated with the use of shock protocols: updates from the National Cardiogenic Shock Initiative. *Catheter Cardiovasc Interv.* 2019;93(7):1173-1183.

Hochman JS, Sleeper LA, Webb JG, et al. Early revascularization in acute myocardial infarction complicated by cardiogenic SHOCK. SHOCK Investigators. Should we emergently revascularize occluded coronaries for cardiogenic shock. *N Engl J Med.* 1999;341(9):625-634.

Kolte D, Khera S, Aronow WS, et al. Trends in incidence, management, and outcomes of cardiogenic shock complicating ST-elevation myocardial infarction in the United States. *J Am Heart Assoc.* 2014;3(1):e000590.

Levine GN, Bates ER, Blankenship JC, et al. 2015 ACC/AHA/SCAI focused update on primary percutaneous coronary intervention for patients With ST-elevation myocardial infarction: an update of the 2011 ACCF/AHA/SCAI guideline for percutaneous coronary intervention and the 2013 ACCF/AHA Guideline for the Management of ST-Elevation Myocardial Infarction. *J Am Coll Cardiol.* 2016;67(10):1235-1250. Erratum in: *J Am Coll Cardiol.* 2016;67(12):1506.

O'Gara PT, Kushner FG, Ascheim DD, et al. 2013 ACCF/AHA guideline for the management of ST-elevation myocardial infarction. A report of the American College of Cardiology Foundation/American Heart Association Task Force on Practice Guidelines. *Circulation.* 2013;127:e362-e425.

Tehrani BN, Truesdell AG, Sherwood MW, et al. Standardized team-based care for cardiogenic shock. *J Am Coll Cardiol.* 2019;73(13):1659-1669.

Thiele H, Akin I, Sandri M, et al. CULPRIT-SHOCK Investigators. One year outcomes after PCI strategies in cardiogenic shock. *N Engl J Med.* 2018;379(18):1699-1710.

Thiele H, Zeymer U, Neumann FJ, et al. Intraaortic balloon support for myocardial infarction with cardiogenic shock. *N Engl J Med*. 2012;367(14):1287–1296.

Unverzagt S, Buerke M, de Waha A, et al. Intra-aortic balloon pump counterpulsation (IABP) for myocardial infarction complicated by cardiogenic shock. *Cochrane Database Syst Rev*. 2015;(3):CD007398.

Wilson-Smith AR, Bogdanova Y, Roydhouse S, et al. Outcomes of venoarterial extracorporeal membrane oxygenation for refractory cardiogenic shock: systematic review and meta-analysis. *Ann Cardiothorac Surg*. 2019;8(1):1-8.

Yancy CW, Jessup M, Bozkurt B, et al. 2013 ACCF/AHA guideline for the management of heart failure: a report of the American College of Cardiology Foundation/American Heart Association Task Force on practice guidelines. *Circulation*. 2013;128(16):e240-e327.

PCI With Left Ventricular Hemodynamic Support

MICHAEL J. LIM

KEY POINTS

- Complex percutaneous coronary intervention (PCI) procedures have become more common as techniques for chronic total occlusions (CTOs), bifurcation, and left main lesions have been developed with improved outcomes.

- Complex PCI can create significant acute risk for hemodynamic collapse in the Cath lab and the placement of prophylactic left ventricular (LV) support can minimize the risk of such an event.

- Multiple percutaneous options for LV support are now available, but they differ in their ease of use, potential complications, and hemodynamic effects.

- Clinical data mainly support the use of the Impella device to support complex PCI.

The performance of percutaneous coronary intervention (PCI) to improve myocardial blood flow to decrease symptoms of angina and potentially improve left ventricular (LV) function has been well established. There exists a large spectrum of potential discussion on this topic from "simple" PCI procedures involving singular lesions of lesser complexity to multivessel PCI, which includes lesions that are chronically occluded or in patients with severely depressed LV function. Regardless, the performance of PCI results in an acute period of myocardial ischemia while balloon inflation impedes forward blood flow in the artery being addressed. Before balloon angioplasty, it was demonstrated in animal models that acute ischemia rapidly decreased the maximum pressure that could be generated in the LV in a given time (the derivative of pressure over time [dP/dT]), that decreased systolic force generated by the ischemic myocardium, that the effects become apparent within seconds of the occlusion of the vessel, and that these changes recurred with reocclusion (i.e., subsequent balloon inflation).

Putting it together, patients with preserved LV function and relatively simple PCI will still have some short-term effects from the procedure within the LV wall, but this is not sufficient to result in prolonged hypotension, impaired cardiac output, or ventricular rhythm disturbances. Patients with impaired function and/or undergoing a PCI procedure to multiple arteries, which potentially increases the amount of acute ischemia that the ventricle is exposed to, may not be able to tolerate the short-term dysfunction within the myocardium—a subset now referred to as "complex PCI" (Fig. 10.1). Thus, to perform PCI on these patients, the LV requires "support" to maintain hemodynamic stability throughout the procedure.

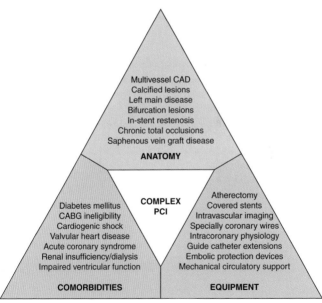

Figure 10.1 Complex percutaneous coronary intervention (PCI) is now defined by a combination of clinical, anatomic, and equipment needs for the procedure. (From Riley R, Henry TD, Mahmoud E, et al. SCAI position statement on optimal percutaneous coronary interventional therapy for complex coronary artery disease. *Cathet Cardiovasc Intervent.* 2020; 96:346-362; Fig. 2.)

Patient Selection

Presently, selection of patients in whom hemodynamic support is used during PCI remains institution dependent. Nevertheless, there are some similar guiding principles that can be found to help with preprocedural planning. The first of these is that these procedures are not recommended to be done on an "ad hoc" basis and there should be a formal Heart Team discussion that is documented within the medical record that goes through the relative merits of this procedure and gains support from the collective team of surgeons and interventional cardiologists. Although these procedures have a higher complication rate than those of standard PCI, they are also potentially associated with greater benefit for the patient, and it is recommended that the goals to be achieved by taking on a supported PCI procedure be defined before the procedure and agreed upon by the Heart Team and the patient.

Currently, there is a single randomized controlled trial (RCT) that has investigated supported PCI: PROTECT II. The findings of this trial will be discussed later in this chapter, but the enrollment criteria can provide information on the types of patients who should be considered (Table 10.1). A suggested algorithm (Fig. 10.2) for decision making in supported PCI procedures illustrates many critical issues. After a Heart Team recommendation on pursuing the procedure, using historical clinical data, understanding the implications of the planned PCI procedure itself (e.g., hemodynamic insult of atherectomy), and assessing invasive hemodynamics has been recommended in an attempt to predict the potential for hemodynamic collapse during the procedure. Typically, baseline LV function has been used as a significant and common element when considering using LV support. When it is felt that alterations to hemodynamics are likely, the prophylactic implantation of an LV support device before performing a PCI is achieved. Operators experienced at these devices also have the ability to implant them relatively quickly when hemodynamic collapse occurs unexpectedly.

Table 10.1

Inclusion Criteria for Patients to Be Considered for PROTECT II	
Patient's EF	**Angiographic Disease**
EF ≤ 35%	Unprotected left main or last patent vessel
EF ≤ 30%	Three-vessel disease

EF, Ejection fraction.

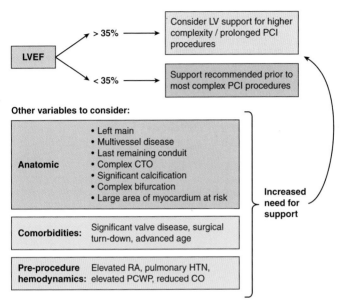

Figure 10.2 Key factors to consider when planning a complex percutaneous coronary intervention (PCI) as to when implementing a left ventricular (LV) support device preprocedure would be most beneficial. The patient's LV ejection fraction remains a key determinate, and anatomic features, patient comorbidities, and invasive hemodynamic findings significantly increase the need for support.

Lesion subsets frequently requiring consideration for support during PCI include left main intervention and patients who have previously undergone bypass surgery with multiple failed grafts. In patients with left main disease, Fig. 10.3 illustrates some of the critical elements involved with successful PCI. Because most lesions involve the distal left main, these interventions frequently involve bifurcation techniques. Thus should the patient have an impaired baseline ejection fraction (EF) or heart failure (e.g., pulmonary capillary wedge pressure [PCWP] > 20 mm Hg), multiple balloon inflations resulting in decreased perfusion to the left coronary system will potentially result in significant hypotension, ventricular dysrhythmias, or loss of pulsatilla of the ventricle, and pre-PCI placement of LV support would be indicated. Patients with prior bypass grafts that have failed often have complex disease within the native vessels that requires multiple stents and sometimes prolonged atherectomy procedures to prepare the vessel, which may also result in similar untoward hemodynamic results as left pain PCI.

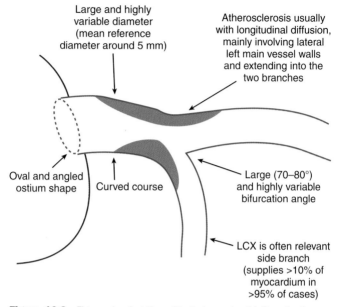

Large and highly variable diameter (mean reference diameter around 5 mm)

Atherosclerosis usually with longitudinal diffusion, mainly involving lateral left main vessel walls and extending into the two branches

Oval and angled ostium shape

Curved course

Large (70–80°) and highly variable bifurcation angle

LCX is often relevant side branch (supplies >10% of myocardium in >95% of cases)

Figure 10.3 Figure showing the critical elements of left main disease that must be considered for procedure planning. The extent of disease, involving the optimum, body, and/or the distal portions of the left main, remains imperative to understand and often requires intravascular imaging to delineate. The curvature of the left main itself and the angle of take-off of the left anterior descending (LAD) and circumflex (LCX) arteries also affect procedural success. (From Burzotta F, Lassen JF, Barning AP, Et al. Percutaneous coronary intervention in left main coronary artery disease: the 13th consensus document from the European bifurcation club. *EuroIntervention.* 2018;14:112–120; Fig. 1.)

Devices Available for Temporary Left Ventricular Support

See Fig. 10.4.

Intra-Aortic Balloon Pump

The intra-aortic balloon pump (IABP) has been the device with the largest usage in the catheterization (Cath) lab for many years. Developed decades ago, the catheter was inserted via a femoral artery with the balloon tip positioned in the most proximal portion

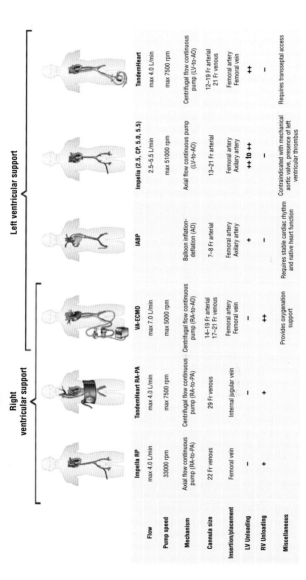

Right ventricular support | **Left ventricular support**

	Impella RP	TandemHeart RA-PA	VA-ECMO	IABP	Impella (2.5, CP, 5.0, 5.5)	TandemHeart
Flow	max 4.0 L/min	max 4.0 L/min	max 7.0 L/min		2.5–5.5 L/min	max 4.0 L/min
Pump speed	33000 rpm	max 7500 rpm	max 5000 rpm		max 51000 rpm	max 7500 rpm
Mechanism	Axial flow continuous pump (RA-to-PA)	Centrifugal flow continuous pump (RA-to-PA)	Centrifugal flow continuous pump (RA-to-AO)	Balloon inflation-deflation (AO)	Axial flow continuous pump (LV-to-AO)	Centrifugal flow continuous pump (LV-to-AO)
Cannula size	22 Fr venous	29 Fr venous	14–19 Fr arterial 17–21 Fr venous	7–8 Fr arterial	13–21 Fr arterial	12–19 Fr arterial 21 Fr venous
Insertion/placement	Femoral vein	Internal jugular vein	Femoral artery Femoral vein	Femoral artery Axillary artery	Femoral artery Axillary artery	Femoral artery Femoral vein
LV Unloading	–	–	–	+	++ to ++	++
RV Unloading	+	+	++	–	–	–
Miscellaneous			Provides oxygenation support	Requires stable cardiac rhythm and native heart function	Contraindicated with mechanical aortic valve, presence of left ventricular thrombus	Requires transseptal access

Figure 10.4 Spectrum of mechanical circulatory support devices currently available and their specific features/attributes. (From Riley R, Henry TD, Mahmoud E, et al. SCAI position statement on optimal percutaneous coronary interventional therapy for complex coronary artery disease. *Cath Cardiovasc Intervent.* 2020;96:346–362; Fig. 3.)

of the descending thoracic aorta. The inflation of the balloon was timed to occur during diastole and, therefore, increases in aortic diastolic blood pressure were noted on arterial line recordings (Fig. 10.5). The deflation of the balloon was timed to occur just before aortic valve opening, and the theory was that this rapid deflation resulted in a lower intra-aortic pressure at the time of early systolic flow from the left ventricle – thus LV "unloading."

Given its long-standing place in the Cath lab, most staff and physicians are very familiar with the setup and use of the device. After insertion, the device is set to inflate and deflate with a trigger from the arterial pressure signal or from an electrocardiogram (ECG) signal. Most consoles have an "auto" mode that is activated to rely on the programmed algorithm for balloon inflation and deflation, but users can change these setting manually. The highest

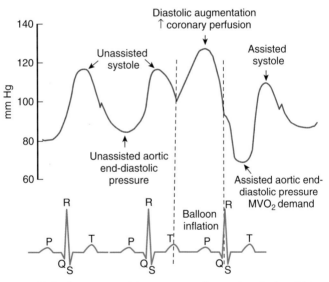

Figure 10.5 Systemic arterial pressure waveform on introduction of intra-aortic balloon pump–assisted diastolic augmentation. The intra-aortic balloon pump inflates at the dicrotic notch, leading to peak-augmented diastolic pressure. As the balloon deflates, assisted end diastolic pressure is seen to be lower than unassisted end diastolic pressure, and assisted systolic pressure is lower than unassisted systolic pressure. Peak diastolic augmentation should be greater than the unassisted systolic pressure, and both assisted pressures should be less than the unassisted pressures. (From Patterson T, Perera D, Redwood SR. Intraaortic balloon pump for high-risk percutaneous coronary intervention. *Circ Cardiovasc Interv.* 2014;7:712–720.)

level of support is achieved with a 1:1 setting, where the balloon inflates and deflates with every heartbeat. Faster heart rates and irregular rhythms result in decreased performance of this device. Anticoagulation with heparin is recommended for all patients, but some patients with increased bleeding risk have been left without heparin while the pump is set at 1:1 and issues have not been observed in terms of thrombus on the balloon.

The device is "weaned" by decreasing support from 1:1 to 1:2, then 1:3, and so on, and observing the patient's hemodynamic response. The speed by which this happens remains operator dependent and monitoring vital signs, cardiac output, and renal output have all been used to determine "stability." Once it has been determined that the IABP is to be removed, the following steps are followed:

1. Remove all anchoring sutures.

2. Disconnect the balloon from the console. Many operators will attach a 60 cc syringe to the balloon port and remove all the air/gas in an attempt to ensure that the balloon is reduced to the smallest profile achievable.

3. The balloon catheter (and sheath) are removed and manual pressure is applied to the femoral artery to achieve hemostasis. Many have advised allowing some "back bleeding" through the arterial site to ensure that no clots or "debris" are retained with the vessel.

4. Manual pressure for 20 to 30 minutes has been standard to achieve complete hemostasis. This is followed by immobilization of the leg and bed rest for 4 to 6 hours afterward.

Nevertheless, as other devices have become available, the total amount of afterload reduction and enhanced cardiac output provided by the IABP has proven to be very minimal (Table 10.2). Its use has continued mainly because of the familiarity that operators and Cath lab staff have with it and the relatively low number of complications associated with insertion and removal secondary to its 7.5 French (F) profile.

TandemHeart

The TandemHeart device was introduced as a percutaneous LV device, and its placement involves cannulation of the femoral artery and femoral vein with subsequent transseptal puncture to position the "inflow" venous cannula within the left atrium (Fig. 10.6A). The "traditional" configuration uses a left atrial cannula that is 21F and connects to an external centrifugal pump. The other connection to the pump is a 15F to 17F cannula in the femoral artery extending to the abdominal aorta. The pump can run at varying speeds to provide up to 5 L/min of blood flow. In the aforementioned configuration, the LV is unloading "indirectly" as blood is taken from the left atrium and pumped back to the abdominal aorta (see Table 10.1). This device requires patients to be anticoagulated, most typically with heparin, with an activated clotting time (ACT) of 400 seconds during insertion and setup. An ACT of 250 to 300 seconds should be maintained for the duration of support.

The device has been shown to have the capability of being used in alternative setups, with the inflow cannula positioned in the inferior vena cava-right atrium (IVC-RA) and the addition of an oxygenation to provide both right ventricular (RV) and LV support with external oxygenation. Because it involves much larger cannulas, most of the complications reported with its use have been access site related. Using best practices for obtaining access remains the best recommendation for minimizing these issues. Furthermore, the size of the cannulas also potentially results in decreased perfusion to the leg and operators must assess antegrade limb perfusion after insertion of this device if the intent is for longer-term support for the patient (see later for tips and techniques to improve antegrade limb perfusion).

Weaning of the device is typically done by decreasing the speed of the pump (RPMs) and monitoring the patient's hemodynamic response. Current best practice involves the use of invasive

Table 10.2

Comparison of Left Ventricular Support Devices			
Device	**Hemodynamic Effects**	**Contraindications**	**Complications**
IABP	↑ Diastolic BP ↑ CO	≥ 2+ AI, aortic dissection	Stroke, limb ischemia, vascular trauma
Tandem-Heart	↓↓ PCWP ↓↓ LV work ↑↑↑ CO ↑↑ MAP	Severe PAD, profound coagulopathy	Vascular trauma, limb ischemia, tamponade, thrombo-embolism
ECMO (V-A)	↑↑↑ CO ↑ Wall stress ↑↑ MAP	Severe PAD (requires surgical insertion)	Bleeding, thromboembolism, hemolysis
Impella	↓↓ LV O$_2$ consumption ↓↓ PCWP ↑↑ CO ↑ MAP	Mechanical AVR, LV thrombus	Limb ischemia, vascular injury, bleeding

AI, Aortic incompetence; *AVR*, aortic valve replacement; *BP*, blood pressure; *CO*, carbon monoxide; *IABP*, intra-aortic balloon pump; *LV*, left ventricular; *MAP*, mean arterial pressure; *PAD*, peripheral artery disease; *PCWP*, pulmonary capillary wedge pressure

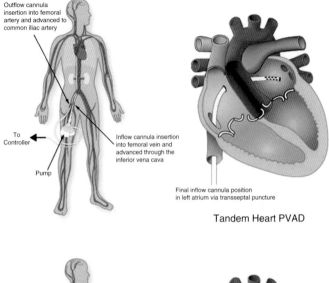

Outflow cannula insertion into femoral artery and advanced to common iliac artery

To Controller

Pump

Inflow cannula insertion into femoral vein and advanced through the inferior vena cava

Final inflow cannula position in left atrium via transseptal puncture

Tandem Heart PVAD

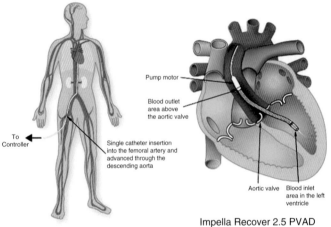

To Controller

Pump motor

Blood outlet area above the aortic valve

Single catheter insertion into the femoral artery and advanced through the descending aorta

Aortic valve   Blood inlet area in the left ventricle

Impella Recover 2.5 PVAD

Figure 10.6 Inflow/outflow configuration for the TandemHeart device (A) and the Impella device (B). (From Kar B, Basra SS, Shah N, et al. Percutaneous circulatory support in cardiogenic shock. *Circulation.* 2012;125: 1809–1817.)

hemodynamics to guide weaning. Once it has been determined that the pump can be removed, operators have either taken the patients back to the Cath lab for decannulation using large-bore access closure techniques to ensure safe removal and hemostasis or taken the patients to the operating room (OR) for direct vascular repair after decannulation.

Extracorporeal Membrane Oxygenation

Extracorporeal membrane oxygenation (ECMO) is a tool that was developed to mimic the heart-lung bypass machine used in the cardiac operating room. There are two different "setups" for ECMO that can be employed: V-V and V-A. V-V ECMO is implemented in patients with arterial oxygenation issues and involves removing blood from a venous cannula, passing it through an external oxygenator, and returning the oxygenated blood to the venous side. For patients requiring LV support, V-A ECMO returns the blood to the arterial system, providing in excess of 5 L/min of flow and does not depend on intrinsic LV function. Initiation of ECMO can be done via surgical vascular "cut-down" procedures or can be done percutaneously using large-bore access techniques and involves the placement of greater than 15F cannula(s). Placing a patient on ECMO requires anticoagulation with heparin. This device has not been used extensively to support complex PCI because it is quite extensive in its setup and personnel requirements to maintain support of the patient while on this device, but it has been used in cardiogenic shock with a growing body of evidence to support its utility.

Impella

As a single catheter, the Impella is placed with the distal "inflow" cannula in the LV and the "outflow" in the ascending aorta. Within the shaft of the catheter resides the "pump," which rotates at a set RPM to move blood from the LV to the aorta and data show that this results in direct unloading of the LV and increased cardiac output and mean arterial pressure (MAP; see Fig. 10.6B). The Impella at this time is not a single catheter, but a family of catheters with varying levels of support, ranging from the 2.5 Device, to the CP, and the 5.0 Device, which all function in a similar manner. There is also an RP device, which is dedicated to support the RV.

Insertion of the Impella has been mostly from the femoral artery, but this device can also be inserted via the axillary artery (Fig. 10.7) or via the femoral vein using the "transcaval" method to

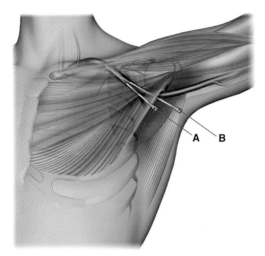

Figure 10.7 Figure illustrating the anatomic landmarks and route for percutaneous access to the axillary artery. Catheter A traverses the pectoralis minor muscle from the anterior chest before entering the vessel. Catheter B runs lateral and inferior to the pectoralis muscles from the anterior axilla.

cross from the abdominal IVC to the aorta when the iliac and femoral arteries are heavily diseased. After insertion, anticoagulation is maintained with IV heparin. The principal contraindications to using this device are the presence of thrombus in the LV or a mechanical aortic valve. There is a rich source of information, including an RCT, to support this device's use to facilitate complex PCI (see later) that exceeds the body of evidence for the other devices to date. Numerous technical advances on using the Impella in this manner have also been published, including the development of a "single access" method in which the 14F Impella sheath facilitates the Impella catheter placement and up to a 7F guiding catheter to perform PCI (Fig. 10.8).

Weaning the device is done by decreasing the "P-level" (i.e., the RPMs that the pump is operating at) and monitoring the hemodynamic response until P-2 has been reached. At that point, the device can be pulled back into the ascending aorta and the pump turned off. The pump can be easily removed through the 14F sheath, and there are varying methods of obtaining hemostasis after sheath removal, including placement of 1 to 2 Perclose devices before the dilation of the femoral artery and placement of the 14F sheath with deployment and tightening of the sutures performed after the sheath has been removed, using multiple Angioseal devices deployed after

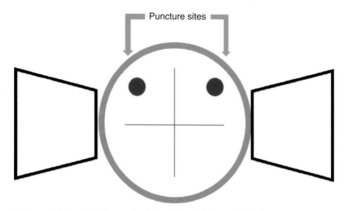

Figure 10.8 (A) Figure depicting the 14 French (F) Impella insertion sheath with the desired "entry" points found in the either upper quadrant of the diaphragm in the sheath. Using a micropuncture needle to penetrate either of these sites with subsequent insertion of up to a 7F sheath has been shown to be a useful method to perform "singe access" protected percutaneous coronary intervention (PCI) procedures. (B) Picture showing guiding catheter and sheath placed through the Impella sheath with the Impella catheter during a "single-access" protected PCI procedure. (From Wollmuth J, Korngold E, Croce K, Pinto DS. The single-access for Hi-risk PCI [ShiP] technique. *Cathet Cardiovascular Intervent.* 2020;1–3; Figs. 2 and 3.)

sheath removal, and using the dedicated large-bore Manta device. Given the 14F sheath used for the Impella CP device (currently the most commonly used), complications from use principally surround access site and closure issues.

Clinical Data for PCI With Left Ventricular Support

When considering the need for placing a patient on LV support before performing complex PCI, several considerations may guide an operator's decision making: ease of use, freedom from complications, and perceived need for the device. As with all decisions in medicine, a risk-benefit decision in favor of what is perceived to be best for the patient is advocated. In terms of complex PCI in a patient at risk, the interventionalist has to protect against periods of significant hypotension, acute myocardial ischemia leading to abrupt increases in pulmonary arterial pressure and pulmonary edema, and the development of ventricular tachycardia or fibrillation as a result of myocardial ischemia, all of which may result in

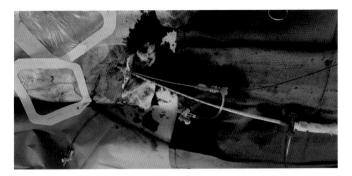

Figure 10.9 A normal left ventricular (LV) pressure volume loop is shown in blue. Emax, representing a load-independent LV contractility, is defined as the maximal slope of the end-systolic pressure-volume point under various loading conditions, known as the end-systolic pressure-volume relationship. Effective arterial elastance (Ea) is a component of LV afterload and is defined as the ratio of LV systolic pressure (LVSP) and stroke volume (SV). (A) Pressure-volume loop in using intra-aortic balloon pump (IABP) demonstrates a mildly decreased LV end-diastolic pressure (LVEDP) and LVSP, leading to a decreased Ea. (B) Pressure-volume loop with Impella device shows a substantially decreased LVEDP, LVSP, and SV. The net effect is a pronounced reduction of LV preload and afterload. (C) Pressure-volume loop with VA-ECMO without LV venting indicates a decreased SV, whereas LVEDP und LVSP are significantly increased with a net effect of substantial increase of LV afterload. (From Kim SH, Bannan S, Behness M, Borggrefe M, Akin I. Patient selection for protected percutaneous coronary intervention: Who benefits the most? *Card Clinics.* 2020;38:507–516; Fig. 1.)

potentially having to abort the revascularization procedure or may result in a patient mortality.

If operators are trying to protect patients from these negative outcomes, a comparison of the device effects on the LV pressure-volume loop can provide insight (Fig. 10.9). Although the IABP may be the simplest device to use, its ability to affect ventricular performance is minimal at best and likely depends on the degree of intrinsic ventricular performance to provide its maximal benefit (not observed during acute ischemia). On the other hand, although ECMO has tremendous ability to provide total-body circulatory support, it also does not have the ability to drastically affect ventricular performance. Thus it is the Impella with its ability to provide blood pressure support and directly unload the LV that has been studied most extensively for support of compelled PCI to date.

The PROTECT II trial represents the only RCT in the arena of supported PCI, randomizing high-risk patients to PCI with IABP support versus Impella 2.5 support. Although the primary outcome of the trial was similar between groups (secondary to an excess of periprocedural troponin elevations in the Impella arm), the curves separated as time from the procedure increased and support the significant improved long-term outcomes in the Impella-supported patients (Fig. 10.10). The trial had an unexpected disproportionate use of rotational atherectomy in the Impella arm, which the investigators believed was because the Impella device provided greater hemodynamic stability that gave the operators more confidence to use atherectomy and likely resulted in the difference in the periprocedural myocardial infarction (MI) rate. More recently, the follow-up PROTECT III study was published and seemed to support these assertions (Fig. 10.11) when using the Impella CP catheter.

Suggestions for Using Impella to Support Complex PCI

After obtaining a consensus Heart Team decision supporting PCI for the patient, the following points of consideration should be followed:

• Preprocedural planning: The long-term improved outcomes seen in the Impella-supported PROTECT II and III patients were

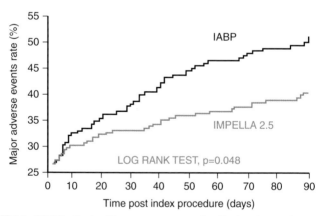

Figure 10.10 Kaplan-Meyer curve representing the long-term outcomes observed in the PROTECT II study. The y-axis represents major adverse events (MAE): all-cause death, myocardial infarction (MI), stroke, transient ischemic attack (TIA), or repeat revascularization. The x-axis is time from the index procedure in days. The yellow line represents patients who underwent the procedure with Impella 2.5 support, whereas the black line represents patients who had intra-aortic balloon pump (IABP) support.

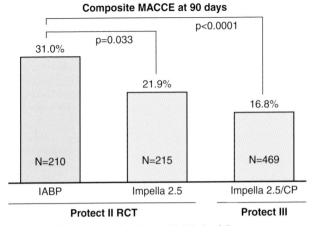

Composite MACCE at 90 days

31.0%		
	p=0.033	p<0.0001
	21.9%	
		16.8%
N=210	N=215	N=469
IABP	Impella 2.5	Impella 2.5/CP

Protect II RCT **Protect III**

N = number of patients with 90-day follow-up

Figure 10.11 Principal finding of the PROTECT III study, which used the Impella CP device to support high-risk percutaneous coronary intervention (PCI) procedures. Shown is a comparison of major adverse cardiovascular events (MACCE) between those patients and the findings from the patients treated in the PROTECT II study, with a lower rate of adverse events that was attributed to better experience with the device and complete revascularization. (Shown as presented at the TCT 2019 meeting.)

believed to be secondary to complete revascularization and PCI techniques that minimized the need for repeat PCI. Thus planning the procedure should emphasize the following:

- Determine access plan:
  - Location of large-bore sheath for support device (femoral vs. alternative access site)
  - Need for second access (e.g., need for two simultaneous guiding catheters) or plan for single-access technique
  - Plan for achieving hemostasis after device removal:
    - Potential that support device required postprocedure and patient transferred to the intensive care unit (ICU) with subsequent weaning and removal
    - Ability to provide antegrade limb perfusion if it becomes compromised
    - Availability of large vessel–covered stents and other equipment needed in case of primary hemostasis method failure

- Preprocedural plan discussed with Cath lab team with definition of roles/tasks for all personnel involved
- Complete revascularization of all significant major epicardial vessels (e.g., aim for lowest residual SYNTAX score after PCI complete). This can be accomplished in a single setting, or in a planned "staged" revascularization with CTOs and other more complex lesion(s) deferred to a separate setting with lower risk given PCI performed with support for the initial procedure (Fig. 10.12).
- Baseline renal function and determination of maximum contrast amount to be delivered to avoid contrast-induced nephropathy
- During the procedure:
  - Use of intravascular imaging (intravascular ultrasound [IVUS] or optical coherence tomography [OCT]) to assess before PCI to evaluate calcification that may require atherectomy, proximal and distal landing zones for stent placement, and ideal stent diameter

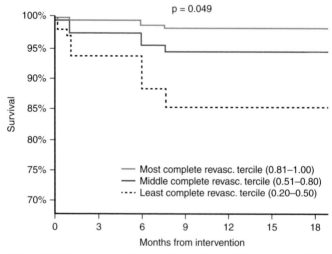

Figure 10.12 As observed from the Roma-Verona Italian registry of high-risk percutaneous coronary intervention (PCI) procedures, this figure shows the differences between patients depending on their completeness of revascularization. (From Burzotta F, Russo G, Ribichini F, et al. Long-term outcomes of extent of revascularization in complex high risk and indicated patients undergoing Impella-protected percutaneous coronary intervention: Report from the Roma-Verona Registry. *J Int Card.* 2019:5243913; Fig. 4.)

- Appropriate lesion preparation with atherectomy and specialty balloons
- Use of intravascular imaging to assure maximal stent area (i.e., expansion) before completion of procedure
- Use of invasive hemodynamics to assist in support device management/decision making
- After the procedure:
  - Patient monitored in unit familiar with care of patients after large-bore sheath implantation
  - Assure appropriate medical therapy prescribed before discharge, including restarting anticoagulation for patients with atrial fibrillation, emphasis on plan for dual-antiplatelet therapy (specific agents and duration), as well as emphasizing guideline-directed medical therapy for coronary artery disease (e.g., statin, beta-blocker, angiotensin-converting enzyme [ACE] inhibitor)
  - Follow-up plan for staged revascularization and/or reassessment of LV function

Key References

Burzotta F, Russo G, Ribichini F, et al. Long-term outcomes of extent of revascularization in complex high risk and indicated patients undergoing Impella-protected percutaneous coronary intervention: report from the Roma-Verona Registry. *J Int Card.* 2019:5243913.

Kim SH, Bannan S, Behness M, Borggrefe M, Akin I. Patient selection for protected percutaneous coronary intervention: who benefits the most. *Card Clinics.* 2020;38:507-516.

Rihal CS, Naidu SS, Givertz MM, et al. 2015 SCAI/ACC/HFSA/STS clinical expert consensus statement on the use of percutaneous mechanical circulatory support devices in cardiovascular care. *J Am Coll Cardiol.* 2015;65:e7-e26.

References

Al-Khadra Y, Alaries C, Darmoch F, et al. Outcomes of nonemergent percutaneous coronary intervention requiring mechanical circulatory support in patients without cardiogenic shock. *Catheter Cardiovasc Interv.* 2020;95:503-512.

Burzotta F, Lassen JF, Barning AP, et al. Percutaneous coronary intervention in left main coronary artery disease: the 13th consensus document from the European bifurcation club. *EuroIntervention.* 2018;14:112-120.

McCabe JM, Kaki AA, Pinto DS, et al. Percutaneous axillary access for placement of microaxial ventricular support devices: The Axillary Access Registry to Monitor Safety (ARMS). *Circ Cardiovasc Interv.* 2021;14. https://doi.org/10.1161/CIRCINTERVENTIONS.120.009657.

O'Neill WW, Kleinman NS, Moses J, et al. A prospective, randomized clinical trial of hemodynamic support with Impella 2.5 versus intra-aortic balloon pump in patients undergoing high-risk intervention. The PROTECT II Study. *Circulation.* 2012;126:1717-1727.

Riley R, Henry TD, Mahmoud E, et al. SCAI position statement on optimal percutaneous coronary interventional therapy for complex coronary artery disease. *Catheter Cardiovasc Interv.* 2020;96:346-362.

Sorajja P, Borlaug BA, Dimas VV, et al. SCAI/HFSA clinical expert consensus document on the use of invasive hemodynamics for the diagnosis and management of cardiovascular disease. *Catheter Cardiovasc Interv.* 2017;89:E223-E247.

Wollmuth J, Korngold E, Croce K, Pinto DS. The single-access for Hi-risk PCI (ShiP) technique. *Catheter Cardiovasc Interv.* 2020;96(1):114–116.

Coils, Plugs, Covered Stents, and Snares

DHAVAL KOLTE • DOUGLAS E. DRACHMAN

KEY POINTS

- Coils, plugs, covered stents, and snares are invaluable components of the interventional "toolbox" with a wide range of emergency and nonemergency applications.

- Coils, vascular plugs, and covered stents can be used effectively for the treatment of coronary or saphenous vein graft (SVG) aneurysms, pseudoaneurysms, and fistulas.

- Coils and/or covered stents are more commonly used in the management of coronary perforations.

- Vascular plugs have been increasingly used in adult structural heart disease interventions for the treatment of paravalvular leak (PVL) in patients with bioprosthetic or mechanical aortic or mitral valve replacement.

- Snares are useful for retrieval of broken or embolized equipment in the coronary or peripheral vascular system and to capture the distal wire tip to create a "rail" to facilitate a variety of coronary and structural procedures (e.g., retrograde chronic total occlusion percutaneous coronary intervention [PCI], paravalvular leak [PVL] closure, transcaval access).

Disclosures:
Dhaval Kolte, MD, PhD, FACC, FSCAI: None
Douglas E. Drachman, MD, FACC, FSCAI: Abbott Vascular (consulting), Boston Scientific (consulting), Atrium Medical (research grant support), Broadview Ventures (consulting), Cardiovascular Systems Inc (consulting).

Coils, plugs, covered stents, and snares are invaluable components of the interventional "toolbox." Although these devices are used for treatment of some uncommon conditions, such as coronary or saphenous vein graft (SVG) aneurysms and pseudoaneurysms, their main applications are in the emergency management of complications that can arise during diagnostic or interventional coronary procedures. As such, it is important for interventional cardiologists to be familiar with these devices and their technical attributes to use them efficiently and effectively in emergency situations. This chapter provides an overview of the various coils, plugs, covered stents, and snares available and some applications for the use of each of these devices.

Coils

Devices

The Concerto Detachable Coil System (Medtronic, Minneapolis, MN) consists of nylon or glycolide/L-lactide copolymer (PGLA) fibered helical or three-dimensional (3D) platinum coils and an instant detacher (Fig. 11.1A–B). The nylon and PGLA fibers increase thrombogenicity of the coils compared with bare metal equivalents, and the LatticeFX technology promotes thrombosis response. The Concerto Helix coils are available in 2 to 20 mm diameter with a minimum microcatheter compatibility of 0.0165 inches (for 2–4 mm diameter coils) or 0.021 inches (for 5–20 mm diameter coils). The Concerto PGLA 3D coils are available in 2 to 18 mm diameter with 0.0165-inch microcatheter compatibility for up to 10 mm coils. The AXIUM Detachable Coils (Medtronic, Minneapolis, MN; see Fig. 11.1C–E) have an outer diameter of 0.014 inches and can be delivered through smaller microcatheters such as Corsair/Caravel (Asahi Intecc USA, Tustin, CA) or Turnpike (Teleflex, Morrisville, NC). The Concerto and AXIUM coils are fully resheathable after complete or partial deployment and are therefore easy to reposition.

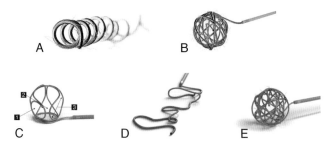

Figure 11.1 Coils. The Concerto Helix (A), Concerto 3D (B), AXIUM PRIME FRAME (C), AXIUM PRIME SOFT (D), and AXIUM MICROFX (E) detachable coils are shown. (Reproduced with permission from Medtronic.)

The AZUR Embolization System (Terumo Interventional Systems, Somerset, NJ) consists of a family of coils: Framing Coil, CX, and Hydrocoil. The AZUR Hydrocoils consist of hydrogel that expands four to five times the original size in the presence of blood to create a mechanical occlusion. The coils are available in diameters ranging from 2 to 20 mm and have a detachable or pushable system. The 0.018-inch coils can be delivered via microcatheters with inner diameter of 0.021 to 0.027 inches, whereas the 0.035-inch coils require diagnostic catheters with inner diameters of 0.038 to 0.047 inches for delivery.

Other peripheral embolization coil systems include the Boston Scientific pushable coils (Boston Scientific, Marlborough, MA), which are available in six shapes (complex helical, VortX, VortX Diamond, straight, figure 8, and multi-loop/two-dimensional [2D] helical) and have highly thrombogenic dense Dacron fibers; the pushable (Nestor, Tornado, MReye, Hilal) or detachable (Retracta, MReye Flipper) fibered embolization coils and microcoils from Cook Medical (Bloomington, IN); and the Ruby Coil Large-Volume and Low-Profile Systems (Penumbra Inc., Alameda, CA).

Applications

Peripheral embolization coils can be used to occlude coronary artery aneurysms, SVG aneurysms, coronary artery fistulas, and left internal mammary artery (LIMA) side branches that cause coronary steal phenomenon in patients with LIMA to left anterior descending coronary artery bypass grafts. For treatment of aneurysms, large-diameter framing/filling coils (e.g., Concerto 3D, AXIUM PRIME FRAME, AZUR Framing/CX, Helical/VortX Diamond, or Ruby Coil) are delivered within the aneurysmal sac. This can be performed directly or using one of the stent-assisted techniques in which a noncovered stent is deployed across the aneurysm and coils delivered into the aneurysm sac through the stent struts or coils delivered via a microcatheter into the aneurysm jailed by a coronary balloon followed by placement of a noncovered stent. Often, occluding the inflow is necessary to achieve complete cessation of flow into the aneurysm sac. This can be accomplished with packing coils (e.g., Concerto Helix, AXIUM PRIME SOFT or MICROFX, AZUR Hydrocoil, VortX, or Tornado) or by deploying a vascular plug in the proximal nonaneurysmal part of the coronary artery (if the distal coronary is known to be occluded or is bypassed), or with the use of covered stents deployed across the aneurysm.

More frequently, embolization coils are used for the management of bleeding from small vessel perforation at the site of vascular access or in a coronary artery. Once a small vessel/branch perforation is identified by angiography, a 0.014-inch workhorse wire is advanced into the branch beyond the site of perforation. A coronary or peripheral microcatheter is then advanced over the wire, through which microcoils (oversized 1–2 mm to the target vessel) may be deployed using either a pushable or a detachable system. A block and deliver (BAD) technique (also known as the "balloon microcatheter technique") has been described in which a balloon is inflated in the vessel proximal to the perforation site to occlude flow, and a microcatheter compatible with at least a 6 French (F) guiding catheter is advanced to the site of perforation over a second parallel guidewire during a very brief deflation of the occluding balloon. A small-volume contrast injection is performed through the microcatheter lumen to confirm persistent extravasation by fluoroscopy, and coils are delivered while maintaining proximal occlusion. The balloon is then deflated, and final angiography is performed to ensure complete cessation of contrast extravasation. In chronic total occlusion (CTO) percutaneous coronary interventions (PCI) via retrograde approach, especially through epicardial collaterals, both antegrade and retrograde coil embolization is often necessary for effective treatment of coronary or collateral perforation (Video 11.1).

Plugs

Devices

The Amplatzer Family of vascular plugs (Abbott Cardiovascular, Plymouth, MN) consist of a disc made of braided nitinol mesh that acts as an embolic agent and promotes clot formation. The disc is attached to a 155-cm long, polytetrafluoroethylene (PTFE)-coated delivery cable with a stainless-steel micro screw, which allows the operator to release the plug into the final position by rotating the cable in a counterclockwise fashion using the supplied torque device. Three types of Amplatzer vascular plugs (AVP) are available in the United States (Fig. 11.2). The AVP is a single-lobe, single-layer device that is available in diameters ranging from 4 to 16 mm that can be delivered through 4 to 6F sheaths. The AVP II is made of a multilayered nitinol mesh designed to increase density and flow disturbance and is available in diameters ranging from 3 to 22 mm compatible with 4F to 7F delivery sheaths. The three lobes of the AVP II create six planes of cross-sectional coverage, resulting in rapid occlusion. The AVP 4 is a bilobed disc designed to reach distal vasculature through tortuous anatomy and can be delivered through an 0.038-inch guidewire compatible diagnostic catheter.

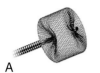 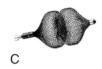

A   B   C

Figure 11.2   Vascular Plugs. The Amplatzer Vascular Plug (AVP) (A), AVP II (B), and AVP 4 (C) are shown. (Amplatzer is a trademark of Abbott or its related companies. Reproduced with permission of Abbott, © 2022. All rights reserved.)

Applications

Although AVPs have a broader range of applications in peripheral endovascular and congenital heart disease interventions, in adults with coronary artery disease, AVPs can be used effectively for the treatment of coronary artery fistulas and coronary artery/SVG aneurysms or pseudoaneurysms. Similarly, in patients with prior coronary artery bypass grafting and failing SVG, after successful PCI of native coronary artery, AVPs can be used to occlude competitive flow via the diseased SVG (Video 11.2). To increase thrombogenicity of the device and prevent migration, it is recommended to oversize the device by approximately 30% to 50% of the target vessel diameter.

AVPs have been increasingly used in adult structural heart disease interventions for the treatment of paravalvular leak (PVL) in patients with bioprosthetic or mechanical aortic or mitral valve replacement. PVL is a serious and underrecognized condition affecting 6% to 15% of surgical prosthetic valves and annuloplasty rings, which—in advanced states—may result in congestive heart failure and/or hemolysis. The majority of aortic PVLs can be closed via the retrograde approach. Closure of mitral PVL may require antegrade (transseptal) or retrograde (transaortic or transapical) approach depending on the location. Cardiac computed tomography and transesophageal echocardiography are used to guide sizing for PVL closure. The choice of device also depends on the shape of the PVL; for a cylindrical leak, AVP II (or Amplatzer Ductal Occluder, Amplatzer Septal Occluder, or Amplatzer Muscular Ventricular Septal Defect Occluder) may be best; for an oval or crescentic leak, the AVP III is ideal. The latter device, however, is not currently available in the United States. For a small leak with significant angulation, AVP 4 is better. Prosthetic leaflet impingement (4%) and device embolization (<1%) are important procedural complications of transcatheter PVL closure.

Covered Stents

Devices

The JOSTENT GRAFTMASTER RX Coronary Stent Graft System (Abbott Cardiovascular, Plymouth, MN) consists of an expandable PTFE (ePTFE) foil membrane sandwiched between two identical stainless-steel stents mounted on a semicompliant balloon (Fig. 11.3A). The stents are available in 2.8, 3.5, 4.0, 4.5, and 4.8 mm diameters and 16, 19, and 26 mm lengths. The 2.8 to 4.0 mm stents can be delivered via a 6F guide, whereas the 4.5 and 4.8 mm stents require a 7F guide catheter. The minimum deployment pressure and rated burst pressure is 15 ATM and 16 ATM, respectively. Maximum stent graft expansion for all sizes is 5.5 mm. Nevertheless, it is important to note that length of the ePTFE foil is shorter than the reported strut length. Thus after expansion of the stent, the ePTFE foil

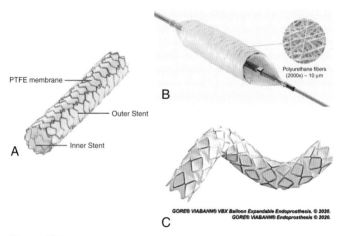

Figure 11.3 Covered Stents. The JOSTENT GRAFTMASTER RX Coronary Stent Graft System (A), PK Papyrus Covered Coronary Stent System (B), and the GORE VIABAHN VBX Balloon Expandable Endoprosthesis (C)* are shown. (Fig. 1A is adapted with permission from Lansky AJ, Yang Y-M, Khan Y, et al. Treatment of coronary artery perforations complicating percutaneous coronary intervention with a polytetrafluoroethylene-covered stent graft. *Am J Cardiol.* 2006;98:370–374. Figures 1B and 1C are reproduced with permission from Biotronik Inc. and W.L. Gore and Associates Inc., respectively. Fig. 1B is protected by copyright [©2020 BIOTRONIK, Inc. All rights reserved]). *See *Instructions for Use* for complete device information, including approved indications and safety information.

may be up to 1.6 mm from each end of the stent graft and the covered length of the stented area may be up to 3.2 mm shorter than the stent length.

In September 2018, the U.S. Food and Drug Administration (FDA) approved the PK Papyrus Covered Coronary Stent System (Biotronik Inc., Lake Oswego, OR) for treatment of coronary artery perforations of native coronary arteries and coronary bypass grafts in vessels 2.5 to 5.0 mm in diameter (see Fig. 11.3B). The PK Papyrus is a cobalt-chromium stent with proBIO (amorphous silicon carbide) coating covered with nonwoven, electrospun polyurethane that creates a thin and highly elastic membrane. The stent is available in 2.5, 3.0, 3.5, 4.0, 4.5, and 5.0 mm diameters and 15, 20, and 26 mm lengths. The 2.5 to 4.0 mm stents can be delivered through a 5F catheter, whereas the 4.5 and 5.0 mm stents require a 6F catheter. Compared with the GRAFT-MASTER, the PK Papyrus covered stents have a smaller crossing profile, greater flexibility, and shorter delivery time.

The GRAFTMASTER and PK Papyrus covered coronary stents are considered humanitarian-use devices (HUD) and are approved by the FDA under the Humanitarian Device Exemption (HDE) Program subject to the Code of Federal Regulations, Title 21, Volume 8 (21 CFR 814). Accordingly, the use of HUDs in the clinical care of patients at a facility requires approval before use by either an Institutional Review Board (IRB) or an appropriate local committee, with the exception of emergency use. In an emergency situation where approval from an IRB cannot be obtained in time to prevent serious harm or death to a patient (e.g., coronary perforation), covered stents can be used without prior approval by an IRB. In such an emergency situation, it is required that the interventionalist provides written notification to the chairman of the IRB within 5 days after the use of the covered stent. Such written notification must include the identification of the patient involved, the date on which the device was used, and the reason for the use.

In addition to the coronary covered stent systems, the GORE VIABAHN VBX Balloon Expandable Endoprosthesis (VBX Stent Graft; W.L. Gore and Associates Inc., Newark, DE) can be used as a covered stent in large aneurysmal coronaries or SVGs (see Fig. 11.3C). The VBX Stent Graft uses the small diameter, ePTFE stent graft technology from the GORE VIABAHN Endoprosthesis. The VBX Stent Graft is available in a range of diameters from 5 to 11 mm and lengths of 15, 19, 29, 39, 59, and 79 mm. The VBX Stent Graft is compatible with 0.035-inch wires and requires a 7 or 8F sheath/catheter to deliver.

Applications

The primary utility of covered stents is in the emergency management of coronary artery perforations (CAP) of native coronary arteries or coronary bypass grafts. CAP is a rare (incidence of 0.3%) but potentially lethal complication of PCI. Chapter 12 provides a comprehensive overview of the management of CAP, whereas here we focus on the use of covered stents in CAP. Once a CAP has been identified by angiography, a balloon should be quickly inflated at or proximal to the site of the CAP to occlude flow. Two techniques to deliver covered stents at the site of the CAP have been described. The single guiding catheter strategy consists of rapid positioning of the covered stent immediately after deflation and retrieval of the occlusion balloon. Delivery of the covered stent can be facilitated with a guide extension (e.g., GuideLiner [Teleflex, Morrisville, NC]), especially in tortuous anatomy. With the availability of the PK Papyrus covered stents, the single guiding catheter technique is the preferred strategy because it is quick and avoids the need for a second arterial access (Video 11.3). In patients with significant hemodynamic compromise, however, a second arterial access and a double guiding catheter strategy ("ping-pong" guiding catheter technique) may be used in which the covered stent is delivered via a second guide catheter across the perforation while the angioplasty balloon is deflated and removed through the first catheter.

Other "off-label" uses of covered stents include for the treatment of coronary or SVG aneurysms or pseudoaneurysms in which a coronary or peripheral covered stent graft is deployed across the aneurysmal segment or neck of the pseudoaneurysm to occlude blood flow into the sac.

Snares

Devices

The Amplatz Goose Neck snares and microsnares (Medtronic, Minneapolis, MN) have a nitinol shaft and a gold-plated tungsten loop (Fig. 11.4A). The snare loop forms a true 90-degree angle, allowing it to remain coaxial to the lumen for proper insertion and successful retrieval or manipulation of atraumatic foreign bodies. The snare kit comes with a Goose Neck snare catheter that has a platinum-iridium radiopaque marker band. The Goose Neck snares are available in diameters ranging from 5 to 35 mm, and the microsnares range from 2 to 7 mm in diameter.

The EN Snare Endovascular System (Merit Medical, Rockland, MA) consists of three interlaced nitinol loops designed to resist prolapse and improve capture by allowing the snare to move as a single-unit through the vessel (see Fig. 11.4B). Platinum strands are incorporated into the EN Snare loops to enhance visualization

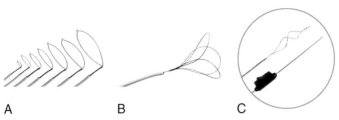

A B C

Figure 11.4   Snares. The Amplatz Goose Neck Snares (A), the EN Snare Endovascular System (B), and the Micro Elite Snare (C) are shown. (Reproduced with permission from Medtronic, Merit Medical, and Teleflex.)

under fluoroscopy. The 6F and 7F snare delivery catheters have a 15-degree curved tip to facilitate vessel navigation. The EN Snares are available in seven configurations with loop diameter sizes ranging from 2 to 45 mm. The ONE Snare Endovascular System (Merit Medical, Rockland, MA) is similar to the Amplatz Goose Neck snares/microsnares.

The Micro Elite Snare (Teleflex, Morrisville, NC) is the only 0.014-inch compatible guidewire-based snare that can be delivered through microcatheters and balloon catheters (see Fig. 11.4C). It has a helical loop design that allows for a smaller profile yet a longer reach than right-angled loops. It is available in 2, 4, and 7 mm diameters and has a handle locking mechanism that facilitates secure capture.

Applications

Snares are used for the manipulation and/or retrieval of atraumatic foreign bodies in the coronary or peripheral vascular system. For example, in case of a kinked sheath or diagnostic/guiding catheter (frequently as a result of overtorquing in the presence of excessive vessel tortuosity) where a guidewire cannot be advanced beyond the kink, a second arterial access is obtained to snare and fix the distal tip of the sheath/catheter (Video 11.4). Securing the distal end of the catheter in this manner may facilitate successful untorquing of the catheter to allow passage of a 0.035-inch or smaller guidewire and subsequent removal of the unkinked catheter. More often, snares are used to retrieve broken or embolized equipment (e.g., catheter or balloon shaft, wire fragment, dislodged/stripped stent, atherectomy device tip). In the event where equipment breaks and embolizes within a coronary artery, whenever possible, wire access through the device should be maintained to provide a direct platform for subsequent retrieval. If the device is separate from the wire, an angioplasty balloon should be inflated as quickly as possible to "pin" the broken fragment against the vessel wall until it can be retrieved to avoid distal or proximal embolization. A microsnare with a loop diameter equal to or 1 mm larger than the target vessel may then be advanced through the guiding catheter distal to the trapped fragment while partially deflating the pinning balloon. The microsnare loop is formed distal to the fragment and retrieved slowly to allow for successful capture and retrieval of the broken device fragment. For retrieval of larger devices (e.g., broken catheter or balloon shaft), a second arterial access and larger than 6F sheath may be necessary to successfully remove the fragment after snaring. Similarly, snares can be used for retrieval of embolized devices in structural heart disease interventions.

Snares are routinely used in various coronary and adult structural heart disease interventions to capture the distal wire tip to create a "rail" to facilitate the procedure. Some examples of this include retrograde CTO PCI, PVL closure, transcaval access, bioprosthetic or native aortic scallop intentional laceration to prevent iatrogenic coronary artery obstruction (BASILICA), and intentional laceration of the anterior mitral valve leaflet to prevent left ventricular outflow tract obstruction (LAMPOON). In transcatheter aortic valve replacement (TAVR), snares can be used for repositioning of self-expanding valves in case of ventricular embolization, to facilitate aortic valve crossing of self-expanding transcatheter heart valve (THV) system, or for externalization of wire after antegrade crossing of the aortic valve (via transapical or transseptal approach) in cases where retrograde crossing is unsuccessful.

Conclusion

Since the first coronary angioplasty procedure was performed by Andreas Gruentzig in 1977, the proliferation of advanced technologies and techniques have permitted treatment of increasingly complex lesions and patients. Correspondingly, the evolution of procedurally associated complications and technical challenges have continued to rise, requiring new devices and techniques to address and resolve such circumstances safely and effectively. Every proceduralist should become familiar with the availability and use of a range of techniques, including the use of coils, plugs, covered stents and snares, to address unforeseen obstacles. Through the judicious use of these technologies, coupled with skill and ingenuity, the interventionalist may treat or potentially avoid complications and improve outcomes for patients.

References

Abdelfattah OM, Saad AM, Kassis N, et al. Utilization and outcomes of transcatheter coil embolization for various coronary artery lesions: single-center 12-year experience. *Catheter Cardiovasc Interv.* 2020;98:1317–1331.

Alkhouli M, Sievert H, Rihal CS. Device embolization in structural heart interventions: incidence, outcomes, and retrieval techniques. *JACC Cardiovasc Interv.* 2019;12: 113-126.

Ando A, Bhopalwala A, Spies C. Transcatheter closure of large bilateral coronary arteriovenous fistulae using Amplatzer vascular plugs. *Int J Clin Cardiol.* 2016;3:080.

Ayub B, Martinez MW, Jaffe AS, Couri DM. Giant saphenous vein graft pseudoaneurysm: treatment with a vascular occlusion device. *Interact Cardiovasc Thorac Surg.* 2012;15:164-165.

Ben-Gal Y, Weisz G, Collins MB, et al. Dual catheter technique for the treatment of severe coronary artery perforations. *Catheter Cardiovasc Interv.* 2010;75:708-712.

Beute TJ, Nolan MA, Merhi WM, Leung Wai Sang S. Use of EN Snare device for successful repositioning of the newest self-expanding transcatheter heart valve. *SAGE Open Med Case Rep.* 2018;6:2050313X18819933.

Eleid MF, Cabalka AK, Malouf JF, Sanon S, Hagler DJ, Rihal CS. Techniques and outcomes for the treatment of paravalvular leak. *Circ Cardiovasc Interv.* 2015;8:e001945.

Gafoor S, Franke J, Bertog S, et al. A quick guide to paravalvular leak closure. *Interv Cardiol.* 2015;10:112-117.

Garbo R, Oreglia JA, Gasparini GL. The Balloon-Microcatheter technique for treatment of coronary artery perforations. *Catheter Cardiovasc Interv.* 2017;89:E75-E83.

Giannini F, Candilio L, Mitomo S, et al. A practical approach to the management of complications during percutaneous coronary intervention. *JACC Cardiovasc Interv.* 2018;11:1797-1810.

Hernandez-Enriquez M, Lairez O, Campelo-Parada F, et al. Outcomes after use of covered stents to treat coronary artery perforations. Comparison of old and new-generation covered stents. *J Interv Cardiol.* 2018;31:617-623.

Kliger C, Eiros R, Isasti G, et al. Review of surgical prosthetic paravalvular leaks: diagnosis and catheter-based closure. *Eur Heart J.* 2013;34:638-649.

Martinez GJ, Valdebenito M, Martinez A, Patel S. Successful percutaneous closure of a ruptured saphenous vein graft aneurysm. *Can J Cardiol.* 2018;34:1370.e1-1370.e3.

Mylonas I, Sakata Y, Salinger MH, Feldman T. Successful closure of a giant true saphenous vein graft aneurysm using the Amplatzer vascular plug. *Catheter Cardiovasc Interv.* 2006;67:611-616.

Nairooz R, Parzynski CS, Curtis JP, et al. Contemporary trends, predictors and outcomes of perforation during percutaneous coronary intervention (From the NCDR Cath PCI Registry). *Am J Cardiol.* 2020;130:37-45.

Qin Q, Chang S, Xu R, et al. Short and long-term outcomes of coronary perforation managed by coil embolization: a single-center experience. *Int J Cardiol.* 2020; 298:18-21.

Spiotta AM, Wheeler AM, Smithason S, Hui F, Moskowitz S. Comparison of techniques for stent assisted coil embolization of aneurysms. *J Neurointerv Surg.* 2012;4: 339-344.

Tarar MN, Christakopoulos GE, Brilakis ES. Successful management of a distal vessel perforation through a single 8-French guide catheter: combining balloon inflation for bleeding control with coil embolization. *Catheter Cardiovasc Interv.* 2015;86: 412-416.

Complications of Percutaneous Coronary Interventions

MICHAEL J. LIM

KEY POINTS

- Complications remain rare during interventional procedures and prediction tools have been developed to help operators appreciate potential risks before the procedure.

- Although avoidance of complications remains the primary goal, keen awareness must exist during the procedure to re-act quickly when complications arise to minimize its impact.

- Access site complications remain the most frequent complications of coronary interventional procedures.

- Cath lab staff and operators must routinely assess prepared-ness for treating complications, including ensuring that everyone is aware of where essential equipment is kept and understands the process of recruiting external help and resources to the lab when needed; it is also important to run "drills" to make sure that staff are skilled in performing key tasks when an emergency arises.

Percutaneous coronary intervention (PCI) is associated with rare but serious complications. Most of the complications are generic to all diagnostic coronary angiography procedures, and some are specific to coronary intervention. Events like death, myocardial infarction (MI), and bleeding occur at higher rates for interventional procedures because there is prolonged procedural time, complexity, and the use of anticoagulation (Tables 12.1 and 12.2). It is critical to understand the possible complications of PCI to provide proper informed consent to the patient. It is also critical to be vigilant and to recognize potential complications at an early

Table 12.1

Event Rates of Diagnostic Versus Percutaneous Coronary Intervention Complications		
Complication	**Event Rate Diagnostic Procedure (%)**	**Event Rate Interventional Procedure (%)**
Death	0.1	1.3
Significant bleed	0.5	5–12
AV fistula	0.75	1.1
Pseudoaneurysm	0.2	1–2
Contrast-induced nephropathy	5	8–57
Periprocedural MI ($>3 \times$ ULN cardiac enzyme)	0.1	8
Air embolism	0.1–0.3	0.1–0.3
Cerebrovascular accident	0.3	0.3
Ventricular arrhythmia	0.4	0.84
Coronary dissection	0.03–0.46	29–50
Aortic dissection	<0.01	0.03
Infection/bacteremia	0.11	0.64
Anaphylactoid reaction to contrast	0.23	0.23
Cholesterol embolization	0.8–1.4	0.8–1.4

AV, Arteriovenous; *MI,* myocardial infarction; *ULN,* upper limits of normal.

Table 12.2

Complications Specific to Percutaneous Coronary Intervention	
Complication	**Event Rate (%)**
No reflow phenomenon	2
Stent thrombosis	2
Vessel perforation	0.84
Stent embolization	0.4–2
Need for emergent bypass surgery	0.15–0.3
Wire fracture	0.1
Stent infection	<0.1 (case reports only)

stage to try to avoid a catastrophic outcome because the most common cause of all post-PCI deaths is from a procedural complication rather than from a preexisting cardiac condition. Fortunately, death is very rare with diagnostic angiography ($<0.1\%$). The mortality rate increases 13 times with the addition of the complexity of PCI to 1.3% (Table 12.3).

Table 12.3

Modes of Death During Percutaneous Coronary Intervention	
Mode of Death	**Event Rate (%)**
Low output failure	66.1
Ventricular arrhythmias	10.7
Stroke	4.1
Preexisting renal failure	4.1
Bleeding	2.5
Ventricular rupture	2.5
Respiratory failure	2.5
Pulmonary embolism	1.7
Infection	1.7

Adapted from Malenka DJ, O'Rourke D, Miller MA, et al. Cause of in-hospital death in 12,232 consecutive patients undergoing percutaneous transluminal coronary angioplasty. *Am Heart J.* 1999;137(4):633; Table 1.

Complications of PCI can occur at any step of the procedure, from the administration of sedation to the transfer as the patient leaves the laboratory. This chapter will discuss many of the possible complications in the order that they might be encountered during the procedure.

Preprocedural Planning and Risk Prediction

Previously, operators in the catheterization (cath) lab attempted to improve outcomes by decreasing access-related complications— mainly by moving toward smaller French (F) sized sheaths and eventually by embracing radial artery catheterizations. Over the past years, the cath lab environment has changed with more widespread adoption of PCI for chronic total occlusions (CTOs) and large-bore femoral access for the insertion of mechanical support devices to support higher-risk and challenging PCI procedures. In taking on these higher-complexity procedures, increasing complications (numerically) logically follow. Therefore it may be worth understanding the contributors to mortality associated with "modern" PCI.

A recent review of PCI procedures revealed that the factors most strongly associated with mortality were salvage PCI procedures, patients in refractory shock, or those undergoing PCI while in cardiogenic shock (Fig 12.1A). Nevertheless, emergency PCI in patients without shock was also strongly associated with mortality, as was PCI performed in patients with advanced chronic kidney disease. As noted in Fig. 12.1B, most of the mortality after PCI is isolated in those at the highest risk. The Society for Cardiovascular Angiography and Interventions (SCAI) also has a risk calculator that can inform treating physicians about procedural risk (http:// scaipciriskapp.org/porc).

All patients who present for PCI with a higher risk for mortality should have a documented discussion with the institution's "Heart Team" (consisting of cardiac surgery, interventional cardiology, and the treating physician[s]) regarding the nuances of proceeding

Predictors (full model)			
Age	Female	Salvage PCI or refractory shock	Number of diseased vessels
CVD	PAD	Cardiogenic shock without salvage	Highest risk lesion- Left main
CLD	CKD	CVI without shock/salvage	Highest risk lesion- Proximal LAD
Prior PCI	Diabetes	Emergency PCI without shock/CVI	CTO
Frailty	Aortic stenosis	Urgent PCI without shock/CVI	In-stent thrombosis
LVEF	SBP	Cardiac arrest - Responsive	
STEMI	Surgical turndown	Cardiac arrest - Unresponsive	

Bedside risk score			
Predictor	**Points**	**Predictor**	**Points**
Age (for every 10-year increase)	1	Salvage PCI or refractory shock	13
CKD stage (GFR)		Cardiogenic shock without salvage	11
Stage 3a CKD (GFR 45–60)	1	CVI without shock/salvage	7
Stage 3b CKD (GFR 30–44)	2	Emergency PCI without shock/CVI	6
Stage 4 CKD (GFR 15–29)	3	Urgent PCI without shock/CVI	3
Stage 5 CKD (GFR 0–14 or dialysis)	3	Cardiac arrest - Responsive	1
		Cardiac arrest - Unresponsive	5

A

Figure 12.1 Predictors of Mortality After Percutaneous Coronary Intervention (PCI). (A) Top portion shows clinical features that were predictive of mortality after PCI, and the lower panel shows relative weight (points) that these factors had in developing the post-PCI mortality risk model. *Continued*

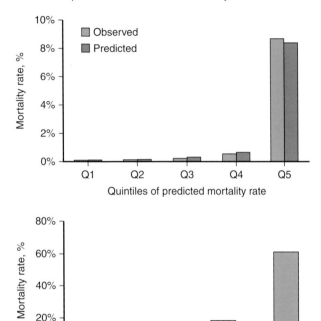

Figure 12.1, cont'd (B) Left shows observed and predicted mortality in patients post-PCI as observed by quintile of risk and right shows the distribution of patients according to risk score. (From Castro-Dominguez YS, Wang Y, Minges KE, et al. Predicting in-hospital mortality in patients undergoing percutaneous coronary intervention. *J Am Coll Cardiol.* 2021;78:216–229; Central Illustration.)

with a catheter-based procedure despite higher risk. Furthermore, the patient, the patient's family, and all the team members in the cath lab should be fully aware of this discussion and the risk of the procedure before proceeding.

Complications

As previously stated, complications in the cath lab remain a rare occurrence, and this creates a barrier to prompt recognition and potential treatment because most in the lab will not have the benefit of experience in complication recognition. Some have advocated for "protocolized" thinking when overall experiential knowledge has difficulty guiding decision making. One such protocol was put together by a group of experienced operators to go through the "basic" steps when a complication is suspected (Fig. 12.2). The key aspect to this flow chart is the importance of assessing the hemodynamic stability of the patient and calling for help early.

To ensure as much preparedness for complications and emergent scenarios as possible, labs should consider conducting "mock" events—practicing the steps needed to deal with potentially catastrophic emergencies and having team members perform their defined roles during the emergency on a regular basis.

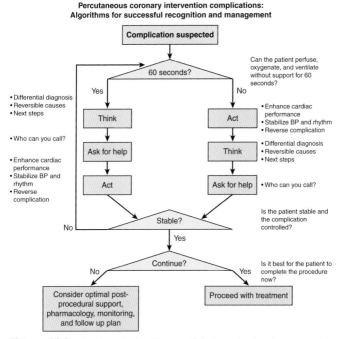

Figure 12.2 Suggested algorithm outlining a step-by-step approach when a complication is suspected in the cath lab. (From Doll JA, Hira RS, Kearney KE, et al. Management of percutaneous coronary intervention complications: Algorithms from the 2018 and 2019 Seattle percutaneous coronary intervention complications conference. *Circ Cardiovasc Interv.* 2020;13[6]:e008962; Fig. 1.)

Box 12.1	**Recommended Equipment and Resources for Managing PCI Complications**
In the Room	Mechanical circulatory support tools/devices (ECMO or Impella)
	ACLS drugs, airway management tools (Crash Cart)
	Defibrillator
	Ability to rapidly call for help (code button)
On a Cart / Immediately Accessible	Pericardiocentesis tray
	Covered stents
	Coils and microcatheters suitable for delivery
	Snares
	Thrombin/microspheres
In-Hospital (with ability to rapidly respond)	Cardiothoracic surgeon and team (including perfusionist)
	Vascular surgeon
	Echocardiography
	Critical Care Team

ACLS, Advanced Cardiovascular Life Support; *ECMO,* extracorporeal membrane oxygenation; *PCI,* percutaneous coronary intervention.
Modified from Doll JA, Hira RS, Kearney KE, et al. Management of percutaneous coronary intervention complications: Algorithms from the 2018 and 2019 Seattle percutaneous coronary intervention complications conference. *Circ Cardiovasc Interv.* 2020;13(6):e008962.

Furthermore, Box 12.1 outlines equipment and resources that every lab should make sure that they have accounted for before performing any PCI.

Vascular Access

The first part of any PCI begins with vascular access. Using the femoral access, the major complications are femoral artery dissections (Fig. 12.3), pseudoaneurysm, arteriovenous (AV) fistula, and retroperitoneal bleeding. As seen in Table 12.1, the incidence of these complications is increased compared with a strictly diagnostic procedure. All arterial complications are markedly reduced (but are not eliminated) using the radial artery access.

Femoral Access Complications

Pseudo-Aneurysm

Often associated with a low puncture, a femoral artery pseudoaneurysm represents a failure of sealing of the initial arterial puncture site, allowing arterial blood to flow into the surrounding tissue. This

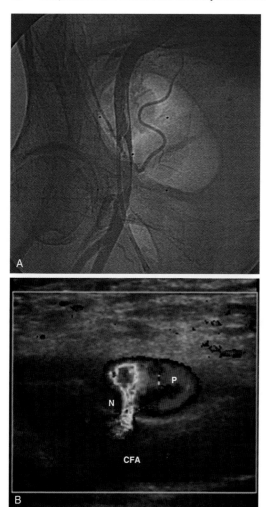

Figure 12.3 (A) Cine angiogram frame of femoral artery dissection. This problem may be associated with limb ischemia or bleeding. It may require surgery but more often can be treated by contralateral access and implantation of iliac stent. (B) Ultrasound picture of a pseudoaneurysm (*P*) arising from the common femoral artery (CFA). The circular color object is the hematoma, which is fed by blood flow from the artery through the characteristic narrow neck (*N*). (From Ahmad F, Turner SA, Torrie P, et al. Iatrogenic femoral artery pseudoaneurysms—a review of current methods of diagnosis and treatment. *Clin Radiol.* 2008;63:1310–1316; Fig. 1.)

forms a pulsatile hematoma that acts as the covering roof over the aneurysm (see Fig. 12.3). Pseudoaneurysms are late appearing, associated with local pain and swelling, and diagnosed with femoral ultrasound with an excellent sensitivity of 94% to 97%. There are multiple risk factors for pseudoaneurysm (Box 12.2).

Small pseudoaneurysms (<2 cm) often close spontaneously within 1 month. In larger pseudoaneurysms, or in small ones that fail to close, active treatment is necessary. The two most common treatment methods are ultrasound-guided compression or thrombin injection. In some hospitals, ultrasound-guided compression is not offered because of increased stress-related wrist injury to the ultrasound technician. Other advantages of thrombin injection over ultrasound compression are seen in Box 12.3.

Thrombin injection can be performed by diluting 1000 U thrombin in a 1-mL syringe with normal saline (final concentration of 100 U per 0.1 mL) and injecting with direct ultrasound visualization through a long 22-gauge needle until thrombus is formed in the pseudoaneurysm cavity and Doppler-detected flow is abolished (Fig. 12.4). Rarely, in very large pseudoaneurysms and those resistant to thrombin injection, vascular surgery is required.

Box 12.2   Risk Factors for Pseudoaneurysm Formation

Procedural Factors

Catheterization of both artery and vein
  Cannulation of the superficial femoral or profunda femoris rather than common femoral
  Inadequate compression after procedure
  More anticoagulation used

Patient Factors

Obesity
  Hemodialysis
  Calcified arteries

Box 12.3   Advantages of Thrombin Injection Compared With Ultrasound Compression for Management of Pseudoaneurysm

Greater technical success (96% vs. 74%)
  Less painful to the patient and technician
  No conscious sedation required
  Effective in patients on anticoagulation
  Can be used in pseudoaneurysms above the inguinal ligament

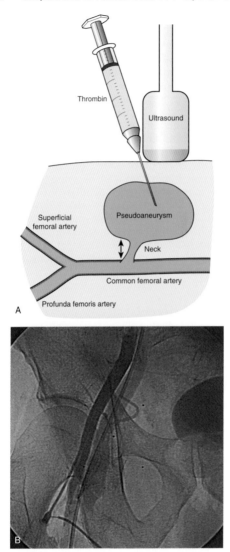

Figure 12.4 (A) Schematic representation of the technique used to inject thrombin into a pseudoaneurysm under ultrasound guidance. (B) Cine angiogram of arteriovenous fistula. Contrast visualized in the vein returning cranially indicates a communication with the artery (i.e., a fistula). Treatment is described in the text. (A, from Ahmad F, Turner SA, Torrie P, et al. Iatrogenic femoral artery pseudoaneurysms—a review of current methods of diagnosis and treatment. *Clin Radiol*. 2008;63:1310; Fig. 3.)

Arteriovenous Fistula

Another complication of vascular access is a femoral AV fistula formation (see Fig. 12.4). This is recognized on physical examination by a palpable thrill or an audible continuous bruit. Unlike pseudoaneurysms, conservative treatment with watchful waiting is the most common treatment modality (90%), which is likely related to the fact that AV fistulae produce low shunt blood flow volumes (160–510 mL/min) compared with most large intracardiac (e.g., left to right) shunts or dialysis shunts (1000 mL/min). One-third of persistent AV fistulae will close during the first 12 months. Most persistent AV fistulae are asymptomatic and do not require repair. Rarely, they can be symptomatic (moderate pain) and, in large patient series, about 10% of AV fistulae will ultimately require surgical repair. AV shunt flows must exceed 30% of the cardiac output to produce symptoms, and therefore it is quite rare to have a truly symptomatic shunt from a femoral AV fistula. The main risk factor for development of an AV fistula is a low femoral arterial puncture, which is responsible for almost 85% of all AV fistulae.

Infection

A rare complication of groin access is systemic infection. SCAI has detailed infection control guidelines for the cardiac cath lab. Proper sterile technique, including hand-washing and use of hats, masks, gown, and gloves, has limited bacterial infections to only 0.64% of interventional cases, with septic complications occurring in only 0.24% of cases. Routine antibiotic prophylaxis is *not* recommended before cardiac catheterization. Nevertheless, if there is any concern for contamination of the femoral sheath (transport between rooms, patient touching site, changing out sheaths in a delayed procedure), it is standard to give 1 g cephalexin as a prophylactic measure. If the patient is allergic, 1 g of vancomycin can be given alternatively.

An equally concerning infectious complication is the exposure of the physicians or staff to the patient's potential pathogens. Universal precautions are to be followed by everyone in the catheterization laboratory. If there is an occupational exposure, proper management per hospital guidelines should be followed. See Box 12.4 for U.S. Public Health Service guidelines.

Bleeding

The last and most dangerous complication of groin access is major femoral bleeding. Large femoral hematomas have an incidence of

> ## Box 12.4 Management of Occupational Exposure to Hepatitis B Virus, Hepatitis C Virus, and HIV
>
> I. Definition: Direct contact with blood or body fluids (including percutaneous injury), contact of mucous membranes, or skin contact, especially if abraded.
> II. Procedure
>   A. Clean site of exposure with soap and copious amounts of water; flush mucous membrane with large quantities of water.
>   B. Victim should report incident promptly, including patient/source information.
>   C. Provide wound care and review with victim tetanus and hepatitis B prophylaxis information.
>   D. Counsel and obtain consent for HIV testing from both victim and patient/source.
>   E. Order the following laboratory specimen with appropriate consent obtained:
>   1. Victim: hepatitis C antibody, hepatitis B surface antigen, HIV
>   2. Patient: hepatitis B surface antigen and core antibody, hepatitis C antibody, ALT, RPR, HIV
>   F. Review hepatitis B vaccination and response status of victim and follow postexposure prophylaxis to hepatitis B protocol.
>   G. If patient is hepatitis C positive or has elevated ALT:
>   1. Follow postexposure prophylaxis to hepatitis B protocol.
>   2. Follow up for anti-HIV therapy per protocol.
>   3. Schedule hepatitis C and HIV testing for 6 weeks, 3 months, and 6 months.

ALT, Alanine aminotransferase; *HIV,* human immunodeficiency virus; *RPR,* rapid plasma reagin.
Adapted from Chambers C, Eisenhauer M, McNicol L, et al. Infection control guidelines for the cardiac catheterization laboratory: Society guidelines revisited. *Catheter Cardiovasc Interv.* 2006;67:85; Table 2.

2.8% compared with a 0.3% incidence of retroperitoneal bleeds. A retroperitoneal hematoma or a significant femoral hematoma (>5 cm) often requires blood transfusions and prolonged hospitalization. More significant bleeds can require surgery, and significant bleeding in relation to PCI has been shown to correlate with mortality. Significant risk factors for major femoral bleeding are listed in Table 12.4.

The bleeding complication of most concern is a retroperitoneal hematoma because large amounts of blood can fill the pelvic cavity, and shock can develop rapidly. If a retroperitoneal bleed is suspected (Box 12.5), volume (crystalloid solutions) should be given, and blood should be ordered immediately for transfusion as soon as available. A vascular surgeon should also be consulted immediately. If the patient remains hemodynamically unstable despite

Table 12.4

Significant Risk Factors for Major Femoral Bleeding	
Risk Factor	**Odds Ratio**
Age >75 vs. <55	2.59
Heparin use after procedure	2.46
Severe renal impairment	2.25
Age 65–74 vs. <55	2.18
Female patient	1.64
Closure device use	1.58
Sheath size 7F–8F vs. <6F	1.53
GP IIb/IIIa use	1.39
Longer procedure duration	1.2

F, French; *GP*, glycoprotein.
Adapted from Doyle B, Ting HH, Bell MR, et al. Major femoral bleeding complications after PCI. *JACC Cardiovasc Interv.* 2008;1(2):202–209.

Box 12.5   Classical Signs and Symptoms of Retroperitoneal Bleed

Hypotension
  Bradycardia
  Back/flank pain
  Groin pain
  Abdominal pain
  Transient response to fluid loading
  Grey Turner sign (bruising along flank) [late appearing]
  Cullen sign (bruising around umbilicus) [late appearing]

---

volume resuscitation, surgery or endovascular repair (covered stent placement) may be needed; this occurs in approximately 16% of patients. Nevertheless, the majority (84%) of cases can undergo a conservative "watchful waiting" strategy because the hematoma usually stabilizes from tamponade of the initial site of extravasation. A computed tomography (CT) scan will be confirmative of the clinical diagnosis and should only be ordered once the patient is stable. Vascular surgeons use the CT scan as a baseline study and as a method to localize the origin of the bleed (if radiographic contrast media is used). Most retroperitoneal hematomas are caused by bleeding from a high puncture of the external iliac artery above the inguinal ligament or inferior epigastric artery. Rarely, bleeding below the inguinal ligament can track between tissue planes and extend into a retroperitoneal accumulation. Bleeding might also rarely extend to the scrotum through extension along the spermatic cord. Most cases of scrotal hematoma can also be managed conservatively with elevation and ice. Rarely, however, large tense scrotal hematomas can cause significant pain and may compromise the viability of the scrotal skin and/or testicle, which would require urgent surgical exploration (Fig. 12.5).

Complications of Radial Access

See Fig. 12.6.

Radial Artery Occlusion

In 2% to 10% of cases, the radial artery may not be found to be patent after radial catheterization procedures; however, in most instances, the consequence of this complication is felt to be quite benign. This is mainly because of the nature of the dual circulation that exists between the radial artery and ulnar artery in supplying the hand with blood flow. When found to be intact by an Allen or Barbeau test before the procedure, circulation is believed to be intact from the ulnar artery through the palmar arch to supply the thumb and first finger with flow, thereby eliminating the

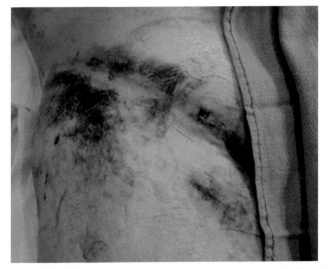

Figure 12.5 Picture of a patient after a cardiac catheterization using femoral access who developed a large hematoma. (Courtesy Dr. Zoltan Turi.)

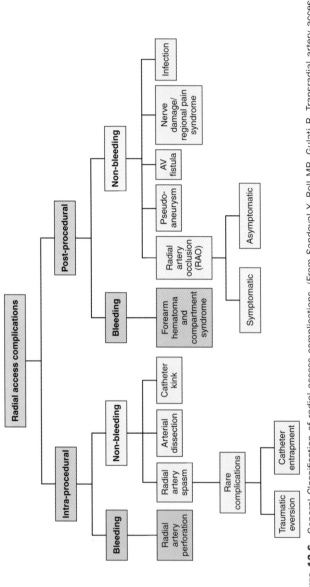

Figure 12.6 General Classification of radial access complications. (From Sandoval Y, Bell MR, Gulati R. Transradial artery access complications. *Circ Cardiovasc Interv.* 2019;12[11]:e007386; Fig. 1.)

complication of hand ischemia should the patency of the radial artery not remain after the procedure. Factors believed to be associated with radial occlusion include lack of adequate anticoagulation, too large a sheath size compared with the vessel size (e.g., consider 5F sheaths for smaller patients and women), prolonged and aggressive post-procedure compression without maintenance of forward flow, and repeat cannulations of the same radial artery.

When the radial artery has been imaged months after a radial catheterization, it has been noted that there is intimal hyperplasia within the radial artery with diffuse narrowing. This has been termed *nonocclusive radial artery injury,* but, again, has not been associated with any serious complications from a patient standpoint.

Radial Artery Spasm

In 12% to 22% of cases, spasm of the vessel may occur and is frequently because of significant $alpha_1$ adrenoceptors within the medial layer of the vessel; it is overcome and minimized using vasodilators (e.g., intraarterial verapamil and/or nitroglycerin). Occasionally, it has been reported that a severe spasm entraps the catheter or long sheath so that it cannot be withdrawn. This diffuse and severe spasm has been managed by increased sedation, sometimes requiring a local nerve block or induction of general anesthesia. Care should be taken to never "force" the withdrawal of a catheter or sheath when resistance has been met because radial artery evulsion has also been reported (Fig. 12.7).

Forearm Bleeding, Hematoma, and Compartment Syndrome

Bleeding within the forearm can arise if a perforation occurs anywhere within the course of the radial artery (Figs. 12.8 and 12.9). This can occur particularly with the use of hydrophilic guidewires (as opposed to nonhydrophilic J-tipped wires), which can advance into small side branches without much appreciated resistance felt by the operator. Furthermore, navigating anatomic variants such as a radial recurrent loop also increases the risk for perforation. Bertrand et al. studied this in a patient population that had all undergone radial artery catheterizations and subsequent interventions and classified the bleeding by grade. Bleeds were characterized as follows – Grade I: superficial hematoma 5 cm or less in diameter (5.3% occurrence), Grade II: superficial hematoma 10 cm or less in diameter (2.5% occurrence), Grade III: hematoma greater than 10 cm but contained below the level of the elbow (1.6% occurrence), Grade IV: hematoma extending above

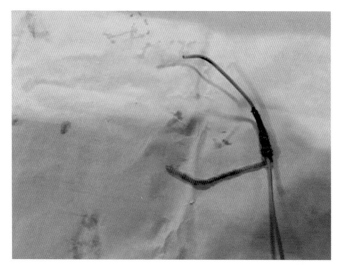

Figure 12.7 A patient underwent catheterization via the right radial approach and a 5 French (F) Tig catheter was used. During manipulation of the catheter, the patient reported severe forearm pain and the procedure was stopped. A 0.035-inch j-tipped wire was placed inside of the Tig catheter, and it was withdrawn, but resistance was noted when it reached the patient's elbow. Additional sedation, intra-arterial calcium channel blockers, and nitrates were delivered. There continued to be resistance when the catheter was pulled, and general anesthesia was induced. The Tig was then able to be slowly pulled back and upon inspection after withdrawal, a 6 to 7 cm length of vascular tissue accompanied the catheter (pictured). Prolonged manual pressure of the brachial artery was performed, and the patient had no long-term complications aside from being found to no longer have a radial arterial pulse. (From Kumar V, Kumar A, Vaddera S, Kumar M. Avulsion of a radial artery during coronary angiogram – a case report. *IHJ Cardiovasc Case Reports.* 2017;1[2]:80–82; Fig. 1.)

the elbow (0.1%), and Grade V: any bleed associated with an ischemic threat to the hand (0% occurrence). The keys to bleeding within the forearm are therefore prevention and recognition. Prevention can be achieved by avoiding hydrophilic straight guidewires for the most part. Bleeding must be recognized in the event of a hematoma or pain within the forearm after the procedure. If the sheath is still in place, angiography can demonstrate extravasation of contrast and thus the location of the bleed. Compression, often achieved with an ACE bandage wrapped around the entire forearm, and avoidance of further anticoagulation are often enough to avoid further complication.

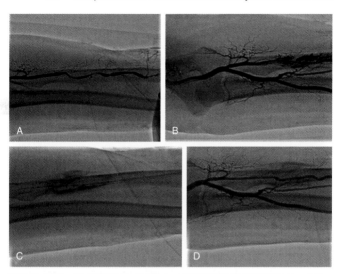

Figure 12.8 Radial Artery Rupture and Salvage During Coronary Intervention Through the Radial Artery. (A) Radial artery angiography through a 2.7 French (F) pressure arterial sheath after generous intraarterial nitroglycerin and verapamil administration, revealing diffuse spasm of the entry site and stenosis of the middle portion of the radial artery. (B) Radial artery angiography through a 6F sheath, revealing rupture of the radial artery. (C) Prolonged balloon inflation. (D) Sealing and stenosis resolution after prolonged balloon inflation. (From Rigatelli G, Dell'Avvocata F, Ronco F, Doganov A. Successful coronary angioplasty via the radial approach after sealing a radial perforation. *J Am Coll Cardiol Interv.* 2009;2[11]:1158–1159; Fig. 1.)

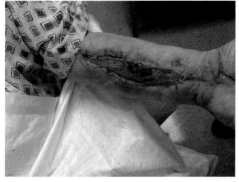

Figure 12.9 Photography of surgical repair with skin graft after compartment syndrome resulting from bleeding into the forearm.

Nevertheless, bleeding into the forearm can result in increased pressure within the fascial planes and resultant compartment syndrome. This would be the most serious complication from radial artery catheterization because it threatens the entire hand and must be recognized and treated emergently in concert with vascular surgery, and so the vascular surgeon should be alerted immediately upon suspecting this potential complication. Measurement of interfascial pressure with a manometer confirms the diagnosis, and fasciotomy with hematoma evacuation remains the only treatment available.

Complications of Vascular Access Closure Devices

Most femoral arterial access sites are closed in the laboratory with percutaneous vascular closure devices. Hemostasis success rates are less than 100% but very high. Each device has failure modes particular to its mechanism of action. Suture fractures or failure to deliver a knot (Prostar, Perclose), clip failure (StarClose), collagen introduction or emboli into the vessel (Angio-Seal), or any failure to seal the puncture site can cause femoral or retroperitoneal bleeding. All vascular complications, including pseudoaneurysm, bleeding and hematoma, infection, arterial stenosis or occlusion, and venous thrombosis, can occur with an incidence of approximately 1% to 5%.

Compared with manual compression, percutaneous closure device complications tend to have a greater incidence of pseudoaneurysms not amenable to ultrasound compression therapy, a greater loss of blood and need for transfusions, a greater incidence of arterial stenosis or occlusion, the need for more extensive surgical repair, and a greater incidence of groin infections. Thus patients treated with vascular closure devices merit as much if not more attention to vascular complications than those treated with manual compression.

Atheroembolism

After vascular access is obtained, the guide catheter is advanced over a guidewire along the aorta to finally seat in the coronary artery of interest. The guidewire protects the vessels from the guide catheter scraping against the aortic wall and causing atheroembolism. This is even more common in larger diameter guide catheters. The guidewire itself can also cause atheroembolism. To minimize atheroembolism, always aspirate blood from the catheter to clear any debris that might have been picked up in transit. If a guide catheter is connected to a Y-connector during advancement, the valve should be cleared before proceeding.

Peripheral atheroembolism with obstruction of small arteries and arterioles by cholesterol crystals is known to produce the cholesterol embolization syndrome (CES), a rare occurrence (incidence of 0.75%–1.4%) using the preceding precautions. Cholesterol emboli are diagnosed by one of three cutaneous signs (Box 12.6 and Fig. 12.10) and an elevated eosinophil count.

Box 12.6 Cutaneous Signs of Cholesterol Embolization Syndrome

Livedo reticularis
    Blue toe syndrome (also known as *purple toe syndrome or trash foot*)
    Digital gangrene

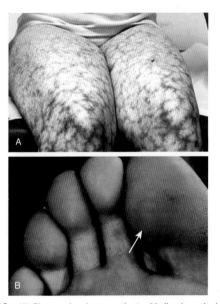

Figure 12.10 (A) Picture showing a patient with livedo reticularis on both legs secondary to the "showering" of emboli after a cardiac catheterization. (B) Picture of a patient's foot depicting the typical findings of cholesterol emboli to the great toe (*arrow*) after cardiac catheterization. (A from Kauke T, Reininger A. Livedo reticularis and cold agglutinins. *N Engl J Med*. 2007;356:284. B from Venzon R, Bromet D, Schaer G. Use of corticosteroids in the treatment of cholesterol crystal embolization after percutaneous transluminal coronary angioplasty. *J Invas Cardiol*. 2004;16[4]:222–223.)

In-hospital mortality is as high as 16% in those patients with definite CES because multiorgan embolization often can lead to multiorgan failure.

Atheroembolism can also cause a cerebral vascular accident (CVA) or transient ischemic attack (TIA). The overall incidence of TIA (0.04%) or CVA (0.25%) is quite low after PCI. There are various multivariate predictors of in-hospital CVA (Table 12.5).

The most common indicator of a periprocedural TIA or CVA is motor or speech deficits. In-hospital death can occur in up to 25% of those with a CVA, but increased mortality is not expected with a TIA. Management follows recommendations of the neurologic consultation. If a stroke occurs during the procedure, consideration should be given for an emergent neurointervention with resultant cerebral angiography and intervention if an ischemic stroke with arterial occlusion is found. If a stroke occurs after the procedure, as confirmed by advanced imaging (Fig. 12.11), thrombolysis can be considered (after hemorrhagic stroke has been ruled out).

Complications Related to Guide Catheters, Balloons, Stents, and Intravascular Devices

The guide catheter itself can cause coronary dissection with or without extension to the aortic root. Guide catheter–related dissection is a rare event with a reported incidence of 0.03% to 0.3%. The

Table 12.5

Independent Predictors of In-Hospital Cardiovascular Accident	
Predictor of CVA	**Odds Ratio**
Thrombolytics before PCI	4.7
Creatinine clearance <40 mL/min	3.1
Urgent or emergent PCI	2.7
Unplanned intra-aortic balloon pump	2.3
IV heparin before PCI	1.9
Hypertension	1.9
Diabetes	1.8

CVA, Cerebrovascular accident; *IV,* intravenous; *PCI,* percutaneous coronary intervention.

Adapted from Dukkipati S, O'Neill WW, Harjai KJ, et al. Characteristics of cerebrovascular accidents after percutaneous coronary interventions. *J Am Coll Cardiol.* 2004;43(7):1161–1167.

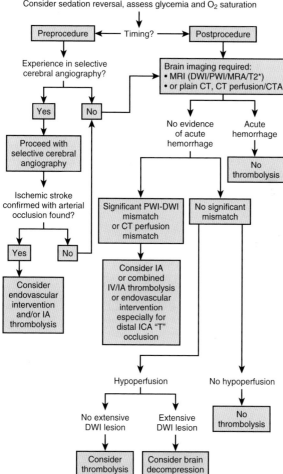

Figure 12.11 Suggested algorithm for the workup and treatment of an ischemic stroke after a catheterization procedure. *CT,* Computed tomography; *CTA,* computed tomography angiography; *DWI,* diffusion-weighted imaging; *IA,* intraarterial; *ICA,* internal carotid artery; *IV,* intravenous; *MRA,* magnetic resonance angiography; *MRI,* magnetic resonance imaging; *PWI,* perfusion-weighted imaging. (Adapted from Hamon M, Baron JC, Viader F, et al. Periprocedural stroke and cardiac catheterization. *Circulation.* 2008;118:678–683.)

mechanism of the dissection is likely because of mechanical trauma to the intima of the vessel (either normal or with plaque) from a catheter that is wedged into the wall rather than lying co-axial in the vessel lumen. A jet of contrast from an abnormally seated catheter can aggravate or produce a coronary dissection. Dissection of the right coronary artery (RCA) from guide catheter trauma is more common than left main dissection because of relative size differences in the ostia. The Amplatz left guide catheters are the most likely to dissect the coronary artery; this is because of their predilection to dive deeply into the artery. Stenting the dissected area remains the standard of treatment. A guide catheter ostial or proximal dissection should be fixed before proceeding to the intended PCI lesion. The rationale is that if the dissection is not fixed, it can propagate forward and cause abrupt vessel closure or propagate backward and cause aortic dissection.

More commonly, coronary dissection is caused by balloon angioplasty trauma. Although microscopic dissections occur with every balloon angioplasty procedure, larger angiographically visible dissections are present in only 30% to 50% of all angioplasty procedures. In the era before stenting, coronary dissection was a significant risk factor for acute or abrupt vessel closure, a rare phenomenon in modern PCI procedures with stents easily sealing the tissue flaps. The classifications of coronary dissections are provided in Table 12.6 and Fig. 12.12.

The incidence of aortic dissection caused by guide catheter trauma is very rare (0.02%–0.07%; Fig. 12.13). Table 12.7 shows a classification scheme for extension of an aortic dissection. Almost all cases of retrograde extension of dissection are from the RCA, although there are a couple of case reports of similar dissection from the left main. Class I and II lesions have a good prognosis and can be treated by stenting of the coronary dissection with close clinical follow-up. It is reasonable to follow the evolution of the dissection

Table 12.6

Classification of Coronary Dissection	
Type of Dissection	**Description**
Type A	Luminal haziness
Type B	Linear dissection
Type C	Extraluminal contrast staining
Type D	Spiral dissection
Type E	Dissection with reduced flow
Type F	Dissection with total occlusion

Dissection type	Description	Angiographic appearance
A	Minor radiolucencies within the coronary lumen during contrast injection with minimal or no persistence after dye clearance.	
B	Parallel tracts or double lumen separated by a radiolucent area during contrast injection with minimal or no persistence after dye clearance.	
C	Extraluminal cap with persistence of contrast after dye clearance from the coronary lumen.	
D	Spiral luminal filling defects.	
E+	New persistent filling defects.	
F+	Those non-A–E types that lead to impaired flow or total occlusion.	
+ May represent thrombus.		

Figure 12.12 Types of coronary artery dissections: NHLBI classification system. (From Safian R, Freed M, eds. *The Manual of Interventional Cardiology*. 3rd ed. Physicians' Press, 2001:389.)

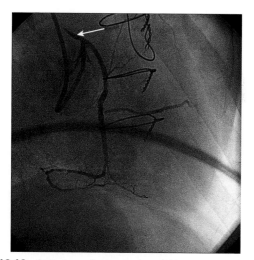

Figure 12.13 Angiogram of an anomalous right coronary artery after the placement of a stent. The arrow is pointing to a contrast stain extending upward from the ostium of the artery representing a dissection of the aorta caused by the guide catheter.

Table 12.7

Classification of Coronary Dissection With Retrograde Extension Into the Aortic Root	
Classification	**Extent of Aortic Involvement in the Dissection**
Class I	Involving the ipsilateral cusp
Class II	Involving cusp and extending up the aorta <40 mm
Class III	Involving cusp and extending up the aorta >40 mm

with imaging modalities (CT or transesophageal echocardiogram [TEE]). If the patient remains stable over the next 24 to 48 hours of hospitalization, they can be safely discharged without the expectation for further complication. To reduce the chance of extension, the systolic blood pressure must be optimally controlled. Nevertheless, antiplatelet therapy should not be suspended with a recently placed coronary stent. Class III lesions generally should be treated surgically and are associated with a high mortality rate.

Contrast Media Complications

Intravascular radiographic contrast media (RCM) can be associated with anaphylactoid reactions and acute renal failure. Fortunately, anaphylactoid reactions are rare, occurring in only 0.23% of procedures. Table 12.8 lists the severity classification for contrast-induced anaphylactoid reactions.

Anaphylactoid Reaction

An anaphylactoid reaction is different from an anaphylactic reaction. An anaphylactic reaction is an immunoglobulin E (IgE)-mediated hypersensitivity reaction requiring prior sensitization of the patient to

Table 12.8

Severity Classification for Contrast-Induced Anaphylactoid Reactions		
Minor	**Moderate**	**Severe**
Urticaria (limited)	Urticaria (diffuse)	Cardiovascular shock
Pruritus	Angioedema	Respiratory arrest
Erythema	Laryngeal edema	Cardiac arrest
	Bronchospasm	

a given antigen. An anaphylactoid reaction does not require prior sensitization and is not antibody mediated. Rather, it is an immediate hypersensitivity reaction caused by direct mast cell activation and/or activation of the kinin and complement cascades. As seen from Table 12.8, the symptoms of the reactions can be similar. Risk factors for an allergic reaction to RCM include prior RCM reaction (up to 60% chance of repeat reaction) and a history of atopy (i.e., asthma, allergic rhinitis, drug allergies, food allergies). Patients are no more likely to have an anaphylactoid reaction than patients with other food allergies. Shellfish allergy involves tropomyosin proteins as the antigen, having nothing to do with iodine content in various shellfish.

Individuals at risk for an anaphylactoid reaction require premedication. Prednisone 60 mg should be given the night before the procedure and the morning of the procedure. Some operators have tried to administer intravenous (IV) Solu-Medrol, but keep in mind that the onset of action of this steroid is like that of orally administered prednisone. If catheterization must be performed without the benefit of oral steroid loading, IV dexamethasone should be used. Benadryl 50 mg IV should also be given up to 1 hour before the procedure. If the first prednisone dose is missed, the glucocorticoid regimen loses its effectiveness. H_1 antihistamines have not been shown conclusively to reduce the risk of contrast-mediated reactions. Low osmolar or iso-osmolar contrast agents are used, which will further decrease the chance of an anaphylactoid reaction compared with the obsolete high osmolar contrast agents.

Treatment of an anaphylactoid reaction depends on the severity of the reaction (Table 12.9). For the most severe reactions, bolus epinephrine is prepared by mixing 0.1 mL of a 1:1000 solution or 1 mL of a 1:10,000 solution diluted in a 10-mL syringe with saline, producing a final concentration of 10 mcg/mL. If a patient has recently taken beta blockers, they might not have an adequate response to epinephrine. In this case, glucagon 1 to 2 mg IV over 5 minutes, then an infusion of 5 to 15 mcg/min, can be given to help reverse the effect of the beta blockade (by activating cyclic adenosine monophosphate [AMP] at a site independent from beta adrenergic agents).

Contrast-Induced Nephropathy

Intravascular contrast media also can put the patient at risk for acute renal failure after PCI. This contrast-induced nephropathy (CIN) is likely caused by acute tubular necrosis. Mehran et al. developed a validated risk-scoring system to predict the likelihood of developing CIN (Fig. 12.14). CIN is typically defined as a relative

Table 12.9

Treatment of Anaphylactoid Reactions in the Cardiac Catheterization Laboratory

Urticaria	Bronchospasm	Facial/Laryngeal Edema	Hypotension/Shock
Diphenhydramine 25–50 mg IV	Oxygen Albuterol Inhaler/nebulizer Diphenhydramine 50 mg IV Hydrocortisone 200–400 mg IV or methylprednisolone 125 mg IV *For severe reaction* Epinephrine bolus 10 mcg/min as needed. An infusion of 1–4 mcg/min might be needed as well.	Oxygen Emergent anesthesia consult for potential intubation. Tracheostomy tray should be available. Diphenhydramine 50 mg IV Epinephrine bolus/drip (as described under bronchospasm)	Epinephrine bolus until BP is maintained; then start infusion (as described previously) 1 L normal saline bolus rapidly (pressure bag). Repeat as necessary. Diphenhydramine 50–100 mg IV Hydrocortisone 400 mg IV or methylprednisolone 125 mg IV

BP, Blood pressure; *IV*, intravenous.

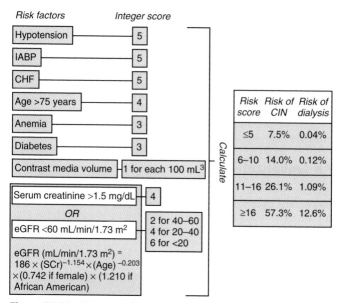

Figure 12.14 Risk score developed by Mehran et al. to predict the likelihood of developing postprocedural contrast-induced nephropathy (CIN). *CHF*, Congestive heart failure; *eGFR*, estimated globular filtration rate; *IABP*, intra-aortic balloon pump.

increase in serum creatinine of greater than 25% or an absolute increase of greater than 0.5 mg/dL. Although it is not uncommon to develop transient increases in serum creatinine, it is rare to need temporary dialysis and even rarer to need permanent dialysis after CIN. The time course of CIN demonstrates an increase in creatinine starting after 12 to 24 hours for most patients, but it may take as long as 48 to 96 hours to peak. Most cases show a return to baseline creatinine by days 3 to 5, but it can take up to 7 to 10 days. Serum creatinine should be routinely obtained at 48 to 72 hours after contrast administration in a high-risk patient.

In high-risk patients, CIN prevention consists of two principles: adequate hydration and limitation of the volume of contrast administered. All other potential therapies, including diuretics, mannitol, dopamine, fenoldopam, n-acetylcysteine, iso-osmolar contrast, or theophylline, have not been consistently proven to work for preventing CIN and should *not* be used. In patients with chronic kidney disease needing coronary intervention, it is highly beneficial to perform the diagnostic angiogram separate from the interventional procedure by at least a week. Determining a preintervention contrast "ceiling" (many operators use 3 x GFR to estimate or others use 2.5 x kg /creat) helps all staff be aware to not exceed this contrast volume and is a useful addition to the preprocedure time-out. Assessing the patient's volume status by measuring their left ventricular end-diastolic pressure before administering contrast can help guide IV hydration strategies before beginning the PCI. Intravascular ultrasound may also be used to perform ultralow contrast PCI procedures and is exceptionally useful in those patients with advanced kidney disease wanting to avoid dialysis.

Air Embolization

Another potential complication of coronary angiography and contrast media injection is air embolization (Fig. 12.15). This is always an iatrogenic complication because of failure to clear the air from the injection manifold system. Automatic contrast injection systems

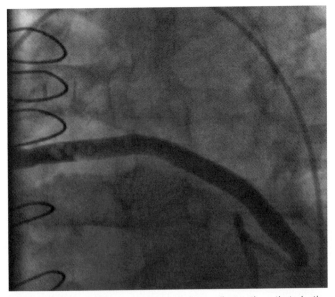

Figure 12.15 Angiogram obtained during a diagnostic catheterization depicting the injection of contrast into a vein graft to the obtuse marginal branch. On close inspection, several round objects can be seen in the proximal portion of this graft that represent air bubbles injected from the guide catheter.

have a much lower rate of air embolism because of built-in air detection sensors. Nevertheless, these systems do not fully eliminate the incidence of air embolism despite their inherent safety mechanisms and are not a replacement for a good manifold technique of aspiration and visual inspection for bubbles. Treatment of coronary air embolism consists of immediate initiation of 100% oxygen by facemask. The oxygen helps to minimize ischemia and produces a diffusion gradient favoring reabsorption of the air. If large bubbles persist, the air can be aspirated by various aspiration catheters.

Arrhythmias

Another general complication of PCI that might occur at any time during the procedure is arrhythmia (either tachycardia or bradycardia). Unstable tachycardias like ventricular tachycardia or ventricular fibrillation are more commonly seen in the setting of an acute MI. Bradycardia is most often seen in RCA occlusions and in use of rotational atherectomy, especially in the RCA. Treatment of arrhythmias should follow standard advanced cardiovascular life support (ACLS) protocols. In general, for unstable patients, it is always good practice to electrically cardiovert tachycardic arrhythmias. For unstable bradycardia, atropine can be given, and transcutaneous pacing can be initiated. These measures can buy time to set up for temporary transvenous balloon flotation pacemaker placement. Transvenous pacemakers should be placed prophylactically for cases of rotational atherectomy in the RCA. If transvenous pacing is not readily available, guidewire pacing (connecting the negative lead to guidewire and positive lead to patient) may be used because it has been shown to be effective.

Many operators have begun to use IV aminophylline before rotational atherectomy procedures to minimize bradycardia and not put in a prophylactic pacemaker. One such prophylactic regimen is shown in Box 12.7.

No Reflow

An acute cessation of coronary flow during PCI can occur as a result of abrupt occlusion or as a consequence of distal failure of outflow (see Fig. 12.16 for a suggested management algorithm). This observation is termed the *no-reflow phenomenon* by some but only in conjunction with microembolization, whereas others reserve the term for myocardial blush grades of 0 or 1 (regardless of coronary thrombolysis in myocardial infarction [TIMI] flow) in the setting of a primary PCI (See Table 12.10 for pharmacologic management).

Box 12.7   Prophylactic Aminophyline for Prevention of RotoBlator Associated Bradycardia/Heart Block

1. Multiply the patient's weight in Kg x 5 = total number mg of aminophylline needed.
2. Mix the above mg into 100 mL normal saline (NS) or dextrose 5% in water (D5W).
3. Set the intravenous (IV) pump at a rate of 300 mL/hr and a volume of 100 mL (to deliver 250 mcg/kg/min).
4. Infuse 10 minutes before atherectomy until the end of the atherectomy portion of the procedure.

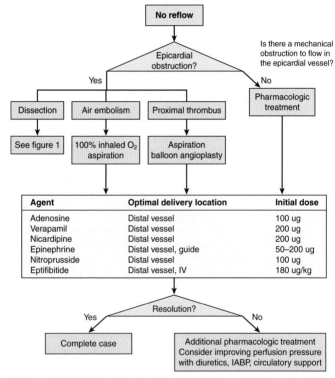

Figure 12.16 Suggested algorithm detailing the critical steps in dealing with No Reflow. (From Doll JA, Hira RS, Kearney KE, et al. Management of percutaneous coronary intervention complications: Algorithms from the 2018 and 2019 Seattle percutaneous coronary intervention complications conference. *Circ Cardiovasc Interv.* 2020;13[6]:e008962; Fig. 4.)

Table 12.10

Pharmacologic Management of No-Reflow Microembolization Syndrome	
Medicine	**Dose**
Adenosine	100 mcg/mL 1–2 mL bolus, reassess flow and hemodynamics
Nitroprusside	100 mcg/mL 1–2 mL IC bolus, reassess
Verapamil	100 mcg/mL 1–2 mL IC bolus, reassess

IC, Intracoronary.

Regardless, the differential diagnosis of no reflow includes severe spasm, dissection, in situ thrombus, plaque rupture, and distal microembolization. If no-reflow is because of thrombus or new plaque rupture, then manual catheter aspiration is appropriate. Additional anticoagulation with IIb/IIIa inhibitors should be started. Rechecking activated clotting time (ACT) levels is prudent. Additional angioplasty and stenting might be necessary to assure a patent vessel and operators should use intracoronary imaging to guide this.

If no-reflow is because of dissection, additional stenting is necessary. If no-reflow is because of severe spasm, intracoronary nitroglycerin doses at a concentration of 100 mcg/mL are given until the vasospasm is relieved. Although intracoronary nitroglycerin can help relieve vasospasm, it has not been shown to be effective in relief of the no reflow phenomenon from distal microembolization.

No-reflow from embolization to the microvasculature is most seen in interventions on saphenous vein grafts and acute MIs. Prophylactic distal embolic filters can help reduce the embolic burden and prevent no reflow.

Coronary Perforation

The incidence of coronary perforation is 0.84% of PCI cases, but its presence is associated with a fivefold increase in in-hospital mortality risk. Coronary perforation can be caused by a wire "exiting" the vessel or by a tear (dissection) in the vessel from balloon angioplasty, stenting, or rotational atherectomy. Table 12.11 shows the classification of coronary perforations.

Class I and II perforations are usually managed conservatively without any specific treatment. Class III perforations are associated with rapid development of tamponade (63%), the need for urgent bypass surgery (63%), and a high mortality rate (19%; see Fig. 12.17 for a suggested management algorithm).

Table 12.11

Class	Description
Classification of Coronary Perforations	
I	Intramural crater without extravasation
II	Pericardial or myocardial blush/staining
III	Perforation >1 mm in diameter with contrast streaming or cavity spilling

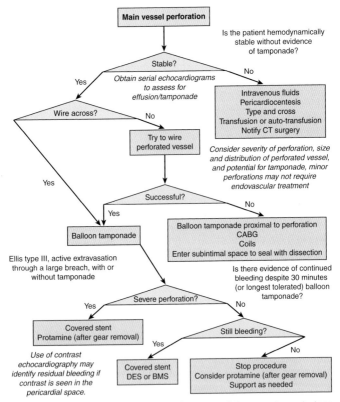

Figure 12.17 Suggested algorithm for appropriate management steps when a perforation of a main coronary vessel is encountered. (From Doll JA, Hira RS, Kearney KE, et al. Management of percutaneous coronary intervention complications: Algorithms from the 2018 and 2019 Seattle percutaneous coronary intervention complications conference. *Circ Cardiovasc Interv.* 2020;13[6]:e008962.)

If the perforation occurred after balloon and stent placement, the balloon should be immediately reinflated to stop further extravasation of blood into the pericardial space. At this point, a pericardial drain can be placed to relieve or protect against tamponade while definitive measures are taken to treat the perforation. Bivalirudin should be discontinued because it will take up to 2 hours to decrease the anticoagulation status to a normal level.

To place a covered stent, obtain contralateral access and, using a second guide catheter, intubate the perforated artery. The first guide catheter can be slightly backed out to allow intubation by the new guide ("ping-pong technique"). A 7F guide is recommended by the package insert to deliver the covered stents, although anecdotally, they have been delivered through 6F guiding catheters as well. Once the second guide is in place, a second guidewire should be used and placed up to the proximal edge of the inflated balloon. The balloon is then briefly deflated as the wire passes down to the distal vessel, and then the balloon is immediately reinflated. Next, a covered stent is placed over the second guidewire to the proximal edge of the inflated balloon. The balloon is deflated, and the balloon and first wire are removed as the covered stent is positioned and immediately deployed. Deployment should be done at higher atmospheres to ensure good apposition of the covered stent. If additional access is not available, a quick exchange of balloon for covered stent can be used as well. Nevertheless, this allows at least 30 to 60 seconds of free coronary flow into the pericardial space, so a pericardial drain must already be in place. As little as 100 mL of an acute effusion can cause chamber compression and hemodynamic collapse. Once the covered stent is deployed and the coronary wire removed, heparin can be immediately reversed. The pericardial drain should be left in place overnight as a precautionary measure. Clinical follow-up with echocardiography is routine for tamponade management.

As opposed to a main vessel perforation, distal vessel perforations are seemingly much more benign but can still result in significant blood loss (see Fig. 12.18 for a suggested management algorithm). To minimize the chance of wire perforation, hydrophilic tipped or stiff wires that are used to get through difficult lesions should be exchanged for workhorse wires with softer hydrophobic tips. If a *distal* perforation from a wire tip occurs, the first step should be balloon tamponade of the vessel at the perforation site. Prolonged (several minutes) inflations with test deflations can be tried over an hour. If balloon tamponade is not successful, the operator must consider distal coil placement, injection of fat, clot, or microspheres. Anticoagulation should *not* be immediately reversed with the wire and balloon in the vessel during the attempted perforation occlusion. Immediate reversal

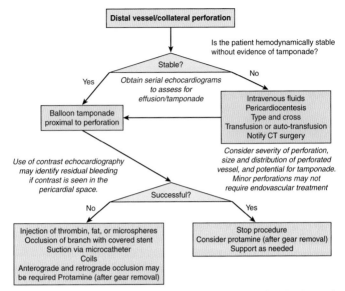

Figure 12.18 Suggested algorithm for management of a distal vessel perforation. (From Doll JA, Hira RS, Kearney KE, et al. Management of percutaneous coronary intervention complications: Algorithms from the 2018 and 2019 Seattle percutaneous coronary intervention complications conference. *Circ Cardiovasc Interv.* 2020;13[6]:e008962.)

could lead to thrombosis throughout the whole vessel, an event that leads to a higher degree of mortality than the perforation itself. Reversal of anticoagulation should be performed after the equipment is removed from the coronary vessel.

Retained PCI Equipment Components

See Fig. 12.19 for management algorithms.

Rarely, fragments of interventional equipment may break off and remain in a coronary artery. This may occur with guidewire tips from both fixed-wire and movable, over-the-wire balloon systems or with distal fragments of various other catheters. These retained intravascular fragments carry the risk for coronary artery occlusion, distal embolization of clot, vessel perforation, infection, and ischemic complications. Dislodgement of stents from the delivery balloons has also been a source of retained interventional equipment.

Removal of intravascular fragments and foreign bodies should be done immediately to avoid the complications just mentioned, as well as incorporation of this material after several days during which the objects become coated and interred within the vessel. There are several techniques for removal of retained intravascular foreign bodies. Baskets, forceps, and snares are available and are manufactured in sizes appropriate for placement within the coronary arteries. Guidewire fracture has an incidence of 0.1%. Most

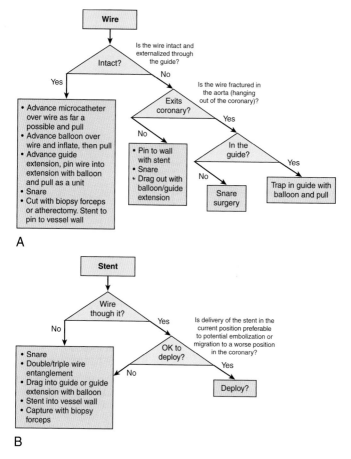

Figure 12.19 Management Steps to Consider When Encountering Retained Equipment. (A) Retained wire. (B) Embolized stent.

Continued

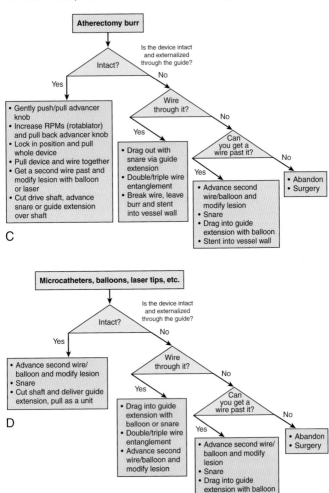

Figure 12.19, cont'd (C) Retained atherectomy burr. (D) Other retained equipment. (From Doll JA, Hira RS, Kearney KE, et al. Management of percutaneous coronary intervention complications: Algorithms from the 2018 and 2019 Seattle percutaneous coronary intervention complications conference. *Circ Cardiovasc Interv.* 2020;13[6]:e008962.)

cases of wire fracture have been reported with the rotational atherectomy wires.

There are multiple options for dealing with a retained wire fragment. A small wire fragment may be left in place and allowed to endothelialize, as a stent would. Dual antiplatelet therapy should be given if a wire is simply left in place.

For a wire fragment more centrally located in the vessel lumen, a stent can be deployed to trap the wire in place and avoid any possibility of further migration.

For a very long wire fragment extending into the guiding catheter, a balloon can be advanced to the end of the guide catheter and inflated, thereby trapping the wire against the side of the guide. At this point, the guide, balloon, and retained wire can be removed together.

For a longer wire fragment that does not extend into the guide, removal with a microsnare catheter may be the best choice. An over-the-wire balloon can be delivered next to a visible end of a retained guidewire (usually only the distal end is visible). A microsnare is then placed through the lumen of the over-the-wire balloon and is used to lasso the retained wire. It can then be pulled into the guiding catheter and subsequently removed. If a microsnare (Fig. 12.20) is not readily available, you can effectively ensnare a retained wire using a two-wire technique. This method is accomplished by placing two new guidewires next to the retained fragment. A single torquing device is placed over both wires, and the Y-connector is left slightly open as the torquing device is spun in one direction. This allows the two wires to form a double helix around each other; this helix will propagate distally and eventually ensnare the retained wire. All wires are then pulled back into the guide together (Fig. 12.21).

Another rare complication is stent dislodgement and embolization, which occurs with an incidence of approximately 0.4%. Stent dislodgement most often occurs in tortuous, calcified vessels. Management options include retrieval, deployment in place, or crushing against the wall of the vessel with a balloon or new stent. Ideally, retrieval should be tried first so that the stent is not placed in an unintended position. Mortality rates as high as 17% have been reported for stent embolizations that are unsuccessfully managed (usually requiring emergent surgery), but they are as low as 0.9% in patients who have successful retrieval of a stent.

Retrieval methods are like those discussed with fractured wire retrieval. Microsnares or dual wires can be used to ensnare and remove the loose stent. Additional methods include advancing a small balloon over the same wire that the undeployed stent is floating on, inflating the balloon past the stent, and then pulling back the balloon, which should shift the free stent into the guide.

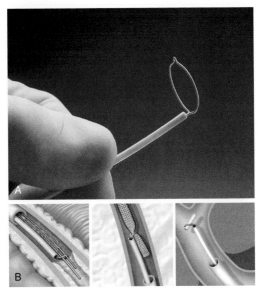

Figure 12.20 (A) Microvena snare for retrieval of intracoronary equipment fragments. (B) *Left panel:* Loop snare is used to capture a stent on second wire. *Middle:* Loop snare can be used to capture free stent. *Right panel:* Loop snare can capture catheter fragments. (Courtesy Microvena Company, Minneapolis, MN.)

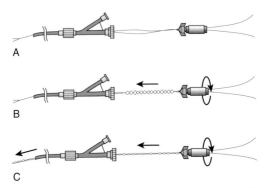

Figure 12.21 (A) Diagram showing two guidewires entering single Y-connector through a single torquing device. (B) The wires are torqued together forming a helix. (C) The helix propagates distally and can be used to ensnare a trapped wire fragment. (From Gurley J, Booth D, Hixon C, et al. Removal of retained intracoronary percutaneous transluminal coronary angioplasty equipment by a percutaneous twin guidewire method. *Cathet Cardiovasc Diagn.* 1990;19:251–256.)

If the stent is dislodged in a large proximal vessel, retrieval with myocardial biopsy forceps can be considered as well. If retrieval is not possible, then "playing the stent where it lies" (i.e., deploying or crushing the stent at that site) is the best option. To attempt to place the stent in its position, a small balloon of similar or longer length than the stent is positioned across the profile of the stent. Initially, this can be attempted with a small 1.5-mm balloon blown up to 1 to 2 atm; this might be enough to capture the stent and move the system to a more desirable spot (to the initial lesion or at least out of the left main). If it cannot be moved, the balloon should be deployed at full atmospheres to dilate the stent as much as possible. A second undeflated balloon equal to the vessel diameter can then be placed to ensure adequate stent apposition. Rarely, a small-diameter balloon will not recross the stent. In this case, a second wire is placed down next to the embolized stent, and another stent is placed adjacent to the embolized stent and is used to crush the loose stent against the arterial wall. In more than 50% of cases of embolization, the stent might be embolized to the peripheral arteries. In these cases, snares or forceps can be used to retrieve the stent if it can be visualized in the periphery.

Stent Thrombosis

Stent thrombosis is a rare but devastating complication of PCI. Mortality rates are reported from 25% to 40%. Stent thrombosis is defined as acute (<24 hours), subacute (within 30 days), late (between 1 month and 1 year), or very late (>1 year). To standardize the definition of stent thrombosis, the academic research consortium divided the criteria for stent thrombosis into definite, probable, or possible (Table 12.12).

Both bare-metal stent (BMS) thrombosis and drug-eluting stent (DES) thrombosis occur most commonly in the acute or subacute time frame. DES, however, also have a higher risk for thrombosis in the late and very late period because of incomplete endothelialization; this provides a strong argument for continuing dual antiplatelet therapy (DAPT) for at least 1 year after DES implantation. Premature discontinuation of DAPT is the greatest risk factor for stent thrombosis. Other risk factors are listed in Box 12.8.

Almost one-third of patients in whom antiplatelet therapy is discontinued prematurely are at risk for stent thrombosis. Because DES require a longer duration of DAPT, it is crucial to decide before the diagnostic angiogram if the patient is an appropriate candidate for long-term DAPT. If a patient cannot afford or cannot take long-term DAPT, or if the patient requires surgery in the next 12 months that would necessitate discontinuation of antiplatelet

Table 12.12

Academic Research Consortium Criteria for Stent Thrombosis	
Definition	**Criteria**
Definite stent thrombosis	Angiographic confirmation of thrombus that originates inside or within 5 mm of the stent, which is associated with symptoms, electrocardiogram (ECG) changes, or biomarker elevation, or pathologic confirmation of stent thrombosis determined at autopsy or from tissue obtained after thrombectomy
Probable stent thrombosis	Unexplained death occurring within 30 days after the index procedure, or a myocardial infarction occurring at any time after the index procedure that was documented by ECG or imaging to occur in an area supplied by the stented vessel in the absence of angiographic confirmation of stent thrombosis or other culprit lesion
Possible stent thrombosis	Unexplained death occurring more than 30 days after the index procedure

---

Box 12.8   Risk Factors for Stent Thrombosis

Premature discontinuation of antiplatelet therapy
   Incomplete stent expansion
   Greater stent length
   Subtherapeutic periprocedural anticoagulation
   Cocaine use
   Prior brachytherapy
   Post-procedure TIMI flow grade <3
   Treatment of bifurcation lesion

TIMI, thrombolysis in myocardial infarction.

---

therapy, using a dedicated stent for which short-DAPT regimens have been proven safe can be considered. Similarly, if the patient currently requires long-term warfarin, or if the patient has a history of major bleeding episodes, they may not be a candidate for long-term DAPT and these issues should be addressed while planning the interventional procedure.

Stent Infection

The rarest complication of PCI is stent infection. There are fewer than 20 case reports of intracoronary stent infection in the literature, which include both DES and BMS. In some cases, mycotic aneurysms are formed at the site of stenting, but other cases present with persistent bacteremia. *Staphylococcus aureus* is the most common microorganism implicated. Stent infection presents within 4 weeks after stent implantation with fever and bacteremia. Typical findings of chest pain, electrocardiogram (ECG) changes, and troponin elevation might be absent. A high degree of suspicion should accompany any fever occurring within 1 month of PCI. Confirmation of the diagnosis may be difficult with imaging. In addition to antibiotic therapy, most cases (>60%) will require surgery. In general, there is up to a 40% mortality rate with stent infection. Strict infection control measures (as discussed in *The Cardiac Catheterization Handbook,* 7e) must be adhered to in the cath lab. Risk factors for bacteremia associated with cardiac catheterization are shown in Box 12.9.

Sudden Hemodynamics Collapse

See Fig. 12.22 for the suggested management algorithm.

The occurrence of a sudden drop in blood pressure during a catheterization procedure is quite rare and the potential causes are widely diverse. Sometimes, the guide catheter pressure becomes damped because it can be pulled into the coronary artery during a complex procedure with multiple manipulations of intracoronary equipment. Equally likely is that a connection became loose in the tubing connecting the guide catheter to the transducer. Neither of these scenarios represents a "true" emergency

---

Box 12.9	**Risk Factors for Bacteremia After Cardiac Catheterization**

Avoidable Risk Factors

Difficult vascular access
    Multiple skin punctures
    Repeated catheterization at the same vascular access site
    Extended duration of the procedure
    Use of multiple PTCA balloons
    Deferred removal of the arterial sheath

Unavoidable Risk Factors

Presence of congestive heart failure
    Patient's age >60

PTCA, Percutaneous transluminal coronary angioplasty.
Adapted from Kaufman B, Kaiser C, Pfisterer M et al. Coronary stent infection: a rare but severe complication of percutaneous coronary intervention. *Swiss Med Wkly.* 2005;135:483–487.

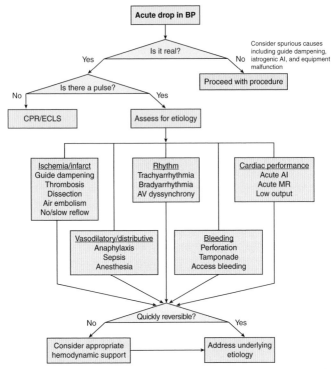

Figure 12.22   Algorithm outlining critical steps when encountering a sudden drop in blood pressure in the catheterization lab. (From Doll JA, Hira RS, Kearney KE, et al. Management of percutaneous coronary intervention complications: Algorithms from the 2018 and 2019 Seattle percutaneous coronary intervention complications conference. *Circ Cardiovasc Interv.* 2020;13[6]:e008962.)

and should be easily troubleshooted. Should these "simple" solutions not be found, however, first attention must be given to determining the patient's true hemodynamic status and a pulse should be assessed. Cardiopulmonary resuscitation (CPR) should be started immediately if a pulse is not appreciated, and team members should all take on dedicated and specific roles because the patient requires immediate resuscitation. Often, resuscitation efforts require the support of anesthesia or another team to place an endotracheal tube, and these personnel should be alerted immediately. Although these efforts remain ongoing, attention must also be given to assessing potential causes for the collapse and treating those believed to be potentially causative as well as quickly reversible. Lastly, all cath labs should have a protocol in place for the administration of mechanical circulatory support—rapid placement of the patient on extracorporeal membrane oxygenation (ECMO) or Impella—to facilitate circulation to the patient's vital organs and assist with resuscitation efforts.

Key References

Amin AP, Caruso M, Artero PC, et al. Reducing bleeding complications in the cath lab: a patient-centered approach. *J Am Coll Cardiol.* 2016;67(suppl 13):84.

Castro-Dominguez YS, Wang Y, Minges KE, et al. Predicting in-hospital mortality in patients undergoing percutaneous coronary intervention. *J Am Coll Cardiol.* 2021; 78:216-229.

Doll JA, Hira RS, Kearney KE, et al. Management of percutaneous coronary intervention complications: algorithms from the 2018 and 2019 Seattle percutaneous coronary intervention complications conference. *Circ Cardiovasc Interv.* 2020;13(6):e008962.

Han C, Strauss C, Garberich R, et al. Prospective decision support tool guides usage of vascular closure devices that reduce bleeding complications, length of stay, and variable costs in high bleed risk patients. *J Am Coll Cardiol.* 2016;67(suppl 13):73.

Naidu SS, Abbott JD, Bagai J, et al. SCAI expert consensus update on best practices in the cardiac catheterization laboratory. *Catheter Cardiovasc Interv.* 2021;98(2):255-276.

Parsh J, Seth M, Green J, et al. The deadly impact of coronary perforation in women undergoing PCI: insights from BMC2. *J Am Coll Cardiol.* 2016;67(suppl 13):179.

Vascular Access for Noncardiac Procedures

YONATAN BITTON-FAIWISZEWSKI • SANJUM S. SETHI •
SAHIL A. PARIKH

KEY POINTS

- Access for noncardiac procedures employs many of the same techniques as access for cardiac procedures with the choice of access site determined by patient-related factors and specific procedural needs.

- Antegrade femoral and tibiopedal access techniques have been developed for lower extremity percutaneous revascularization procedures.

- All operators should be familiar with the techniques for access described within this chapter, regardless of specialty.

Introduction

Endovascular intervention has become the primary approach to treating vascular diseases in many extracardiac territories, with open surgical procedures reserved for refractory or complex cases. These approaches are well established to address both arterial and venous diseases. Current techniques allow for approaching lesions or occlusions in the arteries that supply the leg, pelvic vessels, abdominal organs, upper extremities, and even the carotid arteries. Additionally, endovascular techniques allow for treatment of aortic aneurysms (Table 13.1). Other techniques can be applied to the treatment of deep venous thrombosis, venous compression syndromes, vena cava filter implantation and removal, and treatment of pulmonary embolism, including thrombectomy or catheter-directed lysis. Some standard views for angiography are listed in Table 13.2. The full breadth of these procedural techniques is beyond the scope of this chapter. Because interventional cardiologists that

Table 13.1

Arterial Access and Target Vascular Territories	
Access Segment	**Target Segment**
Retrograde CFA	Arch vessels, renal, mesenterics, ipsilateral iliac
Contralateral CFA ("up and over")	Contralateral iliac, CFA, PFA, SFA, popliteal
Antegrade CFA	Middistal SFA, popliteal, infrapopliteal
Radial	Renal, iliac, CFA, proximal SFA (R2P)
Retrograde popliteal	SFA and iliac
Retrograde tibiopedal	Infrapopliteal, popliteal, SFA

CFA, Common femoral artery; *PFA*, profunda femoris artery; *SFA*, superficial femoral artery

Table 13.2

Common Angulations for Angiography	
Vascular Segment of Interest	**Angulation of Image-Intensifier**
Aortic arch	30–60 degrees LAO
Brachiocephalic vessels (origin)	30–60 degrees LAO
Subclavian	AP, 30 degrees ipsilateral/caudal
Vertebral origin	AP, 30 degrees ipsilateral/cranial
Carotid	AP, 30–60 degrees ipsilateral for bifurcation, lateral
Renal arteries (origin)	0–15 degrees LAO
Mesenteric arteries (origin)	60–90 degrees RAO
Internal/External iliac bifurcation	20/20 degrees contra/caudal
SFA/PFA bifurcation	30–60 degrees ipsilateral oblique
Tibial vessels, trifurcation	30–60 degrees ipsilateral oblique
Foot, pedal arch	AP/10–20 degrees cranial, 30–60 degrees contralateral

AP, Anteroposterior; *LAO*, left anterior oblique; *PFA*, profunda femoris artery; *RAO*, right anterior oblique; *SFA*, superficial femoral artery

perform diagnostic and therapeutic coronary interventions are familiar with primary femoral and radial approaches, which are covered in other chapters, those techniques will not be covered here. Here, we will discuss considerations and approaches to vascular access that may be useful to the endovascular interventionalist.

Femoral Access

The femoral artery remains the mainstay of access for peripheral vascular interventions. The traditional approach involves retrograde access in the common femoral artery, which allows arteriography ("runoff") of the ipsilateral limb and subsequently offers the ability to engage the abdominal aorta and the contralateral iliac artery (Fig. 13.1). Alternatively, the artery can be accessed in antegrade fashion, allowing for in-line access of the vessel to treat lesions involving the ipsilateral limb. This approach is frequently used to treat

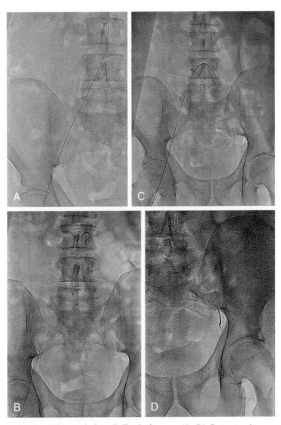

Figure 13.1 "Up and Over" Techniques. (A–D) Retrograde access is gained in the common femoral artery. A crossing catheter (an Omniflush is depicted) is advanced and aortoiliac angiography may be performed. The crossing catheter is used to engage the contralateral common iliac artery and the catheter is withdrawn to "seat the bifurcation." The wire is advanced into the contralateral external iliac and femoral artery. The crossing catheter is advanced over the wire and angiography may be performed of the contralateral limb.

difficult lesions at the level of the distal superficial femoral artery or below, especially in the setting of aortoiliac tortuosity or stenoses. Femoral access is frequently performed using both fluoroscopy and ultrasound guidance to avoid access through calcified plaque and to ensure that a closure device can be used successfully at the termination of the procedure.

Crossing "Up and Over"

Crossing "up and over" for peripheral arteriography remains the standard approach for access because it allows for visualization of the arterial anatomy of both limbs and of the aortoiliac anatomy, the so-called "inflow."

1. Access the common femoral artery (CFA) contralateral to the side of interest. Place a standard sheath for either diagnostic angiography using a modified Seldinger technique.

2. Ipsilateral runoff is frequently performed in advance of iliac crossover. Orient the image intensifier at 30 degrees ipsilateral-oblique to open the femoral bifurcation. This orientation will similarly display the infrapopliteal vessels with minimal overlap when performing distal vessel runoff angiography.

3. Inflow aortography is performed with a catheter inserted through the sheath into the distal abdominal aorta. This can be used to visualize the abdominal aorta (infrarenal or suprarenal if desired) and the aortic and iliac bifurcations. Multiple catheters can be used for this purpose, including Pigtail, Omniflush, and SOS catheters. Have the patient perform an expiratory breath hold under digital subtraction angiography. This can be performed in a straight anteroposterior (AP) projection for a standard view. The common iliac-internal/external bifurcation may also be imaged by positioning the image intensifier 20 degrees contralateral/20 degrees caudal to the bifurcation of interest. Place the image intensifier in a vertical (portrait) orientation, raise the table at maximum height to increase the signal to object distance, and lower the image intensifier to the patient to maximize the field of view. Full opacification can be achieved with dilute contrast (we use 50% contrast diluted with normal saline) and a 20cc rapid injection.

4. There are several catheters available for crossing the iliac bifurcation. For angulated bifurcations, an Imager II (Boston Scientific) or Omniflush (Angiodynamics) offers optimal engagement of the bifurcation because of its shape and presence of radio-opaque tips and simultaneously allows for injection through its side-hole catheter tips. Position the catheter low in the abdominal aorta such that an atraumatic guidewire, commonly a Glidewire or

Glidewire Advantage (Terumo), can engage the contralateral iliac artery. The catheter and wire are withdrawn together (so-called "seating the bifurcation") to allow for firm engagement of the catheter, which allows the wire to be advanced down the contralateral iliac artery.

5. After the contralateral iliac/femoral artery is wired, advance the catheter to the top of the femoral head and angle the image intensifier to 30 degrees ipsilateral-oblique to this limb. Perform runoff angiography. If the decision is made to intervene, then a guiding sheath will need to be inserted. Most contemporary equipment can be delivered through a 6 French (F) or 7F sheath. To perform a sheath exchange, advance a supportive wire through the catheter into a safe distal vessel in the leg of interest and remove the catheter and short sheath. Insert a long braided sheath "up and over" and advance to the desired vascular territory to be intervened upon. For an ostial/proximal superficial femoral artery (SFA) stenosis or occlusion, the sheath would be positioned into the CFA while using the profunda femoris artery (PFA) to position the guidewire as a "rail." Caution should be maintained when wiring the PFA. For most SFA interventions, a 40- to 50-cm sheath is used. Longer sheaths are frequently used when intervening on more distal vessels if inflow is relatively normal.

Antegrade Femoral Access

Antegrade femoral arterial access is used frequently when intervening on distal infrapopliteal lesions when the traditional "up and over" approach may be limited because of the shaft length needed for interventional equipment. This approach can also enhance support to allow for advancement of equipment through difficult lesions because of enhanced "pushability." Patient positioning may be altered to facilitate this approach. A "feet-first" orientation allows for the patient to be positioned on the table such that the normal orientation of the room can still be used without modification to the imaging equipment (Fig. 13.2).

Antegrade access may be obtained with ultrasound guidance with the beam in a longitudinal orientation allowing for visualization of the CFA overlying the femoral head and the femoral bifurcation. This allows for arterial entry at a compressible segment of the vessel when directly visualizing the vessel over the femoral head. It will also allow the operator to direct the access wire into the SFA if the femoral bifurcation is visible. The antegrade approach is best used for mid to distal SFA, popliteal, tibial, and infratibial disease. Standard short 10 cm or braided sheaths can be used. Entry into the

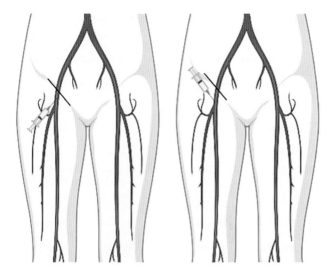

Figure 13.2 Retrograde Versus Antegrade Common Femoral Artery Access. (*Left*) For retrograde common femoral artery (CFA) access, the needle is oriented toward the pelvis. (*Right*) For antegrade access, the needle is oriented toward the foot. The operator may choose to position the patient in a "feet first" orientation on the table, especially when accessing the left CFA antegrade.

CFA may require longer access time; however, studies show that this reduces vascular complications, such as pseudoaneurysm formation, compared with SFA access.

Data from recent studies suggest that vascular closure devices may safely be used in antegrade access, but other work suggests that complications from vascular closure devices in antegrade access occur about fourfold as frequently as they occur in typical retrograde access. Many devices have been used, and so operator experience may vary between centers. Vascular closure devices should be used for antegrade access closure at the discretion and experience of the operator.

Radial

The radial approach for endovascular interventions is being used increasingly as an alternative to the more traditional femoral approach. This approach will allow for quick patient recovery as is comparable to coronary procedures. Limitations of radial access remain, primarily related to working length of available equipment, compatible drug-coated devices and covered stents, and availability of embolic protection filters. Specialty equipment include long-shaft balloons, stents, and atherectomy systems to allow for treatment of lesions from the radial approach. Supplemental Video 13.1 shows an example of introduction of a 119-cm braided slender sheath (R2P, Terumo) from the left radial artery to the right CFA.

Steps for Radial Approach

1. Some operators prefer to use the left wrist for these cases, which minimizes the distance to the abdominal aorta because the innominate artery and aortic arch are bypassed. It therefore shortens the distance to the iliacs, potentially allowing for a greater availability of equipment. Ultrasound examination of the artery is used to confirm the arterial diameter is at least 20 to 25 mm, which is needed for insertion of specialty braided sheaths for this approach.

2. To minimize distance from access to the lesion of interest, the radial artery is frequently accessed more proximally than one would for a coronary procedure. Place a 10- to 11-cm slender sheath into the vessel using a standard technique.

3. Use a JR4 or similarly shaped catheter to engage the descending thoracic aorta. A hydrophilic wire may be useful for engagement of the descending aorta.

4. Exchange wires for an exchange-length guidewire and then change to the catheter to be used in aortography down the abdominal aorta.

5. Similar to inflow aortography described in the previous section, aortography may be performed with a variety of side-hole catheters. We use a long Pigtail catheter or a long multipurpose-shaped catheter with side-holes.

6. Engage and wire each iliac artery and then advance the catheter to the CFA. This allows for complete diagnostic angiography of each limb.

7. A long stiff 0.035-inch guidewire is used to advance the radial intervention sheath (typically, 95, 105, 119 or 149 cm R2P destination sheath, Terumo) proximal to the segment of interest, (e.g., femoropopliteal; as demonstrated in Supplemental Video 13.1). Care should be taken to choose a guidewire of appropriate length, which should frequently be at least 300 cm in length. Watch under fluoroscopy as the sheath traverses the subclavian to the descending thoracic aorta because it will have a tendency to "prolapse" into the ascending aorta. A "push-pull" technique is used to overcome this.

8. After placing the sheath in the segment of interest, proceed with intervention as usual. Specialty long-shaft balloons, stents, and atherectomy systems are available for these purposes.

Tibiopedal Approach

The tibiopedal retrograde approach may be used in a variety of cases. It allows for access to lesions that may be too distal for equipment to reach from typical approaches. It allows for enhanced pushability because of in-line access to the lesion of interest. It also may be useful for chronic total occlusion (CTO) crossing because the distal cap is frequently a more favorable entry point for crossing. We use this approach either as a primary access or as an adjunct to a standard approach.

Steps for Retrograde Access

1. Ultrasound can be used to assess the anterior and posterior tibial arteries to evaluate patency and calcification characteristics. Ideally, access is gained under ultrasound, but if calcification precludes ultrasound imaging, direct puncture under fluoroscopy can also be used. Pre-interventional imaging should also be examined for assessment of anatomy and patency. Caution should be taken in cases where single vessel runoff exists because vascular complication involving the last remaining vessel may threaten the limb.

2. We prefer to access the anterior tibial artery as it crosses the ankle over the dorsum of the vessel and also is compressible, which allows for closure with a radial compression band at termination of the procedure. The posterior tibial artery may also be accessed by placing the patient in a "frog leg" position and closed similarly as the anterior tibial artery. Peroneal arterial puncture is possible under fluoroscopic guidance because ultrasound and palpation are frequently not useful. A generous amount of local anesthetic is administered both to the soft tissue around the vessel and to the adjacent periosteum when accessing the tibial vessels.

3. Once the vessel is punctured, advance an 0.021-inch or 0.018-inch guidewire and insert a tibial access sheath. The sheath only needs to be inserted into the vessel and so does not need to be fully inserted so that the "hub" is against the skin.

4. Standard vasodilator cocktail should be administered through the sidearm of the sheath and subsequent anticoagulation should be administered systemically.

5. Proceed with retrograde lesion crossing and treatment.

Brachial and Axillary Arterial Access

Axillary and brachial artery access have been used since the early days of angiography. In patients with severe aortoiliac disease, which may limit access to the aorta, the axillary and brachial arteries may remain attractive options because of their consistent large size and are frequently relatively spared from the development of atherosclerotic disease. The axillary and brachial arteries have been used as an alternative access site for many years. Although their use has been limited because of complications that may arise both during access and during hemostasis, recent work has demonstrated the feasibility of safe axillary large-bore access for introduction of equipment for mechanical circulatory support. Closure devices have been used in these accesses, including both suture type and collagen-plug type devices having been previously described in addition to simple manual hemostasis. A common technique for hemostasis of an axillary access is the "dry closure" technique, wherein a balloon is advanced from a secondary access site (typically femoral) and inflated at the access site as the equipment is removed to gain hemostasis. Most accesses will have closed after 10 to 20 minutes of balloon inflation. Care should be taken not to oversize a balloon to prevent dissection of the vessel.

Recently percutaneous axillary access has been used to place mechanical circulatory devices with the intent of leaving the device in place for an extended period of time, so that patients can continue to participate with inpatient rehabilitation and ambulation. Larger devices such as an Impella 5.0 (Abiomed) can also be used similarly but are frequently implanted through a surgically placed graft rather than percutaneous access.

Superficial Femoral and Popliteal Arterial Artery Access

Popliteal artery and distal SFA access has been described as a retrograde option for recanalization of complex aortoiliac and proximal femoral disease (Fig. 13.3). Nevertheless, with better equipment and greater operator experience with pedial/tibial access, this access site is not often used. Vascular complications remain high and using this option for retrograde access should be reserved for experienced operators at high-volume centers.

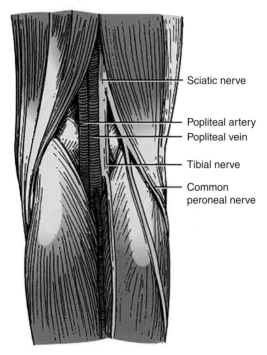

Figure 13.3 Anatomy of the popliteal fossa.

Deep Venous and Large Bore Access

Venous access is frequently used for cardiac and noncardiac procedures. Although superficial venous access is a necessary skill for operators who treat varicose veins and superficial venous reflux, those procedures will not be discussed here.

The deep venous system is frequently accessed in the legs for deep venous thrombectomy and to treat iliac vein compression syndromes. Likewise, large-bore venous access is useful for performing structural heart interventions, cannulating for mechanical circulatory support, including extracorporeal membrane oxygenation (ECMO), and other intravascular procedures, including pulmonary and intravascular/intracardiac thrombectomy/vegetectomy.

For deep venous thrombosis involving the femoropopliteal veins, the distal popliteal vein is accessible under ultrasound while the patient is placed prone on the table (as demonstrated in Supplemental Video 13.2). Large-bore access is obtained to the central venous system typically by the femoral venous or internal jugular vein. For these procedures, the central veins are sufficiently distensible to accommodate insertion of 20F sheath sizes and larger. In the peripheral vascular space, the Dry-Seal sheath (Gore Medical) is a mainstay of large-bore access because these sheaths are available in a variety of sizes and allow for the introduction of a wide range of equipment, including thrombectomy catheters such as the AngioVac (AngioDynamics) and FlowTriever (Inari Medical) systems. These access techniques are used similarly for cannulation for the venous limb of either a venovenous (V-V) or venoarterial (V-A) ECMO circuit or other mechanical support systems including the TandemHeart (TandemLife) and ProTek Duo (CardiacAssist, Pittsburgh PA).

There are several techniques that may be employed for closure of venous access. In the absence of anticoagulation, manual pressure is frequently sufficient to obtain hemostasis for most sheath sizes. In the anticoagulated patient, however, other forms of intra- and extravascular closure are often chosen. The ProGlide (Abbott, Austin Tx) preclose system can be used at time of access as a "preclose" device as is commonly employed for arterial access. For venous accesses ranging from 8F to 12F, a single "preclose" will be effective, whereas for larger-bore accesses, a second suture may be used at the time of access.

The Vascade (Cardiva Medical) is available in sizes that fit 5F, 6F to 7F, and 8F to 12F accesses and are approved for venous closure using an extravascular collagen plug. For larger-bore access, dermal sutures using high tensile suture material, such as 0- Ti-Cron (Covidien), Mersilene (Ethicon) or similar sutures, may be used in several configurations. A "purse-string" stitch has been described as an effective method for extravascular hemostasis and the suture material may be removed 48 to 72 hours after the procedure safely. Similarly, a figure-of-8 stitch is likewise effective in providing hemostasis.

Suture Closure of Large-Bore Access

1. After removing equipment from the large-bore sheath but before removing the access, use a long curved needle to drive high-tensile strength suture material.

2. For the figure-of-8 stitch (Fig. 13.4), the needle enters the skin distal to the access point further from the operator, taking a deep "bite" of dermis and subdermal tissue toward the operator and then exiting the skin. A second similar stitch is made, this

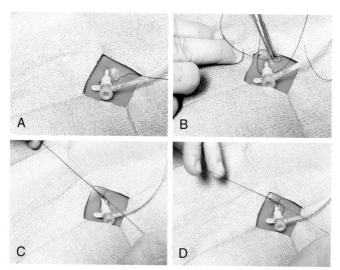

Figure 13.4 **"Figure-of-8" Suture.** (A–D) Start with the needle distal to the sheath and further from you, oriented toward you. Take one "bite," deep enough to grab sufficient dermal tissue. Take a second "bite" with similar orientation but proximal to the sheath, taking care not to capture the vein or sheath with this "bite." Tie the knot and cinch down as the sheath is removed. (Demonstrated on a nonbiologic model.)

time proximal to the access point, again beginning further from the operator and exiting the skin closer to the operator. Care should be taken to be superficial relative to the vein and sheath so as not to tie off the vein with the suture. Cut the needle off. The two ends can now be approximated to form a "figure of 8." Double loop the suture material and cinch down on the skin as the sheath is being removed. The suture should be tied tight but not so tight that it breaks the suture or causes skin necrosis. Several square knots should ensure that the suture does not come loose.

3. For a purse-string stitch (Fig. 13.5), use short, medium-depth "bites" in sequence around the access sheath. Typically, five to seven "bites" are used to traverse the circumference around the access. After the final "bite," cut the needle from the suture material. Double loop the suture and cinch down on the skin as the sheath is being removed. Several square knots will ensure the suture does not come loose. The skin is pulled centrally and becomes "puckered," resembling a coin purse (Fig. 13.6).

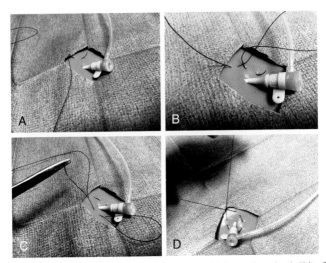

Figure 13.5 **"Purse-String" Suture.** (A–D) Multiple medium-depth "bites" are taken around the sheath in a circular fashion, usually requiring 5 to 7 steps. After completing the circle, tie the suture and cinch down tight as the sheath is removed. (Demonstrated on a nonbiologic model.)

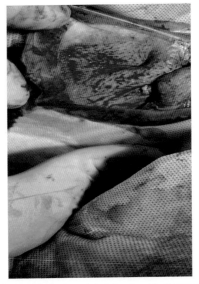

Figure 13.6 Completed "purse-string" suture.

Key References

Bailey SR, Beckman JA, Dao TD, et al. ACC/AHA/SCAI/SIR/SVM 2018 appropriate use criteria for peripheral artery intervention: a report of the American College of Cardiology Appropriate Use Criteria Task Force, American Heart Association, Society for Cardiovascular Angiography and Interventions, Society of Interventional Radiology, and Society for Vascular Medicine. *J Am Coll Cardiol*. 2019;73(2):214-237.

Dawson K, Jones TL, Kearney KE, McCabe JM. Emerging role of large-bore percutaneous axillary vascular access: a step-by-step guide. *Interv Cardiol*. 2020;15:e07.

Harris E, Warner CJ, Hnath JC, Sternbach Y, Darling RC III. Percutaneous axillary artery access for endovascular interventions. *J Vasc Surg*. 2018;68(2):555-559.

Kithcart AP, Beckman JA. ACC/AHA versus ESC guidelines for diagnosis and management of peripheral artery disease: JACC Guideline Comparison. *J Am Coll Cardiol*. 2018;72(22):2789-2801.

Yeow KM, Toh CH, Wu CH, et al. Sonographically guided antegrade common femoral artery access. *J Ultrasound Med*. 2002;21(12):1413-1416.

References

Adnan SM, Romagnonli AN, Elansary NN, et al. Radial versus femoral arterial access for trauma endovascular interventions: a noninferiority study. *J Trauma Acute Care Surg*. 2020;89(3):458-463.

Akkaya E, Sözener K, Rixe J, et al. Venous access closure using a purse-string suture without heparin antagonism or additional compression after MitraClip implantation. *Catheter Cardiovasc Interv*. 2020;96(1):179-186.

Bhimaraj A, Agrawal T, Duran A, et al. Percutaneous left axillary artery placement of intra-aortic balloon pump in advanced heart failure patients. *JACC Heart Fail*. 2020;8(4):313-323.

European Stroke Organisation, Tendera M, Aboyans V, et al. ESC guidelines on the diagnosis and treatment of peripheral artery diseases: document covering atherosclerotic disease of extracranial carotid and vertebral, mesenteric, renal, upper and lower extremity arteries: the task force on the diagnosis and treatment of peripheral artery diseases of the European Society of Cardiology (ESC). *Eur Heart J*. 2011;32(22):2851-2906.

Hwang JH, Park SW, Kwon YW, Min J, Chee HK, Shin JK. Ultrasonography-guided antegrade common femoral artery approach: factors associated with access time. *J Vasc Access*. 2021;22(3):364-369.

Kennedy SA, Rajan DK, Bassett P, Tan KT, Jaberi A, Mafeld S. Complication rates associated with antegrade use of vascular closure devices: a systematic review and pooled analysis. *J Vasc Surg*. 2021;73(2):722-730.e1.

Kumar AJ, Jones LE, Kollmeyer KR, et al. Radial artery access for peripheral endovascular procedures. *J Vasc Surg*. 2017;66(3):820-825.

Norgren L, Hiatt WR, Dormandy JA, et al. Inter-society consensus for the management of peripheral arterial disease (TASC II). *J Vasc Surg*. 2007;45 Suppl S:S5-S67.

Oderich GS, Forbes TL, Chaer R, et al. Reporting standards for endovascular aortic repair of aneurysms involving the renal-mesenteric arteries. *J Vasc Surg*. 2021;73(suppl 1):4S-52S.

Posham R, Young LB, Lookstein RA, Pena C, Patel RS, Fischman AM. Radial access for lower extremity peripheral arterial interventions: Do we have the tools? *Semin Intervent Radiol*. 2018;35(5):427-434.

Ramirez JL, Zarkowsky DS, Sorrentino TA, et al. Antegrade common femoral artery closure device use is associated with decreased complications. *J Vasc Surg*. 2020; 72(5):1610-1617.e1.

Tu T, Toma C, Tapson VF, et al. A prospective, single-arm, multicenter trial of catheter-directed mechanical thrombectomy for intermediate-risk acute pulmonary embolism: The FLARE Study. *JACC Cardiovasc Interv*. 2019;12(9):859-869.

Uceda PV, Feldtman RW, Peralta J, Ahn SS. Endovascular treatment of type 3 and 4 thoracic central vein obstruction in hemodialysis patients. *J Vasc Surg Venous Lymphat Disord*. 2021;9(3):643-651.e3.

Guides, Wires, Balloons, and Stents for Noncoronary Interventions

ANDREW J. P. KLEIN • BEAU M. HAWKINS

KEY POINTS

- Peripheral interventions require a variety of equipment different from coronary interventions and specific for the noncoronary interventional complexity.

- Access site and equipment choices are driven by the specific procedure to be performed and require careful preprocedural planning.

- Most peripheral interventional techniques focus on balloon treatment with adjunctive atherectomy but rarely use stent placement (as opposed to coronary interventions) to maximize outcomes.

Introduction

Peripheral vascular interventions (PVI) are being increasingly performed across a number of vascular beds by a variety of specialists. As with coronary interventions, appropriate patient selection coupled with facile use of equipment facilitates technical success and the achievement of optimal patient outcomes. Although many of the devices used for PVI share similar properties to those used in the coronary tree, important differences exist because of differences in disease location, vessel size, and other

Disclosures:
AJK: None; BMH: Consulting: Baim Research Institute, Research: Behring, Hemostemix, NIH

factors. This chapter reviews commonly used wires, guides, balloons, stents, and other devices for PVI.

General Principles

One can broadly classify PVI into categories based on the lesion site and whether or not the intervention is arterial or venous. Major arterial vascular beds to be considered are the carotid, upper extremity, visceral (renal and mesenteric), and lower extremity. Venous interventions are beyond the scope of this chapter.

As with coronary interventions, most diagnostic peripheral procedures are performed using a vast array of diagnostic catheters. Nevertheless, the majority of peripheral interventional procedures are completed using sheaths as opposed to guiding catheters. The utilization of interventional sheaths allows for use of smaller-bore arterial access (e.g., 5–7 French [F]), increases support to cross rigid and calcified lesions, and facilitates the delivery of devices that are often needed to treat these larger vessels. Peripheral equipment is thus labeled by minimal sheath size and not guide size, which is usually 2F sizes larger. For instance, a peripheral stent that is compatible with a 6F sheath normally requires an 8F guide catheter.

Regarding access location, the common femoral artery (CFA) is most often used to approach and treat peripheral vessels. Indeed, the lengths of existing peripheral equipment allow for most arterial segments to be successfully treated from a transfemoral approach. Many lower extremity arterial interventions can now be safely performed from the radial artery, and interest in this approach is expanding because of perceived improvements in patient safety. For some complex lower extremity arterial interventions, antegrade CFA access or retrograde access (e.g., pedal or popliteal/superficial femoral) is needed. In the case of venous interventions, CFA, popliteal, and jugular approaches are commonly employed.

One of the major differences between PVI and coronary intervention is the varying equipment length and the necessity for different sheath sizes. Sheaths come in varying lengths and French sizes, ranging from 3F to over 24F in diameter, with lengths as short as 4 cm to as long as 200 cm. The optimal length of sheath depends on the distance from the access site to the target lesion. It is advantageous to have the sheath tip parked near the target lesion so that concomitant angiography can be easily performed during each step of the intervention. Typically, a 25-cm sheath is used for ipsilateral common iliac intervention and a 45-cm sheath is often used for crossing over from the CFA to the contralateral CFA to perform femoropopliteal interventions. For popliteal and infrapopliteal lesions, 70-, 90-, and 110-cm sheaths are often used depending on the patient's height. For the radial-to-peripheral (R2P) approach, Terumo has developed several longer sheaths, which can extend from the left radial to the left iliac or CFA on most patients.

With respect to the diameter of the sheath, the risk of bleeding and vessel trauma increases with larger sheaths. Typically, for most arterial interventions outside of endovascular aneurysm repair (EVAR), sheath sizes vary between 5F and 12F. The required sheath size depends on the size of the definitive therapy used to address the lesion. Where stents are to be used, one must be cognizant of the sheath size required to deliver the desired stent, even if the other interventions, such as balloon catheters for angioplasty, are compatible with smaller sheath sizes. Typically, balloon-expandable stents (BES) require larger sheath sizes than self-expanding stents (SES). Covered stents also require larger sheaths than their noncovered counterparts. Depending on lesion location, the choice of sheath size should also account for any possible need for bailout covered stenting in the case of vessel perforation. For example, in aortoiliac intervention, especially if there is a chronic total occlusion (CTO) or marked vessel calcification, most operators use at minimum a 7F sheath to permit covered stent deployments in case of vessel rupture or perforation.

Guidewire selection for PVI is complex and is predicated on the location of the vessel being addressed and on the goal of the procedure (e.g., diagnostic or intervention). There are three major systems based on the caliber in inches of the guidewire being used: 0.014 inches, 0.018 inches, and 0.035 inches. The smaller wires are used mostly in smaller, more delicate arteries, whereas the larger ones are employed in large vessels, such as the iliac arteries and femoropopliteal distributions. Because of the varying equipment lengths for PVI, most operators choose 300 cm length wires. With increasing wire size comes increasing strength, pushability, and torquability but with an increasing risk for vessel trauma and perforation. For smaller, more delicate vessels where perforation could be catastrophic (carotid and renals), 0.014-inch wires are almost always exclusively used.

Guidewires come in a variety of types and are classified into standard workhorse wires, polymer-coated wires for crossing occlusions, and support wires. Each of these subtypes (Tables 14.1–14.3) are available in each size of wire: 0.014 inches, 0.018 inches, and 0.035 inches. Typically, operators will try and cross lesions with a workhorse wire unless the lesion is a CTO, where a polymer-jacketed wire may be required to cross subintimally or through microchannels. Workhorse wires typically have reasonable support and an atraumatic tip, along with adequate steerability to negotiate most vessel bends. In contrast, polymer-jacketed wires are lubricious and slippery and can unknowingly enter into small side branches or into

Table 14.1

Examples of Commonly Used 0.035-inch Guidewires and Performance Characteristics

Producer	Model	Body core	Support	Hydrophilic tip	Flexing point	Main use
Abbott Vascular	Supra Core	Steel	High	No	-	Position
Boston Scientific	Amplatz Super Stiff	Steel	High	No	-	Position
Cordis	AQUATRACK Regular	Nitinol	Low	Yes	3 cm	Crossing
Cordis	AQUATRACK Stiff	Nitinol	Medium	Yes	3 cm	Crossing
Covidien	Stiff Shaft	Nitinol	High	No	-	Position
Terumo	Radifocus M Standard	Nitinol	Low	Yes	3 cm	Crossing
Terumo	Radifocus M Stiff	Nitinol	Medium	Yes	3 cm	Crossing
Terumo	Radifocus M Half-stiff	Nitinol	Medium	Yes	1.5 cm	Crossing
Terumo	Glidewire Advantage	Nitinol	High	Yes	5 cm	Crossing

From Lorenzoni R, Ferraresi R, Manzi M, Roffi M. Guidewires for lower extremity artery angioplasty: A review. *EuroIntervention.* 2015;11(7):799–807.

Table 14.2

Examples of Commonly Used 0.018-inch Guidewires and Performance Characteristics

Producer	Model	Body core	Support	Tip design	Tip weight	Hydrophilic tip	Tapered tip	Flexing point	Main use
Abbott Vascular	Connect	Steel	Medium	Core to tip	4.0 g	Yes	No	–	Crossing
Abbott Vascular	Connect Flex	Steel	Medium	Core to tip	12.0 g	Yes	No	3 cm	Crossing
Abbott Vascular	Connect 250T	Steel	Medium	Core to tip	30.0 g	No	Yes	–	Crossing
Abbott Vascular	Steelcore	Steel	High	Shaping ribbon	–	No	No	–	Position
ASAHI	Treasure 12	Steel	Medium	Core to tip	12.0 g	No	No	–	Crossing
ASAHI	Astato 30	Steel	Medium	Core to tip	30.0 g	No	Yes	–	Crossing
Boston Scientific	Platinum Plus	Steel	High	Core to tip	5 g	No	No	–	Position
Boston Scientific	V-18 Long Taper	Steel	Medium	Core to tip	6 g	Yes	No	–	Crossing
Boston Scientific	V-18 Short Taper	Steel	Medium	Core to tip	8 g	Yes	No	8 cm	Crossing
Boston Scientific	Victory 18	Steel	Medium	Core to tip	12–18– 25–30 g	Yes	No	–	Crossing
Optimed	Plywire	Steel	Medium	Core to tip	–	No	No	–	Position
Terumo	Glidewire Advantage	Nitinol	High	Core to tip	–	Yes	No	1 cm	Crossing

From Lorenzoni R, Ferraresi R, Manzi M, Roffi M. Guidewires for lower extremity artery angioplasty: A review. *EuroIntervention.* 2015;11(7):799–807.

Table 14.3

Examples of Commonly Used 0.014-inch Guidewires and Performance Characteristics

Producer	Model	Body core	Support	Tip design	Tip weight	Hydrophilic tip	Tapered tip	Main use
Abbott Vascular	Command	Steel nitinol	Low	Core to tip	2.8 g	Yes	No	Crossing
Abbott Vascular	Command ES	Steel nitinol	Medium	Core to tip	3.5 g	Yes	No	Crossing
Abbott Vascular	Spartacore	Steel	High	Core to tip	0.9 g	No	No	Position
Abbott Vascular	Winn 40, 80	Steel	Medium	Core to tip	4.8–9.7 g	No	No	Crossing
Abbott Vascular	Winn 200T	Steel	Medium	Core to tip	13 g	No	Yes	Crossing
ASAHI	Regalia XS 1.0	Steel	Low	Core to tip	1.0 g	Yes	No	Crossing
ASAHI	Astato XS 20	Steel	Medium	Core to tip	20.0 g	No	Yes	Crossing
ASAHI	Grand Slam	Steel	High	Core to tip	0.7 g	No	No	Position
Boston Scientific	V-14 Long Taper	Steel	High	Core to tip	3 g	Yes	No	Crossing
Boston Scientific	Victory 14	Steel	Medium	Core to tip	12, 18, 25, 30 g	Yes	No	Crossing
Boston Scientific	Platinum Plus	Steel	High	Core to tip	7.1 g	No	No	Position

Continued on following page

Table 14.3

Examples of Commonly Used 0.014-Inch Guidewires and Performance Characteristics (Continued)

Producer	Model	Body core	Support	Tip design	Tip weight	Hydrophilic tip	Tapered tip	Main use
Cook Medical	Approach CTO 6, 12, 18, 25	Steel	Medium	Core to tip	6, 12, 18, 25 g	No	No	Crossing
Terumo	Glidewire Advantage	Nitinol	High	Core to tip	-	Yes	No	Crossing

From Lorenzoni R, Ferraresi R, Manzi M, Roffi M. Guidewires for lower extremity artery angioplasty: A review. *EuroIntervention.* 2015;11(7):799–807.

the subintimal space. For CTOs, these wires are exceptionally useful for the subintimal dissection/reentry technique. This technique involves the penetration of the CTO intentionally into the subintimal space followed by a support catheter. A small loop is formed with the wire and catheter, and together en bloc they are advanced through the occlusion subintimally until the distal cap, where manipulation of the wire can often result in wire reentry into the true distal lumen. The catheter can then be advanced over this wire, which should be free and mobile if it is true lumen. Most operators will remove the wire and blood should return. Additionally, a pressure can be transduced or contrast injected through the catheter to confirm intraluminal position. If the catheter is in the subintimal space, a characteristic vacuum suction sound will occur upon removal of the wire. The return of blood does not automatically imply the distal catheter is in the true lumen.

Once across the lesion of interest, one may choose to use the workhorse wire or change to a more supportive wire. Changing to a supportive wire facilitates the crossing of the lesion with balloons and stents. Once a strong supportive wire is in place, one can also use the sheath to advance across the lesion. This technique permits one to pull back the sheath, "unsheathing" the device (typically a stent) across the lesion. This technique reduces the chance of the stent coming off the balloon while traversing the lesion. Support wires often have atraumatic tips that lower the risk of downstream wire perforation, but one must be ever vigilant of this possibility as the stiffer wires transfer force more easily.

Finally, PVI differ from coronaries in the issue of working length. In the coronary realm, most guides are 100 cm long. In the periphery, there are numerous options depending on the distance between the access point and the target lesion. Obviously, the longer the distance between these, the less pushability and support exists, given that transmitted force dissipates with increasing distance. One must be ever mindful of the ability to deliver the appropriate equipment to the region of interest with enough support and potential for angiography for accurate placement. For this reason, long 300-cm wires are often used in the periphery to preclude running out of wire length. Balloons and stents come in varying working lengths with short 40-cm working lengths for arteriovenous (AV) fistula work, 80 cm for aortoiliac intervention, 135 cm for femoropopliteal intervention, and a 150-cm length for infrapopliteal intervention. There are also 170 cm and 200 cm working lengths for distal infrapopliteal intervention via the contralateral CFA approach and the advent of even longer working lengths (200 and 250 cm) for the radial approach (R2P).

Balloons

Peripheral interventional balloons come in 0.014-inch, 0.018-inch, and 0.035-inch wire compatible versions with the lowest crossing profile typically being in the 0.014-inch platform. Occasionally, coronary balloons are required to cross especially tight lesions given these balloons have the smallest crossing profile. Regardless of platform, balloon lengths range from 20 mm to 250 mm. With increasing balloon length, there is a noted decrease in crossing profile and therefore one may need a shorter balloon first for vessel prep before use of a longer balloon for definitive therapy. The shaft length of each balloon also varies and the distance to the target lesion must also be considered as previously addressed.

Most balloons in the peripheral space are relatively noncompliant by nature given the calcification that is often present in the peripheral vascular beds. For truly nondilatable lesions, specialty noncompliant balloons coated with Kevlar, for example, or other strong coatings to preclude balloon rupture do exist.

Specialty peripheral balloons including scoring and cutting balloons (Angiosculpt, Cutting, and Chocolate balloons). Fig. 14.1 are often used for vessel preparation or definitive therapy. Although no compelling data suggest these balloons are superior to standard

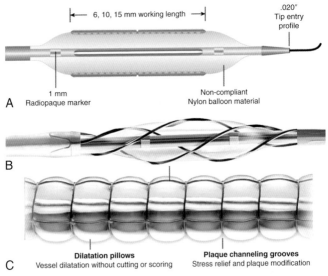

Figure 14.1   Types of Specialty Balloons. (A) Cutting balloon (Boston Scientific). (B) Angiosculpt (Philips Healthcare). (C) Chocolate Balloon (Medtronic).

balloons, operators often use them in cases of nondilatable or calcified, resistant lesions.

Another newer technology for resistant lesions is lithoplasty. The lithoplasty balloon catheters (Shockwave Medical; Fig. 14.2) has been an important advance in the field of peripheral intervention. It uses small emitters within the balloon to pulse soundwaves via a separate generator. The sound energy works in conjunction with low pressure angioplasty to disrupt vessel calcification and facilitate vessel expansion. This soundwave energy approximates the force of a balloon dilated to 50 ATM and has the ability to fracture medial calcification without barotrauma to the endothelium. Because of the nature of the device, distal embolization is infrequent, and most operators do not use distal embolic protection with this device. This technology has recently become available in the coronary vascular bed as well.

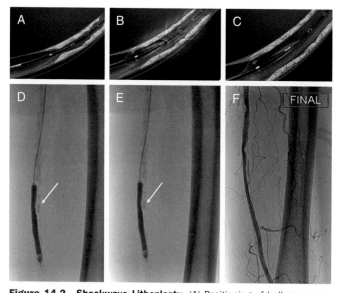

Figure 14.2 Shockwave Lithoplasty. (A) Positioning of balloon across stenosis with emitters placed at areas of high calcium. (B) Inflation of balloon to low pressure with deployment of sound energy fracturing the medial calcification. (C) Full expansion of the balloon after fracture of the calcification (D–E) after crossing subintimally of a calcified sfa inflation of a 6 mm x 60 mm shockwave with balloon expansion being noted after cycle deployment (*arrow*). (F) Final angiography with an adequate angiographic result after balloon angioplasty only.

Drug-coated balloons (DCBs) have been shown to reduce the risk of restenosis in long lesions and in those patients with high risk for restenosis. Currently, because of a metanalysis by Katsanos suggesting an increase in mortality with the use of DCB technology in the form of balloons or drug-eluting stents (DES), there is a US Food and Drug Administration (FDA) warning regarding any drug-coated or eluting technology. For short lesions that have a low risk of restenosis, PTA with non-DCB balloons is likely more than adequate. For longer lesions, CTOs, and patients with risk for factors for restenosis, one must weigh the risks and benefits of drug technology carefully.

Noncoronary Stents

In the coronary realm, all stents are balloon expandable and are mounted on a single shaft length. Most are also now drug-coated. Outside of the coronary beds, stents are divided into balloon-expandable (BES) and self-expanding stents (SES). These two types of stents also have covered and uncovered varieties (Fig. 14.3). BES bare or BES covered stents are effective in treating lesions where radial force and precise deployment are desired (common

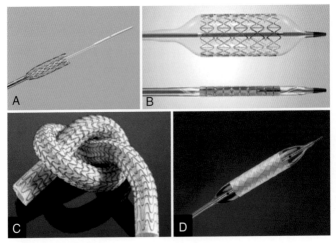

Figure 14.3 Peripheral Vascular Stent Types. (A) Self-expanding stent. (B) Balloon-expandable stent. (C) Self-expanding covered stent. (D) Balloon-expandable covered stent.

iliac, renals, mesenterics, subclavians). These stents are often able to be postdilated 2 mm beyond their listed diameter, which can often be helpful in the required access sheath. For instance, a 9-mm BES can often be delivered through a 7F sheath and postdilated to 11 mm if required, whereas an 11 mm BES would require a 10F sheath. These stents are deployed in the same fashion as coronaries with the caveat that the contrast mixture within the balloon is often diluted to 50/50 with normal saline to enable visualization but also to permit the balloon to deflate in a reasonable time and fashion. This is especially true for longer stents and balloons.

SES bare or SES covered are used when there is vessel-size mismatch (e.g., external iliac artery) and in vessels that are more tortuous and prone to movement. These stents come in varying diameters (4 mm–14 mm) and lengths (20 mm–250 mm). The stent will expand to the diameter listed so a 10-mm stent will deploy to a maximal of 10 mm and conform to the smaller diameter of the distal vessel. Thus one typically oversizes the stent. These stents are then postdilated using a balloon with a 1:1 size to the reference segment. These stents lack radial strength and will conform easily and thus adequate vessel preparation is required before stent deployment. One unique SES, the Supera (Abbott), requires special mention given that the radial strength of this stent is 5 times that of most SES, and this is because of its unique design, which is similar to a Slinky (registered trademark). The deployment of this stent is very unique and novel operators are encouraged to receive training before use.

Both BES and SES come in covered versions. Covered BES (Atrium, ICAST and VBX, Cook) and covered SES (Viabahn, Gore) offer the ability to exclude aneurysms, trap plaque or thrombus that may distally embolize, and permit safe dilatation in calcified vessels where rupture is possible. These stents are invaluable if vessel perforation occurs, and one must plan for this potential because covered stents often require large sheath sizes for delivery. For instance, in the case of CTO revascularization in the iliacs, we recommend at least 7F access in case of perforation, which in this vascular bed can be fatal. Operators must be cognizant of the wire size required for covered stents because not all of them are compatible with 0.035-inch guidewires.

Conclusions

Much of the equipment used for PVI shares similar qualities to that used in the coronary space. Appropriate selection of this equipment tailored to individual vascular beds optimizes the chances of procedural success and optimal patient outcomes.

Key References

Feldman DN, Armstrong EJ, Aronow HD. SCAI consensus guidelines for device selection in femoral-popliteal arterial interventions. *Catheter Cardiovasc Interv.* 2018; 92:124-140.

Feldman DN, Armstrong EJ, Aronow HD, et al. SCAI guidelines on device selection in Aorto-Iliac arterial interventions. *Cathet Cardiovasc Intervent.* 2020;96:915-929.

Gerhard-Herman MD, Gornik HL, Barrett C, et al. 2016 AHA/ACC guideline on the management of patients with lower extremity peripheral artery disease: a report of the American College of Cardiology/American Heart Association Task Force on Clinical Practice Guidelines. *J Am Coll Cardiol.* 2017;69:e71-e126.

Halperin JL, Levine GN, Al-Khatib SM, et al. Further evolution of the ACC/AHA clinical practice guideline recommendation classification system: a report of the American College of Cardiology/American Heart Association Task Force on Clinical Practice Guidelines. *Circulation.* 2016;133:1426-1428.

Katsanos K, Spiliopoulos S, Kitrou P, Krokidis M, Karnabatidis D. Risk of death following application of paclitaxel-coated balloons and stents in the femoropopliteal artery of the leg: a systematic review and meta-analysis of randomized controlled trials. *J Am Heart Assoc.* 2018;7:e011245.

Iliofemoral Peripheral Vascular Intervention

MATTHEW T. FINN • H. KIRAN KUMAR REDDY • SAHIL A. PARIKH

KEY POINTS

- Patients with symptomatic lower extremity peripheral artery disease often present with classical burning, cramping pain made worse with exertion and better with rest (known as "intermittent claudication").

- The symptomatic location is typically one level below the area of arterial stenosis; however, multilevel stenoses are frequently encountered, especially in critical limb ischemia.

- Endovascular intervention for symptomatic claudication has a level I recommendation for iliac interventions and a IIa indication for femoral-popliteal disease in patients not responsive to goal-directed medical therapy and supervised exercise therapy.

- A complex armamentarium of devices exists for the treatment of symptomatic lower extremity peripheral artery disease, including angioplasty, stents, atherectomy devices, specialty/focal force balloons, and drug-coated devices.

Introduction

Guideline-directed treatment of the iliofemoral arterial segments is largely determined by patient presentation and response to medical therapy. First-line treatments for peripheral arterial disease include blood pressure management, antiplatelet treatment, aggressive lipid lowering with statins, and smoking cessation. Additionally, the use of cilostazol and supervised exercise therapy have been associated with significant improvement in functional status and symptoms.

When invasive treatment is indicated, endovascular approaches have become favored in many situations. A study of the Medicare population in the United States demonstrated that endovascular treatments occur at four times the rate of open surgical treatment. In recent years, technological advancements have dramatically diversified the treatment options available to achieve procedural and technical success, with an overall goal of enhancing longer-term patency. Despite these advances, durability of interventions may still be limited because of the complex array of forces caused by flexion, extension, and rotation of joints in each of these vascular segments.

Patient Evaluation and Noninvasive Assessment

Iliac obstructive disease classically manifests as thigh and buttock claudication. It may also present with sexual dysfunction if the obstruction occurs proximal to the origin of the internal iliac artery, which supplies much of the pelvic vasculature. Iliac stenosis also frequently mimics spinal stenosis or lumbosacral spine disease (pseudoclaudication). Classically, more upright posture will worsen symptoms (i.e., walking down a hill), suggesting pseudoclaudication because of postural compression of the nerve roots involved. Pseudoclaudication can be improved with leaning forward, whereas ischemic claudication will be improved with rest. In contradistinction, femoral stenosis manifests as exertional symptoms in the thigh, calf, or foot (burning, cramping pain). Pulses will be diminished below the level of the stenosis on exam.

Pulse volume recordings (PVR) and ankle brachial indices (ABI) can be useful in determining the presence, severity, and location of vascular stenoses (Fig. 15.1). In patients with equivocal testing, exercise may be added to enhance the sensitivity of the test and to garner additional prognostic data. Standardized protocols can help discern progressive disease.

Ultrasound studies are routinely ordered to investigate symptomatic patients with abnormal ABI studies when revascularization or anatomic delineation is required. Increases in peak systolic Doppler velocity are used to grade stenosis severity (Fig. 15.2a) and, when correlated with clinical symptoms, may trigger further evaluation and treatment. The ratio of the affected segment compared with the upstream segment is helpful in quantifying this change. Change in phase of Doppler waveforms may also be useful when interpreting ultrasound studies with proximal aortoiliac disease, which may not have been evaluated specifically on femoropopliteal-focused ultrasonography (see Fig. 15.2b).

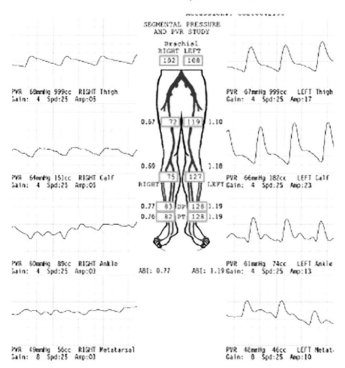

Figure 15.1 Positive resting pulse volume recording in the right leg with loss of phasicity from the proximal thigh with worsening at the ankle.

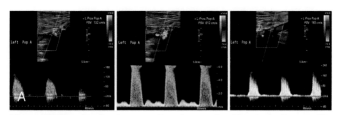

Figure 15.2A Popliteal artery subtotal stenosis with velocity "step up" in stenotic area.

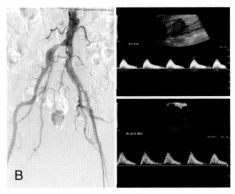

Figure 15.2B Phasicity change to parvus et tardus waveform in the external iliac artery (EIA) and right mid superficial femoral (Rt SFA MID).

Claudication Versus Chronic Limb-Threatening Ischemia

The distinction in patient presentation between claudication and chronic limb-threatening ischemia (CLTI; also commonly referred to as critical limb ischemia [CLI]) warrants discussion because treatment approaches and goals are very different between the groups. In patients with claudication, the primary goal is primarily symptom reduction. This goal can often be accomplished via supervised exercise programs with the addition of cilostazol. CLTI is defined as rest pain or tissue loss/gangrene lasting longer than 2 weeks and associated with abnormal hemodynamic findings. The nomenclature of CLTI has recently changed based on the Society of Vascular Surgery (SVS) guidelines from the classic term "critical limb ischemia" to emphasize the chronicity of the presentation. When CLTI is diagnosed, revascularization (either surgical or endovascular) with goal-directed medical therapy carries a level I recommendation by the 2016 American Heart Association (AHA/American College of Cardiology (ACC) guidelines. Conversely, revascularization for claudication should be performed after inadequate response to goal-directed medical treatment (strength of recommendation IIA).

An additional treatment distinction must be clarified when comparing approaches to treatment of claudication with CLTI. In patients with claudication, invasive intervention can often be approached in a stepwise manner, treating inflow (aortoiliac) lesions first before moving to outflow (femoropopliteal). The goal in CLTI, however, is restoration of in-line flow to the affected area (via surgical or endovascular means) to enhance the probability of wound healing.

Selective Angiography, Carbon Dioxide Imaging, and Vascular Ultrasound

Contrast Angiography

Fluoroscopic angiography with use of iodinated contrast remains the gold standard for invasive assessment of peripheral arterial disease. Digital subtraction angiography (DSA) is often used to remove bony or dense tissue structures to enhance vascular visualization. A half and half mix of saline and contrast is usually used with DSA to reduce dye exposure and diminish patient discomfort associated with contrast injection into the distal vascular beds.

Carbon Dioxide Angiography

Carbon dioxide (CO_2) angiography can enable endovascular angiography with the potential for dramatically reducing or eliminating contrast dye exposure (Fig. 15.3A–C). CO_2 may also be useful for individuals at high risk for severe contrast allergies. Successive CO_2 injections should be spaced apart by 2 to 3 minutes because multiple rapid injections can lead to intestinal ischemia. Visualization of infrapopliteal vessels may be limited with CO_2 injections. In such scenarios, one can switch the system to contrast injections for enhanced distal vessel visualization or, in the absence of severe proximal disease, CO_2 injection can be done via a catheter placed more distally.

Intravascular and Extravascular Ultrasound

Intravascular ultrasound (IVUS) can aid in assessment of vascular pathology, enable accurate vessel sizing, and assist in postintervention assessment (Fig. 15.4). Preintervention IVUS for vessel sizing can be especially useful in vessels at the extremes of size both large and small in which visual estimation may be challenging. IVUS can also assess the severity of vascular calcification and help determine the need for more complex treatments for lesion preparation (e.g., use of focal force balloons, lithotripsy, or atherectomy). Postintervention imaging can assess adequacy of vessel expansion, note lesion coverage, and assess complications such as dissection or intramural hematoma.

Intraprocedural use of extravascular ultrasound has obvious applications for vascular access. Nevertheless, it has also been used to aid in intraluminal wiring during complex chronic total occlusion (CTO) wire crossing. Experienced operators have demonstrated the feasibility of avoiding fluoroscopy during intervention, thereby reducing radiation exposure to patients and staff.

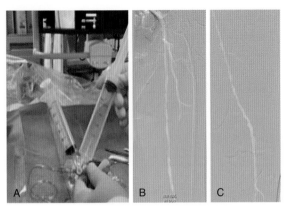

Figure 15.3 (A) CO_2 tubing set up with syringe and two-way stop cock. (B) A diseased common femoral artery and proximal superficial femoral artery seen with CO_2. (C) A diseased distal superficial femoral and popliteal artery demonstrated with CO_2.

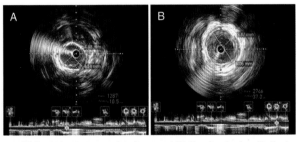

Figure 15.4 Using intravascular ultrasound (Philips, Amsterdam, Netherlands) for distal (A) and proximal (B) reference measurement. These images represent vessel sizing from the external elastic lamina measured as opposed to lumen measurement.

Endovascular Revascularization of the Iliofemoral Segments

Procedural Antithrombotic/Anticoagulant Management

Procedural Antithrombotic Treatment

Unfractionated heparin (UFH) is often used for procedural anticoagulation during iliofemoral interventions because of easy reversibility if required with protamine sulfate. Bivalirudin may also be used for peripheral intervention and has the advantage of not requiring monitoring of activated clotting time. Bivalirudin is not readily reversible.

As for antiplatelet therapy, the standard of care for most patients is to preload with aspirin monotherapy before peripheral vascular intervention. The role of preloading with P2Y12 antagonists or the use of intraprocedural parenteral antiplatelet therapy is not well studied, and the AHA/ACC guidelines make no specific recommendations for postendovascular intervention treatments. The European Society of Cardiology (ESC) 2017 guidelines give a IIa recommendation for dual antiplatelet therapy for a period of at least a month followed by long-term treatment with single antiplatelet (either low-dose aspirin or clopidogrel 75 mg/day). This recommendation is derived from recent drug device trials, which used dual antiplatelet therapy for 1 to 3 months after endovascular intervention. Some variation of this duration of dual antiplatelet therapy has largely become the standard of care after an intervention.

More recently, the VOYAGER PAD randomized trial compared aspirin alone with low-dose rivaroxaban plus aspirin 81 mg after peripheral intervention and demonstrated a reduction in major adverse cardiac and limb events at 3 years in the low-dose rivaroxaban plus aspirin 81 mg arm. Nevertheless, there was a low rate of stenting overall in the trial (30%), which may limit its generalizability.

Cilostazol, which is recommended for symptom reduction before intervention, is frequently discontinued in the United States after endovascular intervention given expectant symptomatic improvement postprocedure (analogous to nitrates in coronary interventions). Several studies have suggested that cilostazol may decrease angiographic restenosis after endovascular intervention when combined with aspirin compared with aspirin monotherapy. Despite this emerging evidence, cilostazol has not been widely adopted by societal guidelines because of an absence of large randomized data supporting its use.

Working Wire Size and Changing Between Systems

An important consideration in peripheral interventions is size of the working wire used after lesion crossing. In coronary artery interventions, 0.014 inches is the standard wire size. In peripheral intervention, however, operators use crossing catheters to change between wire sizes to enable compatibility of specialty balloons and atherectomy equipment. See Table 15.1 for a list of wire sizes associated with various commonly used devices.

Table 15.1

Endovascular Device and Wire Compatibility			
Device	0.035-inch	0.018-inch	0.014-inch
Semi-compliant peripheral balloons[a]	Yes	Yes	Yes
Drug-coated balloons[a]	Yes	Yes	
Scoring/Sculpt/ Kevlar balloons[a]	Yes	Yes	Yes
Shockwave			Yes
SpiderFx Filter			Yes
Emboshield Nav6			Yes
Peripheral IVUS (Boston Scientific and Philips)	Yes	Yes	Yes
Bare-metal stents[a]	Yes	Yes	Yes
Supera bare-metal stents		Yes	
Eluvia DES	Yes		
Zilver DES	Yes		
Tacks	Yes		
Covered stents[a]	Yes	Yes	Yes
Atherectomy		Rotarex, Diamond-back 360 (viper with 0.018" tip and 0.014 working segment)	Yes (Laser, Rotablator, Jet stream, Phoenix, Ocelot, Pantheris, HawkOne, Diamondback 360

[a]Size varies based on individual specifications by manufacturer. Note: list is not comprehensive.
Device manufacturers: Dorado (B-D), SpiderFx (Medtronic), Emboshield and Supera (Abbott), Eluvia (Boston Scientific), Zilver (Cook).
DES, Drug-eluting stent; IVUS, intravascular ultrasound.

Iliac Intervention

Endovascular treatment of patients with symptomatic obstructive iliac disease is supported with a level I recommendation in the 2016 AHA and ACC guidelines for the treatment of peripheral arterial disease because of the high clinical success rates and long-term patency of these procedures. Aortoiliac disease has been classified into four subsets (A-D) by the Trans-Atlantic Inter Society Consensus Classification (TASC). Lesions that are TASC A through

Type A lesions

- Unilateral or bilateral stenoses of CIA
- Unilateral or bilateral single short (≤3 cm) stenosis of EIA

Type B lesions

- Short (≤3 cm) stenosis of infrarenal aorta
- Unilateral CIA occlusion
- Single or multiple stenosis totaling 3–10 cm involving the EIA not extending into the CFA
- Unilateral EIA occlusion not involving the origins of internal iliac or CFA

Type C lesions

- Bilateral CIA occlusions
- Bilateral EIA stenoses 3–10 cm long not extending into the CFA
- Unilateral EIA stenosis extending into the CFA
- Unilateral EIA occlusion that involves the origins of internal iliac and/or CFA
- Heavily calcified unilateral EIA occlusions with or without involvement of origins of internal iliac and/or CFA

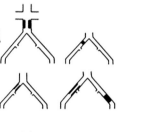

Type D lesions

- Infra-renal aortoiliac occlusion
- Diffuse disease involving the aorta and both iliac arteries requiring treatment
- Diffuse multiple stenoses involving the unilateral CIA, EIA, and CFA
- Unilateral occlusions of both CIA and EIA
- Bilateral occlusions of EIA
- Iliac stenoses in patients with AAA requiring treatment and not amenable to endograft placement or other lesions requiring open aortic or iliac surgery

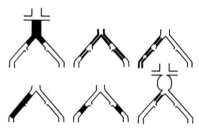

Figure 15.5 TASC II categories for guiding iliac interventions. *AAA*, Abdominal aortic aneurysm; *CIA*, common iliac artery; *TASC*, Trans-Atlantic Inter-Society Consensus. (From Norgren L, Hiatt WR, Dormandy JA, Nehler MR, Harris KA, Fowkes FGR. Inter-society consensus for the management of peripheral arterial disease [TASC II]) *J Vasc Surg.* 2007;45(Suppl S):S5–S6.)

C are typically amenable to endovascular intervention, whereas TASC D lesions may be considered for surgical revascularization (Fig. 15.5).

Iliac lesion severity is not only assessed angiographically but may also be evaluated with pullback gradients across the lesion to demonstrate hemodynamic significance. A translesional mean gradient of 10 mm Hg with hyperemia has been shown to be hemodynamically significant.

Techniques

Access in iliac interventions can be varied. Typically, common iliac lesions are approached from ipsilateral access and external iliac lesions are approached from up-and-over contralateral access or upper extremity access. In the case of aortoiliac ostial lesions, we recommend dual femoral access with a wire protecting the contralateral iliac in the event of carinal shift or geographic miss after unilateral intervention. Left radial access can also be used in common and external iliac stenoses via long specially designed radial sheaths (i.e., Terumo R2P™ sheath 119 cm in length); however, typically only 6 French (F) compatible devices can be used limiting some therapeutic options.

When addressing iliac interventions, it is important to understand the role of percutaneous transluminal angioplasty (PTA) with provisional stenting and the choice of bare-metal stenting versus covered endoprosthetic stenting. Additionally, options are available for balloon expandable (BES) versus self-expanding stents (SES). Iliac disease is often addressed with a stent-based strategy to limit recoil and prevent abrupt closure. Nevertheless, a study following patients to 5 years showed no difference in patency for low-complexity TASC A/B lesions when a PTA with provisional stenting was done compared with a primary stenting strategy. Therefore, in the absence of significant gradient or flow-limiting dissection, it is reasonable to do PTA alone.

When stenting is deemed necessary, several device types are available for consideration. BES have good radial strength and allow for precise placement. BES can also be readily postdilated to larger sizes when needed (with limitations based on individual device specifications; Fig. 15.6). SES are felt to conform better to tortuous vessels and offer enhanced flexibility, but they often have less radial strength and less precision with deployment location. SES have been shown to have greater patency than BES in iliac interventions. These devices are available as uncovered bare-metal and covered endoprosthetic stents. In head to head comparison between uncovered and covered endoprosthetic stents, there was no difference in restenosis or occlusion except in more complex lesion subsets (TASC C and D lesions) where covered endoprosthetic stents performed better. The use of covered endoprostheses are common in heavily calcified disease for prevention of perforation. Nevertheless, operators must take care to ensure accurate covered stent deployment to avoid inadvertent exclusion of side branches with attendant risk for endoleak.

Common Femoral Artery Intervention

The common femoral artery (CFA) has classically been reserved for surgical therapies given the concern for compromise of the

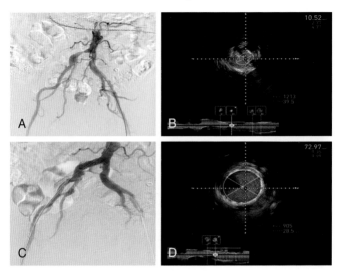

Figure 15.6 Iliac Intervention. (A) Severe right common iliac stenosis seen via contralateral injection. (B) Pre-intervention intravascular ultrasound (IVUS). (C) Open-cell bare-expandable stent (BES) placed via ipsilateral side through long cordis (Santa Clara, CA) Brite Tip Sheath. (D) Postintervention IVUS.

profunda femoris artery, which is a major supplier of collaterals and can prevent acute limb ischemia in patients with significant superficial femoral disease. Furthermore, the desire to avoid stenting the CFA may limit options for reaccess of the artery for future interventions. SES are preferred if stenting is elected. Despite the preference for surgical therapy, a recent French study showed no difference in the 2-year rate of target lesion revascularization with a higher rate of postprocedure complications in the surgical arm. Additional studies using vascular mimetic scaffolds are underway. Fig. 15.7 demonstrates a possible endovascular approach to avoid stenting the CFA. Note if there is disease involving the profunda ostium, we commonly wire it before ballooning to ensure the vessel does not become compromised. Extra care should be taken when wiring the profunda with hydrophilic wires because there are many small perforators that can be prone to perforation.

Superficial Femoral and Popliteal Intervention

The femoropopliteal segments are the most frequent sites of arterial stenosis in the lower extremity. Lesions in this territory can be

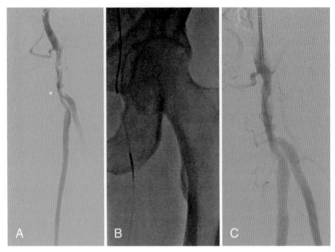

Figure 15.7 (A) Common femoral stenosis represented by (*). (B) HawkOne LS atherectomy system (Medtronic, Minneapolis, MN) (C) Angiogram after ballooning with a drug-coated balloon.

approached with endovascular or surgical intervention in patients with claudication refractory to medical management and supervised exercise therapy or in the setting of CLTI. The AHA/ACC guidelines recommend surgery as a reasonable alternative to refractory symptomatic claudication in those with acceptable operative risk and with an adequate venous conduit. The TASC anatomic characterizations (Fig. 15.8) have also been applied to guide treatment decisions between endovascular and surgical therapies.

Crossing Techniques

Using the aforementioned alternative access approaches, options for peripheral intervention can allow numerous options for lesion crossing. Historically, 0.035-inch wires, particularly hydrophilic wires (e.g., Glidewire TM) have been used as frontline. Increasingly, however, the use of lower profile 0.018-inch and 0.014-inch wires has become more common. Coupled with crossing catheters used in pairs as "mother-daughter" systems, a host of techniques are available for lesion crossing. Adjunctive tools such as vascular "roadmap" angiography and IVUS may assist in the timely and atraumatic traversal of complex stenoses.

CTOs present particular challenges to the endovascular operator, involving up to 50% of clinically important lesions. Longer segment CTO (>15–20 cm), multiple occlusions, and those CTOs

Type A lesions
- Single stenosis ≤10 cm in length
- Single occlusion ≤5 cm in length

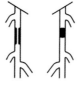

Type B lesions
- Multiple lesions stenoses or occlusions), each ≤5 cm
- Single stenosis or occlusion ≤15 cm not involving the infrageniculate popliteal artery
- Single or multiple lesions in the absence or continuous tibial vessels to improve inflow for a distal bypass
- Heavily calcified occlusion ≤5 cm in length
- Single popliteal stenosis

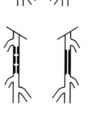
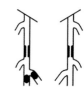

Type C lesions
- Multiple stenoses or occlusions totaling >15 cm with or without heavy calcification
- Recurrent stenoses or occlusions that need treatment after two endovascular interventions

Type D lesions
- Chronic total occlusions of CFA or SFA (>20 cm, involving the popliteal artery)
- Chronic total occlusion of popliteal artery and proximal trifurcation vessels

Figure 15.8 TASC II Categories for guiding femoral interventions. *AAA,* Abdominal aortic aneurysm; *CIA,* common iliac artery; *SFA,* superficial femoral artery; *TASC,* Trans-Atlantic Inter-Society Consensus. (From Norgren L, Hiatt WR, Dormandy JA, Nehler MR, Harris KA, Fowkes FGR. Inter-society consensus for the management of peripheral arterial disease [TASC II]) *J Vasc Surg.* 2007;45(Suppl S):S5–S6.)

involving the ostial segments near large branch points require special consideration because of increased complexity.

Based on lesion assessment, algorithms have been proposed for vascular crossing. One such example is the Chronic Total Occlusion Crossing Approach Based on Plaque Morphology (CTOP) Classification (Fig. 15.9a), which has been used with a crossing algorithm (see Fig. 15.9b) to standardize the approach to vascular occlusions

Recent reports have advocated alternate access sites (radial or pedal) for successful lesion crossing. Some peripheral arterial disease centers have begun using primary pedal access without

CTOP classification

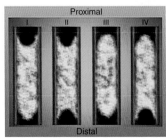

Cranial to caudal evaluation:

Type I: two concave caps

Type II: concave proximal, convex distal

Type III: convex proximal, concave distal

Type IV: two convex caps

A

Figure 15.9A Chronic total occlusion crossing approach based on plaque morphology (CTOP) classification.

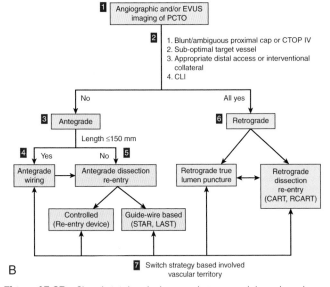

B

Figure 15.9B Chronic total occlusion crossing approach based on plaque morphology (CTOP) classification. Algorithm for chronic total occlusion use with algorithm for crossing femoropopliteal and below-the-knee occlusions. *CART,* Controlled antegrade retrograde tracking; *CLI,* critical limb ischemia; *EVUS,* extravascular ultrasound; *LAST,* limited antegrade subintimal tracking; *RCART,* reverse CART; *STAR,* subintimal tracking and reentry. (From Banerjee S, Shishehbor MH, Mustapha JA, et al. A percutaneous crossing algorithm for femoropopliteal and tibial artery chronic total occlusions [PCTO algorithm]. *J Invasive Cardiol.* 2019;31[4]:111–119. Used with permission.)

antegrade imaging as their primary treatment strategy. This approach may have limitations in those individuals with limited below-the-knee run off or if larger devices are needed.

Atherectomy

Adjunctive atherectomy in lower extremity interventions has been touted to enhance lumen gain, ease device passage, reduce dissection, and decrease the need for stenting. Despite this, no compelling evidence exist regarding their role to enhance long-term patency or reduce morbidity or limb events. Their role in lesion preparation, therefore, is important for operators to understand because a variety of device types and mechanisms of action are marketed in the United States and Europe. Available devices and general indications for use are discussed in Table 15.2 and Fig. 15.10.

These devices may be associated with increased rates of complications, such as distal embolization, abrupt closure, and perforation. Many devices are frequently used with distal embolic protection filters. Notably, atherectomy is generally not recommended by the guidelines in the iliac vessels where the risk of vascular perforation can have more dire consequences.

Percutaneous Transluminal Angioplasty, Focal Force/Specialty Balloons, and Drug-Coated Balloons

In cases of endovascular intervention, after successful lesion crossing has been achieved, ballooning to expand the lesion is typically performed. Predilatation balloon sizing may be guided by IVUS as previously mentioned.

PTA remains the mainstay of lesion preparation techniques for femoropopliteal disease. Several principles of optimal PTA have emerged over the decades to optimally dilate lesions while minimizing flow-limiting dissections so as obviate bailout stenting. For example, prolonged inflation times (i.e., >3 minutes) at lower pressures with longer balloons more closely matching lesion lengths (i.e., using one longer balloon rather than using a short balloon with multiple side-by-side inflations) seem to have improved outcomes with PTA alone.

Table 15.2

Atherectomy Device Summary

Device	Mechanism	Rail Guidewire Size (inches)	Sheath Size	Eccentric calcium	CTO lesion with subintimal segment	Thrombotic lesions efficacy	ISR lesions
Excimer Laser	monochromatic light to dissolve/soften plaque	0.014	6F	Yes	Yes	Yes	Yes
Rotablator	rotational	specialty wire: tapered wire with 0.014 spring tip	Depends on burr size. 6F sheath generally acceptable				
JetStream	Rotational	0.014	7F	Yes		Yes	Yes
Phoenix	Rotational	specialty wire: 0.014	5F–7F depending on device size	Yes			
Ocelot	Rotational - OCT image guided	0.014	6F	Yes	Yes		

Pantheris	Directional-OCT image guided	0.014	7F or 8F	Yes	Yes
SilverHawk	Directional	0.014	6F or 7F	Yes	Yes
TurboHawk	Directional	0.014	6F–8F	Yes	Yes
HawkOne	Directional	0.014	7F	Yes	Yes
Diamondback 360	Orbital	0.14 with 0.18 tip	4F 1.25 mm burrs 5F 1.25 mm, 1.75 mm burrs and all radial compatible burrs 6F 2.0 mm Burr	Yes	
ShockWave	Lithotripsy	0.014	M5 device 3.5 –6.0 6F; 6.5 – 7.0 7F S5 device 3.0 –4.0 5F	Yes	Yes

BTK, Below the knee; CTO, chronic total occlusions; F, French; ISR, in-stent restenosis; OCT, optical coherence tomography.

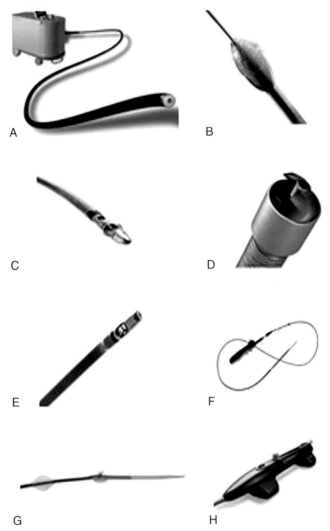

Figure 15.10 Atherectomy/Plaque Modification Devices Available in the United States. (A) Excimer laser. (B) Rotablator. (C) Jetstream. (D) Phoenix. (E) Rotarex. (F) HawkOne. (G) Pantheris. (H) Diamondback360. (I) ShockWave. Images compliments of their respective device companies (see text). (Adapted from Finn MT, Ingrassia JJ, Parikh SA. Plaque modification in endovascular procedures in patients with infrainguinal disease. *Interv Cardiol Clin.* 2020;9[2]:125–137. Used with permission.)

In refractory or highly calcified lesions, specialty focal force balloons are available such as cutting or scoring balloons. The role of these balloons is not well-studied. These devices may prevent dissections by avoiding balloon slipping or by inducing controlled plaque fracture. The ShockWave intravascular lithotripsy balloon has recently been approved by the U.S. Food and Drug Administration (FDA) for peripheral intervention in the United States. Shockwave has been shown to be safe and effective in dilating heavily calcified vessels.

Paclitaxel drug-coated balloons (DCBs) in the periphery have recently been the subject of considerable controversy. Although the devices have been shown to significantly improve patency compared with PTA alone, a 2018 meta-analysis observed a higher mortality with the use of DCBs. The results of this meta-analysis were called into question because of large numbers of patients being lost to follow-up and concerns for subsequent selection bias. Clarifying manufacturer-led safety studies, large-scale Medicare studies, and a large randomized trial have failed to show a difference in mortality with DCB compared with PTA.

Stent Types and Alternative Stent Technologies in Femoropopliteal Disease

Bare-Metal Stents

In many patients, suboptimal post-PTA results (recoil, flow-limiting dissection, subintimal wire course) will require vascular stenting. The Randomized Study Comparing the Edwards Self-ExpandIng LifeStent Versus Angioplasty-alone In LEsions INvolving The SFA and/or Proximal Popliteal Artery (RESILIENT) randomized trial evaluated bare-metal stents versus PTA with a highly superior patency at 3 years (75.5% vs. 41.1%; $p < .001$) in the stenting group. A registry evaluating the Supera nitinol woven stent (Fig. 15.11A; Abbott, Chicago, IL) reported a greater than 85% 1-year patency without a single stent fracture event. Subsequent studies have tempered these results by showing lower patency rates in longer lesions and those with smaller minimal stent areas.

Drug-Eluting Stents

Drug-eluting stents are commonly used in the peripheral interventions of the femoral popliteal segments with the goal of improving patency in lesions requiring vascular stenting. The Zilver paclitaxel drug-eluting stent (see Fig. 15.11B, Cook Medical, Bloomington, IN)

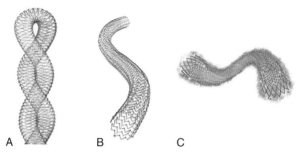

Figure 15.11 (A) Supera Bare Metal Stent (Abbott, Chicago, IL). (B) Zilver Paclitaxal Eluting Stent (Cook, Bloomington, IN). (C) Eluvia Paclitaxal Eluting Stent (Boston Scientific, Marlborough, MA). Images obtained with permission from respective companies. Supera is a trademark of Abbott or its related companies. Reproduced with permission of Abbott, © 2022. All rights reserved.

demonstrated superior patency at 5 years (66.4% vs. 43.4%; $p < .001$) compared with control bare-metal stents. This study was followed by IMPERIAL, which compared the second-generation Eluvia drug-eluting stent (see Fig. 15.11C, Boston Scientific, Marlborough, MA) to Zilver and met criteria for noninferiority and even crossed the threshold for superiority, although this analysis was performed posthoc.

Alternative Stent Technologies: Covered Stents and Tacks

Covered stents are available as self-expandable or balloon-expandable endoprostheses (useful in undilatable lesions to avoid perforation). A retrospective cohort study of stent graft use with the Viabahn SES (Gore Medical, Newark, DE) in the above-the-knee vasculature demonstrated a 1-year patency of 81.7%.

The Tack endovascular stent (InTack Vascular, Wayne, PA) is a 6-mm nitinol stent used to "tack down" significant dissections. The tacks were evaluated in a single-arm trial examining the device after PTA, with a primary patency rate of 79.3% at a year.

Complication Management

Embolization

Several complications can occur during endovascular treatment of the femoropopliteal segments. Distal embolization with poor runoff can lead to limb-threatening ischemia. This may be of particular concern if the patient has limited lower extremity runoff before the intervention.

Distal embolization can occur with atherectomy and, therefore, one may use embolic protection (Emboshield Nav6, Abbott or SpiderFx, Medtronic, Minneapolis, MN), although some devices and access approaches prohibit their use (i.e., atherectomy with retrograde pedal access or radial to pedal approach). On occasion, these filters can become filled with debris, limiting downstream visualization beyond the filter. When this occurs, one may place a curved crossing catheter or coronary diagnostic catheter near the opening of the filter and aspirate the debris. One may then recapture the filter with the retrieval catheter with subsequent aspiration and back-bleeding of the sheath to ensure removal of all particulate debris.

Despite these techniques, distal embolization can still occur. In these scenarios, one may deliver vasodilators into or beyond the area of decreased flow (typically nicardipine, verapamil, or nitroprusside). Wiring the affected vessel and using a mechanical thrombectomy device (i.e., Pneumbra Cat 6, 3 or Cat Rx [Pneumbra, San Francisco, CA], Export [Medtronic], Pronto [Teleflex, Wayne, PA], QuickCat [Philips, Amsterdam, Netherlands], or Fetch2 [Boston Scientific]) for particulate aspiration may also improve results. If this is unsuccessful, pedal access can be obtained for distal aspiration and administration of vasodilators. Alternative diagnoses can also be considered, such as distal dissection, if flow is failing to improve.

Perforation

Given hydrophilic wires are commonly used to cross lesions in peripheral interventions, occasionally they can move into small branches and lead to wire perforations. In these cases, one can balloon proximally to decrease flow to the area and place a blood pressure cuff inflated above the patient's diastolic blood pressure over the affected area. A period of 15 to 20 minutes will typically resolve the perforation; however, in some situations, anticoagulation may need to be reversed. For more severe perforations, the branch vessel can be coiled or excluded with a properly sized covered stent.

Large vessel perforations can occur when dilating heavily calcified vessels. These are often addressed by prolonged balloon inflation, sometimes with adjunctive external compression either manually or with a blood pressure cuff. If this is unsuccessful, covered stent endoprostheses are useful. When using a covered endoprosthesis for this application, it is important to recognize the sheath size required may necessitate up-sizing, depending on the stent specifications. Furthermore, attention should be paid to avoid covering large branches or collaterals. Decisive action need be taken with arterial perforation given the possibility of compartment syndrome.

Conclusion

The treatment of peripheral arterial disease in the iliofemoral segments has become increasingly nuanced; however, in the claudicant, the mainstay of therapy remains optimal medical treatment and supervised exercise. For those patients who fail to improve with conservative therapies, a wide array of endovascular and surgical approaches can be used for the successful relief of obstructive iliofemoral disease.

Key References

Aboyans V, Ricco JB, Bartelink MEL, et al. 2017 ESC Guidelines on the Diagnosis and Treatment of Peripheral Arterial Diseases, in collaboration with the European Society for Vascular Surgery (ESVS): Document covering atherosclerotic disease of extracranial carotid and vertebral, mesenteric, renal, upper and lower extremity arteries Endorsed by: the European Stroke Organization (ESO) The Task Force for the Diagnosis and Treatment of Peripheral Arterial Diseases of the European Society of Cardiology (ESC) and of the European Society for Vascular Surgery (ESVS). *Eur Heart J.* 2018;39(9):763-816.

Bailey SR, Beckman JA, Dao TD, et al. ACC/AHA/SCAI/SIR/SVM 2018 appropriate use criteria for peripheral artery intervention. *J Am Coll Cardiol.* 2019;73:214-237.

Gerhard-Herman MD, Gornik H, Barrett C, et al. 2016 AHA/ACC guideline on the management of patients with lower extremity peripheral artery disease: a report of the American College of Cardiology/American Heart Association Task Force on Clinical Practice Guidelines. *J Am Coll Cardiol.* 2017;69(11):e71-e126.

Gerhard-Herman MD, Gornik HL, Barrett C, et al. 2016 AHA/ACC guideline on the management of patients with lower extremity peripheral artery disease: executive summary: a report of the American College of Cardiology/American Heart Association Task Force on Clinical Practice Guidelines. *J Am Coll Cardiol.* 2017;69(11): 1465-1508.

Olin JW, White CJ, Armstrong EJ, Kadian-Dodov D, Hiatt WR. Peripheral artery disease: evolving role of exercise, medical therapy, and endovascular options. *J Am Coll Cardiol.* 2016;67:1338-1357.

References

Armstrong EJ, Brodmann M, Deaton DH, et al. Dissections after infrainguinal percutaneous transluminal angioplasty: a systematic review and current state of clinical evidence. *J Endovasc Ther.* 2019;26(4):479-489.

Banerjee S, Shishehbor MH, Mustapha JA, et al. A percutaneous crossing algorithm for femoropopliteal and tibial artery chronic total occlusions (PCTO Algorithm). *J Invasive Cardiol.* 2019;31(4):111-119.

Finn MT, Ingrassia JJ, Parikh SA. Plaque modification in endovascular procedures in patients with infrainguinal disease. *Interv Cardiol Clin.* 2020:9(2):125-137.

Gouëffic Y, Della Schiava N, Thaveau F, et al. Stenting or surgery for de novo common femoral artery stenosis. *JACC Cardiovasc Interv*. 2017;10(13):1344-1354.

Gray WA, Keirse K, Soga Y, et al. A polymer-coated, paclitaxel-eluting stent (Eluvia) versus a polymer-free, paclitaxel-coated stent (Zilver PTX) for endovascular femoropopliteal intervention (IMPERIAL): a randomised, non-inferiority trial. *Lancet*. 2018;392:1541-1551.

Guez D, Hansberry DR, Gonsalves CF, Eschelman DJ, Parker L, Rao VM. Recent trends in endovascular and surgical treatment of peripheral arterial disease in the medicare population. *J Vasc Surg*. 2020;71:2178.

Katsanos K, Kitrou P, Spiliopoulos S, Diamantopoulos A, Karnabatidis D. Comparative effectiveness of plain balloon angioplasty, bare metal stents, drug-coated balloons, and drug-eluting stents for the treatment of infrapopliteal artery disease. *J Endovasc Ther*. 2016;23:851-863.

Katsanos K, Spiliopoulos S, Kitrou P, Krokidis M, Karnabatidis D. Risk of death following application of paclitaxel-coated balloons and stents in the femoropopliteal artery of the leg: a systematic review and meta-analysis of randomized controlled trials. *J Am Heart Assoc*. 2018;7(24):e011245.

Klein WM, van der Graaf Y, Seegers J, et al. Dutch iliac stent trial: long-term results in patients randomized for primary or selective stent placement. *Radiology*. 2006;238(2):734-744.

Krankenberg H, Zeller T, Ingwersen M, et al. Self-expanding versus balloon-expandable stents for iliac artery occlusive disease: the randomized ICE trial. *JACC Cardiovasc Interv*. 2017;10(16):1694-1704.

Mwipatayi BP, Sharma S, Daneshmand A, et al. Durability of the balloon-expandable covered versus bare-metal stents in the Covered versus Balloon Expandable Stent Trial (COBEST) for the treatment of aortoiliac occlusive disease. *J Vasc Surg*. 2016; 64(1):83-94.e1.

Nordanstig J, James S, Andersson M, et al. Mortality with paclitaxel-coated devices in peripheral artery disease. *N Engl J Med*. 2020;383(26):2538-2546.

Perry M, Callas PW, Alef MJ, Bertges DJ. Outcomes of peripheral vascular interventions via retrograde pedal access for chronic limb-threatening ischemia in a multicenter registry. *J Endovasc Ther*. 2020;27(2):205-210.

Zen K, Takahara M, Iida O, et al. Drug-eluting stenting for femoropopliteal lesions, followed by cilostazol treatment, reduces stent restenosis in patients with symptomatic peripheral artery disease. *J Vasc Surg*. 2017;65(3):720-725.

Zhang H, Li X, Niu L, et al. Effectiveness and long-term outcomes of different crossing strategies for the endovascular treatment of iliac artery chronic total occlusions. *BMC Cardiovasc Disord*. 2020;20(1):431.

Aortic, Renal, Subclavian, and Carotid Interventions

PARTHA SARDAR • JOSE D. TAFUR • CHRISTOPHER J. WHITE

KEY POINTS

- Endovascular aneurysmal repair (EVAR) for abdominal aortic aneurysm (AAA) is a minimally invasive procedure that involves the placement of a bifurcated or tubular endoluminal stent graft over the AAA to exclude the aneurysm from arterial circulation suitable for patients at increased perioperative risk for open surgical repair (OSR).

- In patients with symptomatic atherosclerotic renal artery stenosis (RAS), renal artery stenting is reasonable for hemodynamically significant RAS causing resistant (refractory) hypertension despite guideline-recommended medical therapy, declining renal function, and those with cardiac destabilization syndromes.

- A moderately severe (indeterminate) RAS (50%–70%) should have the lesion's hemodynamic significance confirmed. Renal artery stenting with an optimally sized bare-metal stent is the revascularization procedure of choice.

- The indications for subclavian artery stenosis revascularization are subclavian steal syndrome, coronary-subclavian steal syndrome, and arm claudication.

- Carotid artery stenting with embolic protection device is recommended as an alternative to carotid endarterectomy in average-surgical-risk symptomatic patients when the anticipated risk of periprocedural stroke or mortality is less than 6%.

- Carotid artery stenting may be considered in highly selected asymptomatic patients with 60% or greater angiographic stenosis.

Introduction

The technical skills necessary to perform coronary intervention are transferable to the peripheral vasculature. Proper selection and management of peripheral vascular patients, however, require specific training and a knowledge base obtained (preferably) in a formal fellowship training program. Appropriate preparation and training include understanding the value of a multidisciplinary team approach.

Abdominal Aortic Interventions

Abdominal Aortic Aneurysm

An aortic diameter greater than 3.0 cm is generally considered aneurysmal. An aortic size index (ASI), determined by formulas that adjust for age and/or body surface area, is more predictive of clinical events. The incidence of abdominal aortic aneurysm (AAA) is much higher in men than in women. The prevalence is 41 to 49 per 100,000 men and 7 to 12 per 100,000 women. The risk factors for development of AAA include smoking, older age, hyperlipidemia, hypertension, and family history (Table 16.1).

Table 16.1

A: Risk Factors for the Development of Abdominal Aortic Aneurysm	
Risk Factor	**Odds Ratio (OR)**
History of smoking	3.59 (3.0–4.28)
Family history	1.88 (1.58–2.24)
Age	1.52 (1.44–1.62)
Hyperlipidemia	1.46 (1.29–1.65)
Hypertension	1.14 (1.02–1.26)
B: Rates of Rupture Based on Aneurysm Diameter	
Maximal Diameter	**5-Year Rupture Rate**
<4.0 cm	2%
4.0–4.9 cm	3%–12%
5.0–5.9 cm	25%
6.0–6.9 cm	35%
>7.0 cm	75%

(Adapted from Lederle FA, Johnson GR, Wilson SE, et al. Relationship of age, gender, race, and body size to infrarenal aortic diameter. The Aneurysm Detection and Management [ADAM] Veterans Affairs Cooperative Study Investigators. *J Vasc Surg.* 1997;26:595–601.)

Detection

Most aortic aneurysms are diagnosed incidentally on abdominal imaging performed for unrelated indications. Physical examination can be helpful if an AAA is large (>5.5 cm). Abdominal ultrasonography is the most commonly used imaging modality for diagnosis and follow-up, which has sensitivity and specificity approaching 100% for an aortic diameter greater than 3.0 cm. Computed tomographic angiography (CTA) is the modality of choice for planning of endovascular or surgical intervention because it provides low interobserver variability and helps determine the anatomic eligibility for endovascular repair.

For asymptomatic patients, the U.S. Preventive Services Task Force recommends one-time screening for AAA with abdominal ultrasonography in men older than 65 with a smoking history (Table 16.2). Screening is recommended to be selective in men who have never smoked and not recommended for women who have never smoked. There is insufficient evidence to make a recommendation for screening in women who have a smoking history or a family history of AAA.

Indications for Intervention

Symptomatic AAA

There are three main clinical presentations of AAA: (1) rupture or impending rupture, (2) embolic or thrombotic complications, and (3) compression of adjacent structures because of mass effect.

Table 16.2

United States Preventive Services Task Force (USPSTF) Recommendations for Abdominal Aortic Aneurysm Screening	
Population	**Recommendation**
Men aged 65–75 years who have ever smoked	The USPSTF recommends one-time screening for abdominal aortic aneurysm (AAA) with ultrasonography in men aged 65–75 years who have ever smoked.
Men aged 65–75 years who have never smoked	The USPSTF recommends that clinicians selectively offer screening for AAA in men aged 65–75 years who have never smoked rather than routinely screening all men in this group.
Women aged 65–75 years who have ever smoked	The USPSTF concludes that the current evidence is insufficient to assess the balance of benefits and harms of screening for AAA in women aged 65–75 years who have ever smoked.
Women who have never smoked	The USPSTF recommends against routine screening for AAA in women who have never smoked.

The classic clinical triad of AAA rupture includes sudden on-set of abdominal or lower back pain, pulsatile abdominal mass, and hypotension; however, this triad is present in less than 40% of patients. The prognosis of ruptured AAA is very poor with an in-hospital mortality of around 40% to 50%. It is estimated that 80% of the mortality from AAA is secondary to rupture, highlighting the importance of early detection and intervention.

Asymptomatic AAA

The decision to treat an asymptomatic AAA should include the risk of rupture, the procedural risk, and the patient's life expectancy. The maximum aneurysmal diameter is currently accepted as the most primary determinant of the risk of rupture. In general terms, the risk of rupture increases substantially when the diameter is greater than 5 cm (Fig. 16.1). Additionally, rapidly expanding aneurysms defined as a greater than 1 cm increase in diameter over 1 year represent a higher risk of rupture and constitute an indication for intervention. The operative mortality of elective open AAA is reported to be between 5% and 8%.

Aneurysm repair can be accomplished using open surgical repair (OSR) or endovascular aneurysm repair (EVAR) techniques. The choice between OSR and EVAR should be individualized, taking into account the patient's age, risk factors for perioperative morbidity and mortality, anatomic factors, and the experience of the surgeon. EVAR is associated with a lower risk of perioperative morbidity compared with OSR for asymptomatic, symptomatic, and ruptured AAA. Long-term mortality after elective AAA repair, however, is not significantly different between the techniques.

Endovascular Aneurysm Repair. Conceptually, during EVAR, an endoluminal stent graft connects the proximal "normal" nondilated portion of the aorta proximal to the aneurysm to the distal nondilated arteries, therefore excluding the aneurysm from the circulation. Excluding the aneurysm decreases the pressure on the wall and lowers the risk of rupture. With contemporary techniques, including custom-made fenestrated and branched devices, most patients can be considered candidates for EVAR in experienced endovascular centers.

The EVAR-1 and Dutch Randomized Endovascular Aneurysm Repair (DREAM) trials randomized patients who were suitable for both EVAR and OSR, showing similar 2-year all-cause mortality but lower aneurysm-related deaths for the EVAR group (4% vs. 7%; $p = .04$ in EVAR-1 and 2% vs. 6% in DREAM). Since then, EVAR has gained significant acceptance as the treatment of choice for most asymptomatic AAAs requiring repair. A recent systemic review and meta-analysis, however, have demonstrated that although the hazard of all-cause and aneurysm-related death within 6 months of surgery

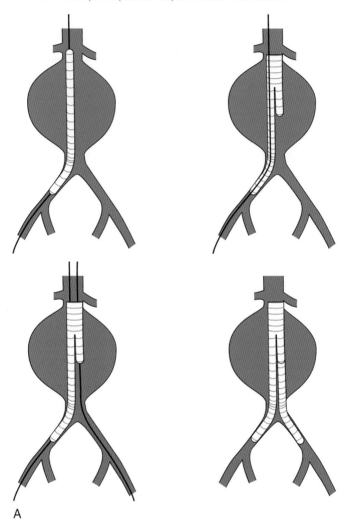

A

Figure 16.1 (A) Procedural steps for endovascular aneurysm repair (EVAR). See text.

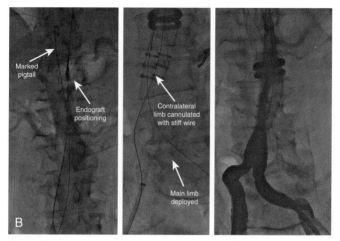

Figure 16.1, cont'd   (B) Example of EVAR with Ovation device. (Courtesy Stephen Jenkins.)

was significantly lower after EVAR, with further follow-up, the pooled hazard estimate moved in favor of OSR; in the long term (>8 years), the hazard of aneurysm-related mortality was significantly higher in patients who underwent EVAR. The risk of secondary intervention, aneurysm rupture, and death caused by rupture was significantly higher after EVAR. These data have led the British National Institute for Health and Care Excellence (NICE) to issue a recommendation that patients should not be offered EVAR if OSR is suitable.

Moreover, not all patients are anatomically suitable for EVAR. Preprocedural planning is the cornerstone of a successful procedure. CTA is the modality of choice for anatomic evaluation before endovascular repair. The critical anatomic elements that determine the patient's suitability for EVAR are:

1) A patent superior mesenteric artery (SMA) or celiac trunk: The inferior mesenteric artery is usually excluded with the graft. One of the worse complications of EVAR is ischemic colitis, which occurs in less than 2% of elective cases. The risk of colon necrosis is higher if the patient has had previous abdominal surgery that interrupts the collateral circulation from the SMA and celiac arteries or if there is significant preexisting stenosis of these arteries.

2) An infrarenal neck diameter of less than 32 mm and greater than 10 to 15 mm in length is needed to appropriately land the proximal end of the graft and create a complete seal. The most

common reason for a patient with AAA to be considered unsuitable for EVAR is the anatomy of the proximal aortic neck. In a series of 526 patients, EVAR performed in subjects with a hostile neck—defined as length less than 10 mm, angle greater than 60 degrees, diameter greater than 28 mm, or more than 50% circumferential thrombus or calcification—was associated with higher rates of intraprocedural type I endoleak (poor edge sealing).

3) No more than 90 degrees of circumferential calcification or mural thrombus in the infrarenal neck: This would interfere with appropriate anchoring and sealing of the device.

4) The minimal diameter of the external iliac arteries is large enough to allow the passage of the device (Currently 14 French [F]).

5) Distal fixation requires 10 to 15 mm in length of normal vessel in the common iliac segment, similar to that required for proximal fixation.

6) The diameter of the common internal iliac artery should be less than 20 mm. If this is not the case, an additional cuff is required to extend the graft into the external iliac artery with coiling of the internal iliac artery (see later).

Available Devices. Presently, several devices have received U.S. Food and Drug Administration (FDA) approval for the treatment of AAA in the United States (Table 16.3). The overall performance among the available devices is similar.

Table 16.3

Currently Available Endovascular Aneurysm Repair Devices in the United States				
Company	Device	Largest Main Body Diameter (mm)	Delivery System Profile	Fixed Location
Cook Medical	Zenith Flex	36	20, 23, 26 F	Suprarenal
Endologix	Powerlink	28	21 F	Infrarenal
W.L. Gore & associates	Excluder AAA endoprosthesis	28.5	18 F	Infrarenal
Medtronic Vascular	Endurant	36	16, 18, 20 F	Infrarenal
TriVascular	Ovation Prime	30	15 F	Suprarenal

AAA, Abdominal aortic aneurysm; *F*, French.

The basic EVAR system includes three main components: a delivery system, a stent graft, and iliac extensions. Advanced devices can be used in challenging anatomy, such as fenestrated, branched, or chimney grafts.

Preprocedural Evaluation. Preprocedural risk assessment should be performed in EVAR patients because there is a small risk that the endovascular repair may need to be converted to an OSR. Before endograft placement, antibiotic prophylaxis is recommended within 30 minutes of the skin incision. Prophylactic renal artery stenting may be considered in selected patients with severe renal artery stenosis and preexisting renal insufficiency. Hypogastric (internal iliac) artery embolization also can be considered in selected patients. A small study suggested use of preoperative methylprednisolone as a prophylaxis for acute flu-like postimplantion inflammatory syndrome.

Technique. There is some variation in technique depending on the type of endograft used. There is, however, a common workflow for most EVAR procedures:

1. Aortogram: After bilateral femoral access is obtained, a marked pigtail is inserted through the contralateral side to the main graft and positioned just above the level of the renal arteries. A digital subtraction angiogram is performed and the level of the lowest renal artery is identified.

2. Embolization of internal iliac artery when necessary: If the common iliac arteries are aneurysmal, the distal limb of the device can be anchored in the external iliac artery. However, collateral flow into the ipsilateral internal iliac artery can result in a type II endoleak (see later). Prophylactic embolization with coils of the internal iliac artery can be performed during EVAR or in a staged manner before the procedure.

3. Introduction and deployment of the endograft: Once the lowest renal artery is identified, the sheath containing the endograft is positioned just below it. It is important to adjust the angulation of the x-ray camera to be perpendicular to the plane of the infrarenal aorta for appropriate positioning (see Fig. 16.1). The pigtail used for aortography should be removed before deployment. Postpositioning ballooning is often required and depends on the device used.

4. Deployment of the contralateral limb: For modular endografts, one needs to deploy a separate iliac limb graft in the contralateral side. A wire should be introduced into the main limb of the endograft via the contralateral femoral artery. Once the wire is successfully placed in the suprarenal aorta through the already deployed endograft, the sheath with the iliac endograft is advanced into the main body of the endograft. The final step is to deploy the contralateral limb.

5. Dilation of the endograft: Although stent grafts are self-expanding, balloon expansion of the proximal and distal attachment sites should be performed, as well as the junction of the modular components.

6. Completion angiogram: A completion angiogram with a power injector is performed at completion of the procedure and identifies endoleaks.

Endoleaks

Immediate type I and type III endoleaks are generally treated with additional ballooning or the placement of additional endograft components (Fig. 16.2; Table 16.4).

Postoperative Care

Postoperative care includes pain control, fluid therapy, peripheral pulse exam assessment at regular intervals, and resumption of antithrombotic therapy.

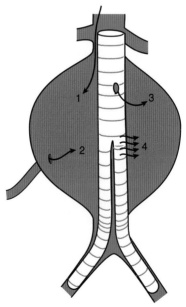

Figure 16.2 Classification of endoleaks.

Table 16.4

Classification of Endoleaks			
Type	**Definition**	**Causes**	**Treatment**
1	Arises from the distal and proximal attachment sites	Undersizing of the stent, poor sealing, neck dilatation, and stent migration	Postdilatation of the stent
2	Retrograde filling of the aneurysmal sac from lumbar or internal iliac arteries that were excluded with the endograft	Collateral circulation	Benign course. If needing treatment, translumbar embolization or surgical ligation
3	Limb separation or fabric wear	Mainly occur with modular grafts at the sites of attachment	Regrafting
4	Extravasation through graft material	Because of porosity of the fabric material	Benign course, usually aneurysmal sac thrombosis without clinical consequence
5	Endotension: Space between aortic graft and the native aorta has elevated pressure without demonstrable endoleak	Missed endoleaks, thrombosed endoleaks, hygroma, infection	Unknown

Complications

Complications related to EVAR occur in 10% of cases, including vascular access bleeding, technical failure, endoleak, and open conversion.

Surveillance After EVAR

EVAR offers the advantage of lower perioperative morbidity but is associated with a concern for device-related complications, such as endoleaks, migration of the stents at the aortic and iliac landing zones, graft thrombosis, and separation of the device components. Because of these potential complications, lifelong surveillance is mandatory. Current standard of care includes serial studies at 1, 6, 12 months, and yearly thereafter. Since the advent of EVAR, this has largely been accomplished with serial CTA with delayed images. Compared with CTA, duplex ultrasonography (DU) is cost effective and has no risk of contrast and radiation exposure. The reported specificity of endoleak identification by DU is high (89%–97%).

Renal Artery Interventions

Renal artery stenosis (RAS) is the most common cause of secondary hypertension. It affects 25% to 35% of patients with secondary hypertension, is associated with progressive renal insufficiency, and causes cardiovascular complications, such as refractory heart failure and flash pulmonary edema. A critical issue is the appropriate patient selection for interventional procedures.

Clinical Syndromes Associated With RAS

Renovascular Hypertension

Resistant hypertension is defined as blood pressure above goal on three different classes of antihypertensive medications, ideally including a diuretic drug. Current American Heart Association (AHA)/American College of Cardiology (ACC) guidelines recommend renal artery stenting for RAS with accelerated, resistant, or malignant hypertension; hypertension with unilateral small kidney; and hypertension with medication intolerance (Class IIa, LOE B).

Ischemic Nephropathy

RAS is a potentially reversible form of renal insufficiency. In 73 patients with chronic renal failure (estimated glomerular filtration rate [eGFR] < 50 mL/min) and clinical evidence of RAS, renal stenting demonstrated an improved renal function in 34 of 59 patients (57.6%). Current AHA/ACC guidelines and appropriate use criteria recommend renal artery stenting for patients with ischemic nephropathy if they have progressive chronic kidney disease (CKD) with bilateral RAS (Class IIa, LOE B), progressive CKD with RAS to a solitary functioning kidney (Class IIa, LOE B), or CKD with unilateral RAS (Class IIb, LOE C; Fig. 16.3).

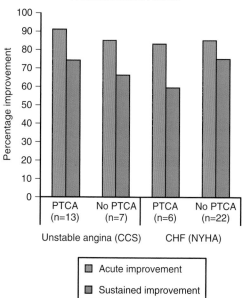

SYMPTOMS AFTER RENAL ARTERY STENTING IN PATIENTS PRESENTING WITH UA/CHF

Figure 16.3 Improvement in cardiac destabilization syndromes after renal artery revascularization. (From Khoshla S, White CJ, Collins TJ, Jenkins JS, Shaw D, Ramee SR. Effects of renal artery stent implantation in patients with renovascular hypertension presenting with unstable angina or congestive heart failure. *Am J Cardiol.* 1997;80:363–366.)

Cardiac Destabilization Syndromes

The most widely recognized example of a cardiac destabilization syndrome is "flash" pulmonary or Pickering syndrome. In patients with either congestive heart failure (CHF) or an acute coronary syndrome (ACS), successful renal stent placement resulted in a significant decrease in blood pressure and symptom improvement in 88% (42 of 48) of patients. For those patients who presented with unstable angina, renal artery stenting improved the Canadian Class Society (CCS) symptoms at least by one regardless of concomitant coronary intervention (see Fig. 16.3). Current AHA/ACC guidelines recommend renal artery stenting for RAS with recurrent, unexplained heart failure decompensation, or sudden unexplained pulmonary edema (Class I, LOE B) and for hemodynamically significant RAS and medically refractory unstable angina (Class IIa, LOE B).

Diagnostic Testing

Doppler Ultrasound Evaluation

Significant RAS is associated with a peak systolic velocity (PSV) greater than 180 cm/sec and a ratio of the PSV of the stenosed renal artery to the PSV in the aorta that is greater than 3.5. PSV greater than 395 cm/s and renal artery ratio (RAR) greater than 5.1 are the most predictive of angiographically significant in-stent restenosis (ISR) in more than 70% of cases.

Computed Tomographic Angiography

CTA can provide high-resolution cross-sectional imaging of RAS while supplying three-dimensional angiographic images of the aorta, renal, and visceral arteries, allowing localization and enumeration of the renal arteries, including accessory branches. CTA can be used to follow patients with prior stents to detect ISR, an advantage over magnetic resonance angiography (MRA) in which metallic stents generate artifact.

Magnetic Resonance Angiography

This imaging modality allows for localization and enumeration of the renal arteries and characterization of the stenosis. Limitations for MRA include the association of gadolinium with nephrogenic systemic fibrosis when administered to patients with an eGFR of less than 30 mL/1.73m^2. Metal also causes artifacts on MRA and, therefore, it is not a useful test for patients with prior renal stents.

Treatment Strategies

Medical Management of RAS

The appropriate use recommendations for RAS intervention are based on expert consensus and evidence, including the randomized CORAL trial (Stenting and Medical Therapy for Atherosclerotic Renal-Artery Stenosis), which recommends best medical therapy as the initial treatment for a newly diagnosed patient. Medical management of atherosclerotic vascular disease involves blood pressure control, lipid-lowering therapy, an antiplatelet agent, and lifestyle advice, including dietary counseling, smoking cessation, and physical activity.

The CORAL trial found that the primary composite endpoint (death from cardiovascular or renal causes, myocardial infarction [MI], stroke, hospitalization for CHF, progressive renal insufficiency, or the need for renal replacement therapy) in patients with RAS (>60% diameter stenosis) did not differ when comparing an initial strategy of medical therapy (MT) with MT plus renal artery stenting in patients with hypertension and RAS. All patients received, unless contraindicated, the angiotensin II type-1 receptor blocker candesartan with or without hydrochlorothiazide, and the combination agent amlodipine–atorvastatin, with the dose adjusted on the basis of blood pressure and lipid status. It is important to note that the CORAL trial does not apply to patients with resistant or refractory hypertension. CORAL did not investigate patients in whom medical therapy had failed to control blood pressure.

Renal Artery Surgery

Surgical repair of RAS was the only available revascularization option before renal artery angioplasty. Today, percutaneous, catheter-based therapy has largely replaced surgical renal revascularization for RAS because of the increased morbidity and mortality associated with surgery.

Renal Artery Stenting

Renal artery stenting is the standard of care for patients with hemodynamically significant renal artery stenosis (>70% angiographic diameter renal artery stenosis or 50%–70% stenosis with a significant translesional gradient) who also have: (1) resistant or uncontrolled hypertension and the failure of three antihypertensive drugs, one of which is a diuretic, or hypertension with intolerance to medication; (2) ischemic nephropathy; and (3) cardiac destabilization syndromes. This population was not addressed by the CORAL trial.

Despite excellent angiographic outcomes achieved with renal stenting, there is a mismatch between angiographic (>97%) and clinical (~70%) success for controlling hypertension and renal dysfunction. Technically, renal artery stent placement is highly successful and safe. In a meta-analysis of 14 studies (678 patients) evaluating renal artery stenting for either hypertension or CKD, the procedure success rate was 98% (95% confidence interval [CI], 95%–100%). The clinical response rate for hypertension, however, was only 69%, with a cure rate of 20% and improvement in blood pressure in 49% (Fig. 16.4A). Renal function improved in 30% and stabilized in 38% of patients with an overall favorable response rate of 68% (see Fig. 16.4B). The mismatch between angiographic success and clinical response may be explained by (1) treatment of nonobstructive RAS lesions (visually overestimating the stenosis severity) or (2) symptoms (hypertension or CKD) that were not caused by RAS (i.e.,

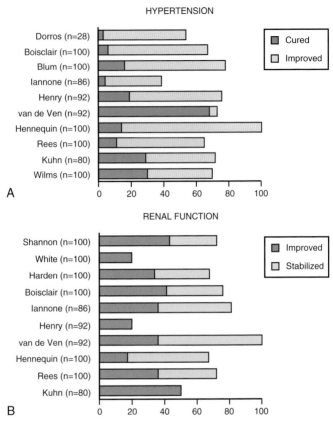

Figure 16.4 Summary of initial reported series in terms of improvement of (A) hypertension and (B) renal function after renal artery revascularization. Despite a technical success of >95%, clinical outcomes did not match technical success. This suggests that selection of patients is crucial to obtaining clinical benefit.

essential hypertension). The key to successful clinical outcomes is to identify which patients are likely to benefit from intervention.

Several recent randomized clinical trials have attempted to determine the clinical benefit of renal artery stenting. The STent Placement and Blood Pressure and Lipid-Lowering for the Prevention of Progression of Renal Dysfunction Caused by Atherosclerotic Ostial Stenosis of the Renal Artery (STAR) and Angioplasty and Stenting for Renal Artery Lesions (ASTRAL), trials were flawed by poor design and the inability to objectively assess the severity of the RAS. They failed to select patients with hemodynamically significant RAS lesions that would cause renal hypoperfusion and included inexperienced operators, resulting in an unusually high complication rate.

Selecting Patients Likely to Benefit From Revascularization

The "Achilles heel" of renal artery revascularization is that angiography is a very uncertain and unreliable "gold standard" for determining the hemodynamic severity of moderate RAS. When a single operator performed visual estimation of angiographic diameter stenosis in patients with moderate RAS (50%–90% diameter stenosis), the correlation was poor between the angiographic diameter stenosis and resting mean translesional pressure gradient ($r = 0.43$; $p = .12$); hyperemic mean translesional pressure gradient ($r = 0.22$; $p = .44$); and renal fractional flow reserve (FFR; $r = 0.18$; $p = .54$). Therefore physiologic assessment should always be performed in patients with moderate RAS lesions.

Translesional Pressure Gradients

As per the ACC/AHA/SCAI (Society for Cardiovascular Angiography and Interventions)/SIR (Society of Interventional Radiology)/SVM (Society for Vascular Medicine) 2018 Appropriate Use Criteria document (Fig. 16.5), a stenosis in the range of 50% to 69% by visual estimation is considered significant if there is a resting or hyperemic systolic translesional gradient of at least 20 mm Hg or a mean gradient of at least 10 mm Hg (measured with a $\leq$5F catheter or pressure wire), hyperemic gradients of the same magnitude, or an FFR of less than 0.8.

Renal Artery Fractional Flow Reserve

Renal artery FFR correlates well with other hemodynamic parameters of lesion severity and in some series has proven to be a better predictor of clinical response. Hyperemia for measurement of renal FFR is induced with a 32-mg intrarenal bolus of papaverine or 50 mg/kg intrarenal bolus of dopamine. In one study, renal FFR was measured after renal stent placement in 17 patients with refractory hypertension and moderate to severe (50%–90% stenosis) unilateral RAS. At 3 months after intervention, 86% of patients with an abnormal renal FFR experienced improvement in their BP, compared with only 30% of those with normal renal FFR ($p = .04$).

Chronic kidney disease		
	AUC Score	
Indications	Continue or intensify medical therapy	Renal stent placement (primary stenting)–Atherosclerotic lesions
Hemodynamically significant RAS (with a severe [70%–99%] RAS or 50%–69% RAS with hemodynamic significance)		
1. • Unilateral smaller kidney (<7cm pole to pole)	A (9)	R (2)
2. • Accelerating decline in renal function • Unilateral RAS	A (9)	M (4)
3. • Accelerating decline in renal function • Bilateral RAS or a solitary viable* kidney with RAS		A (7)

*Viable is pole to pole kidney length ≥7cm.
A = Appropriate; AUC = Appropriate use criteria; M = May be appropriate; R = Rarely appropriate; RAS = Renal artery stenosis.

A

Hypertension		
	AUC Score	
Indications	Continue or intensify medical therapy	Renal stent placement (primary stenting)–Atherosclerotic lesions
Hemodynamically significant RAS (with a severe [70%–99%] RAS or 50%–69% RAS with hemodynamic significance)		
4. • New onset • New mdeical management	A (9)	R (1)
5. • Well-controlled blood pressure on ≥2 anti-hypertensive medications	A (9)	R (1)
6. • Uncontrolled on <3 antihypertensive medications	A (9)	R (3)
7. • Failure to control blood pressure on 3 maximally tolerated medications, 1 of which is a diuretic		M (6)

A = Appropriate; AUC = Appropriate use criteria; M = May be appropriate; R = Rarely appropriate; RAS = Renal artery stenosis.

B

Figure 16.5 American College of Cardiology (ACC)/American Heart Association (AHA)/Society for Cardiovascular Angiography and Interventions (SCAI)/Society of Interventional Radiology (SIR)/Society for Vascular Medicine (SVM) 2018 Appropriate Use Criteria for Renal Artery Stenosis.

	Cardiac destabilization	
	AUC Score	
Indications	Continue or intensify medical therapy	Renal stent placement (primary stenting)– Atherosclerotic lesions
Hemodynamically significant RAS (with a severe [70%–99%] RAS or 50%–69% RAS with hemodynamic significance)		
8. • Recurrent heart failure • Uncontrolled on maximal medical therapy		**M (6)**
9. • Sudden-onset flash pulmonary edema		**A (7)**
10. • Uncontrolled on <3 antihypertensive medications		**M (6)**

A = Appropriate; AUC = Appropriate use criteria; M = May be appropriate;
R = Rarely appropriate; RAS = Renal artery stenosis.

C

Figure 16.5, cont'd

Technical Aspects of Revascularization

There are several important technical and procedural considerations to prevent complications during renal stenting. Selective renal angiography should be preceded by nonselective abdominal aortography. The catheter-in-catheter or no-touch techniques should be used to minimize contact with the aortic wall and injury to the renal ostium during guiding catheter engagement (Fig. 16.6). Aggressive preprocedure hydration and limiting contrast volume are helpful to prevent the development of contrast-induced nephropathy (CIN).

Radial Access

The radial approach for renal stenting represents a valuable tool to reduce access-site complications and improve patient's comfort. This approach might be useful in renal arteries with natural downward angulation. However, the operator needs specific technical skills and knowledge of device compatibility. Both radial arteries are suitable for renal intervention. Depending on the configuration of the aortic arch, the left radial access allows for a shorter distance to renal arteries. The right radial approach is more comfortable for the operator and radiation exposure is less compared with the left. The use of 125-cm long guiding catheters with 150-cm

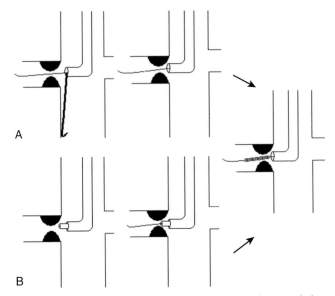

Figure 16.6 No-touch technique. (A) Catheter in catheter technique. (B) From radial access.

balloon/stent shafts are appropriate for almost all patients, whereas the 100-cm long catheters and 135-cm long balloon/stent shafts may not reach the renal arteries in taller patients or in patients with excessive aortic arch tortuosity. Fig. 16.7 shows an example of renal artery stenting via right radial access.

Embolic Protection Devices

Atheroembolism has been associated with an increase in morbidity and a dramatic reduction in 5-year survival compared with patients who had no evidence on biopsy of renal atheroembolization (54% vs. 85%, $p = .011$). Because atheroembolism is a potential complication of renal artery stenting, investigators have looked for the role of embolic protection devices (EPDs) in optimizing outcomes after renal intervention. Distal protection may be complicated, however, by a proximal bifurcation of renal arteries, which would require two EPD devices and an 0.035-in lumen balloon/stent catheter. A randomized controlled trial (RCT) of 100 patients undergoing renal artery stenting were assigned to an open-label EPD or use of abciximab in a 2×2 factorial design. A positive interaction was observed between treatment with abciximab and embolic protection. Renal

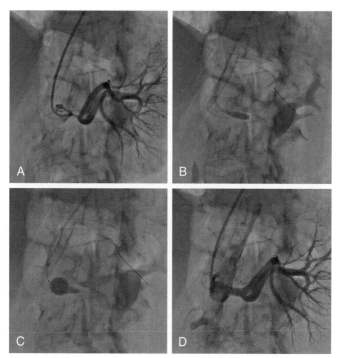

Figure 16.7 Renal intervention via right radial access. (A) Diagnostic angiogram. (B) A 6-mm Herculink stent deployment. (C) Ostial postdilation with Flash balloon. (D) Final result.

artery stenting alone, stenting with EPD, and stenting with abciximab were associated with similar and modest declines in eGFR at 1-month follow-up (−10, −12, −10 mL/min/1.73m² eGFR change, respectively); however, the group treated with both EPD and abciximab was protected from a decline in eGFR and was superior to the other three groups (+9 mL/min/1.73m² eGFR change; p < .01). At present, we reserve the use of EPDs with renal stenting to patients with impaired renal function.

Stent Sizing With Intravascular Ultrasound

Intravascular ultrasound (IVUS) can provide precise anatomic characterization of the atherosclerotic plaque. IVUS guidance during renal artery stent placement resulted in additional lumen enlargement not considered necessary at angiography. In a series of

363 renal artery interventions, follow-up angiography was available in 102 patients (34%) at an average of 303 days. Larger-diameter arteries were associated with a significantly lower incidence of angiographic restenosis. The restenosis rate was 36% for vessels with a reference diameter less than 4.5 mm compared with 16% in vessels with a reference diameter of 4.5 to 6 mm ($p = .068$) and 6.5% in vessels with a reference diameter greater than 6 mm ($p < .01$). IVUS provides a more accurate way to measure vessel diameter than two-dimensional angiography, allowing the operator to safely maximize the stent size. Visual estimate tends to underestimate the size of the vessel, which can translate into higher rates of ISR.

Drug-Eluting Stent Versus Bare-Metal Stent

Restenosis after stent angioplasty of atherosclerotic RAS is a limitation, especially in small-diameter renal arteries. Recent reports suggest that with optimal deployment techniques, restenosis rates of less than 11% can be achieved when followed up to 60 months when using bare-metal stents (BMS).

The GREAT study (Palmaz Genesis Peripheral Stainless Steel Balloon Expandable Stent, comparing a Sirolimus Coated with an Uncoated Stent in REnal Artery Treatment) was a prospective, multicenter study of angiographic patency of drug-eluting renal artery stents placed in 105 patients with atherosclerotic RAS. The binary restenosis rate was 6.7% for sirolimus-eluting stents (SES) versus 14.6% for the BMS ($p = .30$). At 1-year follow-up, the clinical patency was 88.5% in the BMS and 98.1% in the drug-eluting stent (DES) group ($p = .21$). There is no clinical difference between BMS and DES for RAS at this time.

Restenosis Lesions

The durability of renal artery interventions is limited by the development of ISR and the need for secondary or tertiary renal interventions. Two meta-analyses of renal artery intervention have demonstrated mean restenosis rates after stent placement of 16% and 17% at 2 and 5 years follow-up, respectively. Renal stents have excellent long-term patency rates, with cumulative primary patency of 79% to 85% and a secondary patency of 92% to 98% at 5 years. A larger reference vessel diameter (RVD) and larger acute gain (post-stent minimal lumen diameter) after stent deployment are associated with a lower incidence of restenosis. The restenosis rate for smaller renal arteries (RVD ≤ 4.5 mm) was 36% compared with a restenosis rate of 6.5% for larger renal arteries (RVD > 6.0 mm).

The optimal treatment of renal artery ISR is uncertain. The use of covered stents in the renal arteries has been reported in the management of complications including perforation. Polytetrafluoroethylene (PTFE)-covered stents and DES may offer a way to treat recurrent renal artery stenosis. In a series of patients diagnosed having their at least second ISR after renal artery stenting, covered stents had 17% (1/6) ISR at a mean follow-up of 36 months whereas DES were free of ISR (0/10).

Follow-Up

Patients should be followed clinically in terms of blood pressure control with laboratory results to monitor renal function and surveillance Doppler ultrasonography (DUS) imaging at 1 month, 6 months, and 1 year and annually thereafter recommended to evaluate stent patency. DUS is the recommended imaging technique to screen for ISR. DUS surveillance monitoring for renal stent patency should take into account that a stented artery is less compliant than a native artery and that PSV and RAR obtained by DUS are higher for any given degree of arterial narrowing within the stent; therefore obtaining a postprocedure DUS is reasonable to establish a new baseline PSV.

Subclavian Interventions

Subclavian and innominate artery (S/IA) obstruction is an important cause of symptomatic extracranial cerebrovascular disease and may be associated with significant morbidity. Symptoms include those associated with posterior cerebral ischemia (vertebrobasilar insufficiency [VBI]) because of reversal of flow in the vertebral artery (subclavian steal syndrome [SSS]), angina pectoris because of reversal of flow in an internal mammary arterial graft (coronary-SSS), and arm ischemia because of claudication related to exercise or distal embolization.

Although the technical success of surgical revascularization is high, major complications include stroke in 0.5% to 5%, perioperative death in 2% to 3%, and an overall complication rate of 13% to 19%. A systematic review and meta-analysis found angioplasty and stenting for subclavian artery stenosis was significantly superior to angioplasty alone for maintenance of patency at 1 year, as indicated by absence of events (odds ratio [OR] 2.37, CI 1.32–4.26) without significant complication rates for either procedure.

Diagnosis of Subclavian/Innominate Artery Stenosis

Screening for S/IA disease is easily performed by obtaining bilateral arm blood pressure in the office. A systolic blood pressure difference of at least 15 mm Hg is highly (≥90%) specific for diagnosing subclavian stenosis, and this physical finding has proven to be an independent predictor of adverse cardiovascular events, including mortality.

Noninvasive studies include DUS, CTA, and MRA. Doppler can measure velocities and direction of flow in the subclavian artery and in the vertebral artery, therefore providing information about the underlying pathophysiologic process. Reversal of flow in the vertebral artery is seen in cases of SSS. CTA and MRA can provide more anatomic detail, including the aortic arch anatomy, and can give precise determinations of anatomic relations of the diseased segments to the ostia of the vertebral and internal mammary arteries (IMAs).

Indications for Revascularization

Subclavian Steal Syndrome

The diagnosis of SSS requires the presence of neurologic symptoms usually triggered by arm exercise with all of the following: (1) evidence of S/IA occlusion or marked stenosis, (2) retrograde vertebral flow, and (3) patency of both the vertebral and basilar arteries.

Coronary-Subclavian Steal Syndrome

In patients with prior coronary artery bypass surgery (CABG) using the IMA, hemodynamically significant subclavian stenosis proximal to the origin of the IMA causes reversal of flow through the IMA and "steal" flow from the coronary vasculature during upper extremity exercise. Coronary and graft angiography can demonstrate retrograde flow in the involved IMA during selective angiography of the grafted coronary artery. Simultaneous coronary and cerebrovascular ischemia have also been reported.

Arm Claudication

Upper extremity claudication is far less common than lower extremity claudication. However, lifestyle-limiting exertional symptoms, especially in the dominant hand, can be successfully treated with subclavian stent placement.

Technical Considerations

Vascular Access

Access site selection depends on the nature of the obstructive lesion. Femoral access offers an advantage in better visualizing the ostium at the aortic arch. For occlusions, a dual approach may be necessary. In such circumstances, femoral access helps identify the ostium of the artery and a wire placed in the ipsilateral upper extremity can help identify the target. Radial access is a good alternative to brachial

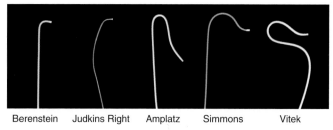

| Berenstein | Judkins Right | Amplatz | Simmons | Vitek |

Figure 16.8 Catheter shapes most used for engagement of the great vessels.

access; however, the placement of large stents (average 6 mm) often requires 6F or 7F systems, which limits the use of the radial artery to a select group of patients.

Angiography

Selective angiography of the innominate or left subclavian artery from a femoral approach can be accomplished most of the times with a JR4 or Berenstein diagnostic catheter. For patients with type III aortic arch, alternative "shepherd's crook" catheters like the Vitek or Simmons may be required (Fig. 16.8). After selective engagement of the S/IA, at least two orthogonal views are recommended. The bifurcation of the right subclavian artery and right common carotid artery is best evaluated in the right anterior oblique (RAO) projection; the origins of the right IMA and the right vertebral artery are better visualized in the left anterior oblique (LAO) projection. On the left side, the origin of the left IMA and the left vertebral artery can be visualized in the anteroposterior (AP) projection. Digital subtraction angiography (DSA) can be used to better delineate the vascular anatomy without overlying bony structures; however, it requires adequate breath holding to prevent motion artifacts.

Stenting

The choice of guiding catheter and/or sheath is largely dependent on the aortic arch anatomy. A coronary guiding catheter may allow for easier access to the ostia of the subclavian artery in patients with challenging anatomy or ostial lesions; however, it requires at least an 8F lumen to deliver the equipment necessary for subclavian stenting and a larger sheath in the femoral artery. On the other hand, a guide-sheath like a Shuttle sheath will require a smaller arterial puncture to deliver the same equipment (6/7F) but is less steerable in engaging the ostium of the subclavian artery.

A 0.035-in wire is preferred for delivery of interventional equipment; however, in some circumstances, when the lesion is heavily calcified with severe stenosis or there is an occlusion, a 0.014-in or 0.018-in wire can be used. In some cases of occlusion or severe stenosis, a femoral approach can be challenging, and the operator may not be able to cross the lesion. A retrograde approach via the brachial or radial access can be considered. On some occasions, it is necessary to use both antegrade and retrograde routes to cross the lesion.

Once the lesion is crossed, balloon angioplasty is usually performed before stenting to facilitate stent delivery and provide some information about the size of the vessel. The subclavian artery usually ranges from 6 to 8 mm in diameter. Balloon angioplasty alone is rarely performed as the use of BMS achieves patency rates of 97% at 12 months and 75% at 10 years compared with restenosis rates of 15% to 20% with balloon angioplasty alone. Covered stents may be necessary to treat complications like vessel rupture or subclavian artery aneurysms.

When the stenosis is proximal to the vertebral arteries and IMAs, balloon-expandable stents are preferred over self-expanding stents for precision in placement and the need for stronger radial force in this vascular structure. It is important to know that the proximal subclavian artery is an intrathoracic structure, and its rupture may manifest with intrathoracic hemorrhage. An example of subclavian stenting is shown in Fig. 16.9.

In-Stent Restenosis

The management of ISR largely depends on the presumed etiology. Geographic miss is a common cause of ISR, especially when the

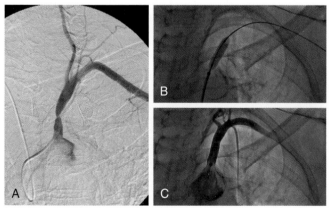

Figure 16.9 (A) Diagnostic angiography via right radial access using a Simmons 2 catheter. (B) Stent deployment in left subclavian artery through a shuttle sheath. (C) Final result.

lesion involves the true ostium. Restenting with appropriate ostial coverage is required in those situations. When there is suspected underexpansion based on angiography or IVUS, aggressive stent dilation with high-pressure balloons is recommended and provisional restenting is preserved for unsatisfactory results. When neither of these situations is present, repeated angioplasty with vascular brachytherapy or drug-eluting balloons are available options, although there is no current evidence to support its use.

Complications

The major risk of S/IA intervention is distal embolization. Embolization may occur in the ipsilateral digits or in the posterior circulation via the vertebral artery. During innominate artery intervention, potential embolization to the anterior cerebral circulation may occur via the right common carotid artery (CCA). Additionally, a challenging arch is a risk factor for embolic complications because it requires more manipulation.

Carotid Interventions

Epidemiology and Natural History

Atherosclerotic carotid artery disease is responsible for 80% of new noncardioembolic strokes. Carotid plaque most often causes cerebrovascular events because of plaque rupture with atheroembolization, rather than carotid artery occlusion (<20% of ischemic strokes) with thrombosis (Fig. 16.10).

The natural history of carotid artery stenosis depends on the presence of symptoms (transient ischemic attack [TIA], stroke, amaurosis fugax). Symptomatic patients have a 5- to 10-fold risk of stroke compared with asymptomatic patients. Asymptomatic patients with carotid artery stenosis outnumber symptomatic patients by 4:1. Because the majority (≥80%) of ischemic strokes have no warning symptoms, the management of asymptomatic carotid atherosclerosis with revascularization or medical therapy is important.

Asymptomatic Patients

Two RCTs (Asymptomatic Carotid Atherosclerosis Study [ACAS] and the Asymptomatic Carotid Surgery Trial [ACST]) showed that carotid endarterectomy (CEA) reduced the incidence of ipsilateral stroke in patients with asymptomatic carotid artery stenosis by 60% or more when compared with 50% reduction by medical therapy (e.g., aspirin) alone. However, CEA did not reduce overall stroke and death and did not show any benefit in women or in patients older than 75 years of age. It is important to note the medical therapy

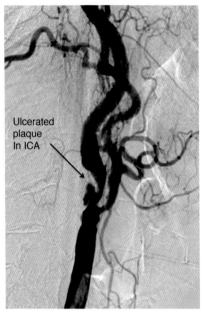

Ulcerated
plaque
In ICA

Figure 16.10 Catheter angiography of right carotid artery in a patient with recent transient ischemic attack. There is ulcerated plaque at the origin of the internal carotid artery.

provided in these trials (aspirin) has significantly improved nowadays. Currently, the risk of progression of an asymptomatic carotid artery stenosis to occlusion with modern medical therapy is very low (see Fig. 16.14).

Symptomatic Patients

The natural history of symptomatic carotid artery stenosis was reflected in the medical arm of the randomized North American Symptomatic Carotid Endarterectomy Trial (NASCET). The risk of stroke increases with severity of stenosis, and the 3-year risk of ipsilateral stroke in symptomatic patients with stenosis greater than 80% was 26.5%; however, as the stenosis approaches total occlusion (95%–99%), the risk of ipsilateral stroke goes down to 17.2%.

Clinical Presentation

Symptoms of carotid artery stenosis include ipsilateral transient visual defects (amaurosis fugax) from retinal emboli; contralateral weakness or numbness of an extremity or the face, or of a combination of these; visual field defect; dysarthria; and, in the case of dominant hemisphere involvement, aphasia. The National Institutes of Health Stroke Scale (NIHSS) should be performed in all symptomatic patients to quantify the neurologic deficit, which correlates with outcome.

Anatomic Imaging

DSA is the gold standard for defining carotid anatomy with the NASCET method of stenosis measurement the most widely accepted methodology (Fig. 16.11). Invasive cerebral catheter-based angiography carries a risk of cerebral infarction of 0.5% to 1.2%; therefore noninvasive imaging should be the initial strategy for evaluation. Carotid duplex imaging, transcranial Doppler imaging, CTA, and MRA are the noninvasive methods of assessment. Duplex imaging is the best initial choice given its safety profile, low cost, and wide availability. Cerebral and cervical imaging should define the aortic arch and the circle of Willis (Fig. 16.12).

Medical Therapy

Medical therapy for carotid atherosclerosis should focus on preventing stroke and stabilizing atherosclerotic lesions to prevent plaque rupture and atheroembolization. Blood pressure control, cholesterol lowering, and antiplatelet medications, including aspirin and clopidogrel, play a significant role in both primary and secondary prevention of stroke in patients with carotid artery disease. There is uncertainty regarding the best therapy for asymptomatic carotid artery disease, a question to be addressed by the CREST 2 study.

Surgical Therapy to Prevent Stroke

Asymptomatic Patients

Although there have been large RCTs comparing CEA with antiplatelet (aspirin) therapy in the treatment of at least moderate (≥50%–60%) carotid stenosis in patients without focal neurologic symptoms, the benefit of surgery was significant across varying degrees of stenosis (60%–90% stenosis). However, CEA did not reduce overall stroke and death and did not show any benefit in women or in patients older than 75 years of age.

Symptomatic Patients

Current AHA/ASA guidelines recommend CEA in symptomatic patients with stenosis of 50% to 99% if the risk of perioperative

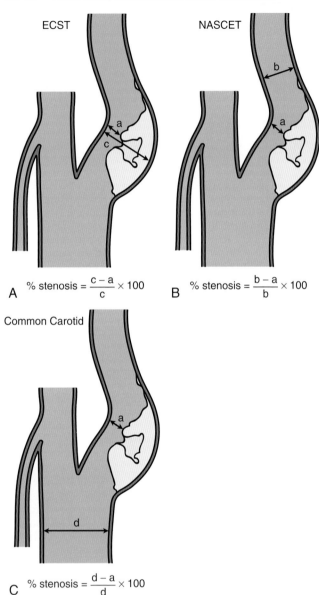

Figure 16.11 Methods of grading carotid artery stenosis in different trials.

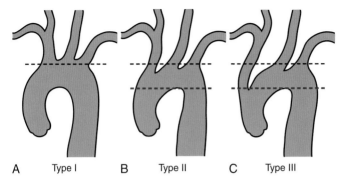

Figure 16.12 Aortic arch types.

stroke or death is less than 6%. In asymptomatic patients, guidelines recommend CEA for stenosis of 60% to 99% if the perioperative risk of stroke is less than 3% and life expectancy is at least 5 years. Some have recommended delaying revascularization in asymptomatic patients until the stenosis has reached 80%, but the evidence from ACST demonstrated equal benefit for moderate and severe stenosis.

Carotid Artery Stenting

Clinical Evidence

For carotid artery stenting (CAS) to become a routine and commonly used procedure, clinical trial data must justify its performance relative to the standard, CEA. When interpreting data on carotid stenting, it is important to realize that a patient who is at high risk for surgery is not necessarily at increased risk for stenting (and vice versa). Features that place a patient at increased risk for complications from CEA and CAS are summarized in Table 16.5.

High Surgical Risk Patients

The Stenting and Angioplasty with Protection in Patients at High Risk for Endarterectomy (SAPPHIRE) trial compared high surgical risk (HSR) patients treated with CEA with those treated with CAS. In that trial, 334 patients with a symptomatic stenosis of 50% or greater or an asymptomatic stenosis of 80% or greater (~30% were symptomatic) were randomized to either CEA or CAS. The primary endpoint of death, stroke, or MI at 30 days plus ipsilateral stroke or death from neurologic cause between day 31 and 1 year occurred

Table 16.5

High-Risk Features for CAS and CEA			
High-Risk Features for CAS		**High-Risk Features for CEA**	
Clinical Features	**Angiographic Features**	**Comorbidities**	**Anatomic Features**
Age ≥ 75/80	≥ 2 acute (90 degree) bends	Age ≥ 80	Lesion C2 or higher; below clavicle
Dementia	Circumferential calcification	Class III/IV CHF or angina	Prior neck surgery (including ipsilateral CEA) or radiation
Bleeding disorder	Intracranial microangiopathy	Left main or ≥ 2 vessel CAD	Contralateral carotid occlusion
Multiple lacunar strokes	Evidence of thrombus	Urgent heart surgery	Tracheostoma
Renal failure	Poor vascular access	LVEF ≤ 30% MI within 30 days Severe chronic lung disease Severe renal disease	Contralateral laryngeal nerve palsy

CAS, Carotid artery stenting; *CEA*, carotid endarterectomy; *CHF*, congestive heart failure; *LVEF*, left ventricular ejection fraction; *MI*, myocardial infarction.
(Adapted from Bates ER, Babb JD, Case DE, Jr., et al. ACCF/SCAI/SVMB/SIR/ASITN 2007 clinical expert consensus document on carotid stenting: a report of the American College of Cardiology Foundation Task Force on Clinical Expert Consensus Documents [ACCF/SCAI/SVMB/SIR/ASITN Clinical Expert Consensus Document Committee on Carotid Stenting]. *J Am Coll Cardiol.* 2007;49:126–170; and Roubin GS, Iyer S, Halkin A, Vitek J, Brennan C. Realizing the potential of carotid artery stenting: Proposed paradigms for patient selection and procedural technique. *Circulation.* 2006;113:2021–2030.)

in 12.2% of patients in the stenting group and 20.1% in the CEA group (*p* = .004 for noninferiority). The 30-day stroke and death rate among the asymptomatic patients was 4.6% for the CAS group and 5.4% for the CEA group. At 3 years, there were no differences between the CEA or CAS groups.

Average Surgical Risk Patients

Large RCTs in average or usual surgical risk patients have compared CAS with CEA. Three of these trials were conducted in Europe and were compromised by allowing very inexperienced CAS operators to participate in the trials and not requiring EPDs to be used.

The Carotid Revascularization Endarterectomy versus Stenting Trial (CREST) is the largest ($n = 2502$) RCT published that looks at CAS with EPD compared with CEA in patients at average risk for surgery and includes both symptomatic ($n = 1321$) and asymptomatic ($n = 1181$) patients. Over 10 years of follow-up, there was no significant difference in the rate of the primary composite endpoint of periprocedural stroke, death, or MI or follow-up ipsilateral stroke between the two groups (11.8% vs. 9.9%). For average-surgical-risk asymptomatic carotid stenosis patients enrolled in the symptomatic Carotid Trial (ACT-1), stenting was noninferior to endarterectomy with regard to death, stroke, or MI within 30 days after the procedure or ipsilateral stroke within 1 year (3.8% vs. 3.4%). When taken together, the message from large RCTs is that CAS with EPD is a reasonable alternative to CEA for average-surgical-risk patients but, as with CEA, only when performed by experienced operators.

Transcarotid Artery Revascularization

Transcarotid artery revascularization (TCAR) combines endovascular strategy with surgical principles of neuroprotection. The carotid artery is accessed through a short incision at the base of the neck over the proximal ipsilateral CCA with the ENROUTE transcarotid neuroprotection and stenting done with a stent system (Silk Road Medical, Inc, Sunnyvale, Calif). The Safety and Efficacy Study for Reverse Flow Used During Carotid Artery Stenting Procedure (ROADSTER) multicenter trial reported acute device and technical success of 99% and an overall stroke rate of 1.4% with TCAR.

In patients elected for carotid intervention, the following factors may favor TCAR over CAS: unfavorable peripheral arterial access and inability to use a cerebral protection device.

Contraindications

Contraindications to CAS include visible thrombus within the lesion detected on preoperative imaging (e.g., ultrasound, angiography) or intraoperative imaging, severe plaque calcification, circumferential carotid plaque, and severe carotid tortuosity.

Technical Aspects of Carotid Stenting

Baseline Aortography and Cerebral Angiography

Vascular access is most commonly obtained from the femoral artery, although brachial or radial access may be used. Before selective angiography, an arch aortogram is performed with a pigtail catheter placed in the proximal ascending aorta to define the anatomy of the aortic arch, which is critical to the success of the stent procedure. This is done in the 45-degree LAO position with a large-format image intensifier (12-inch to 16-inch) using DSA (15 cc per second for 3 seconds) and a power injector.

Once the morphology of the aortic arch is determined, catheters are chosen for selective angiography of the cervical arteries supplying the brain (right and left carotid and vertebral arteries) and the cerebral vasculature. For a type I arch, Berenstein or Judkins Right (JR) catheters are often used. For type II or III arch morphologies, shepherd's crook–shaped catheters (i.e., Simmons or Vitek catheters) may be best (see Fig. 16.11).

Angiograms are obtained to delineate the anterior and posterior circulation supplying the brain. The intracranial and extracranial portions of each vessel are studied. Generally, two orthogonal views of each are obtained, one in the AP projection and one in the lateral projection. Alternatively, some operators use rotational angiography. It is important to demonstrate the circle of Willis to define any baseline abnormalities. DSA may be performed with a 50/50 mix of saline and contrast. An external reference object is used with carotid angiograms to accurately measure the diameter of the artery.

Internal Carotid Intervention

The steps for internal carotid intervention are summarized in Fig. 16.13. A diagnostic catheter is used to engage the CCA, and a road map angiogram is made of the carotid bifurcation. A 0.035-in. stiff angled hydrophilic glidewire is advanced into the external carotid artery, and the diagnostic catheter is advanced over the wire into the CCA. The glidewire is exchanged for a 0.035-in. stiff Amplatz wire over which an 8F guiding catheter or a 6F sheath may be advanced to the CCA. Care must be taken to avoid plaque disruption with wires and catheters, and, at this point in the procedure, the plaque in the internal carotid artery should remain untouched.

Because of the very low incidence of stroke complicating CAS, demonstrating clinical benefit for any EPD in an RCT is difficult. Two meta-analyses support the use of EPDs. The risk-to-benefit assessment intuitively favors using a protection device. One simply has to retrieve a filter full of debris to realize the empirical benefits relative to the rare complications associated with an EPD. At the present time, optimal practice should include the use of an EPD, one that the operator is most comfortable using.

EPDs are standard of care in the United States, and several types exist (Fig. 16.14). If the distal EPD will not cross the lesion, the stenosis may be crossed with a conventional 0.014-in guidewire

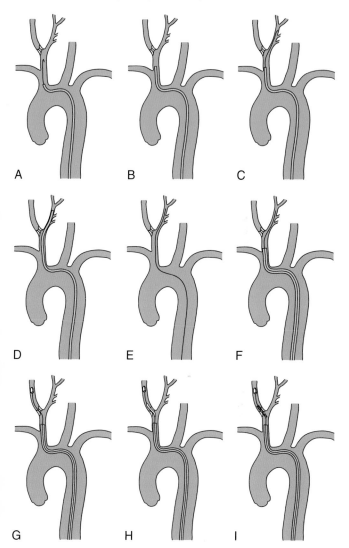

Figure 16.13 Internal carotid artery stenting step by step.
Continued

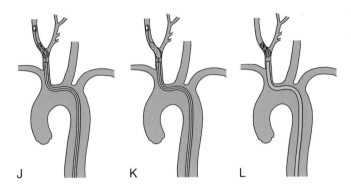

J   K   L

Figure 16.13, cont'd

and subsequently predilated with a small (2.5 mm) balloon. Then the EPD may be placed. After distal EPD deployment, the lesion is often predilated with an undersized coronary balloon, typically 3 to 4 mm in diameter. A self-expanding stent is then placed across the lesion. The stent is typically sized to fit the CCA. There is no demonstrated benefit for using tapered stents. It is common practice, when treating an internal carotid bifurcation lesion, to place the stent across the ostium of the external carotid artery.

There are two types of self-expanding stents: closed-cell and open-cell. Open-cell stents are more flexible and may better navigate tortuous vessels. Closed-cell stents are more rigid but may better "cover" atherosclerotic plaque. Although some evidence suggests that the frequency of embolic complications in symptomatic patients is lower with closed-cell stents, others have found no significant correlation between stent design and outcomes. Typical stent sizes are 6 to 10 mm in diameter and 2 to 4 cm in length. Gentle postdilation with an up to 5-mm balloon is often performed to improve stent apposition with the vessel wall. There is no benefit to aggressive postdilation because restenosis and late loss are very low in the carotid artery. Balloons are conservatively sized ($\leq$ 1:1) to minimize vessel trauma/dissection, plaque embolization, and stimulation of the carotid sinus. A poststent carotid diameter stenosis of up to 50% is an acceptable result.

An alternative to distal embolic protection is proximal protection. Two devices are available: the Gore flow reversal system (W L Gore, Flagstaff, AZ) and the Mo.Ma system (Medtronic, Minneapolis, MN). Both are positioned in a similar fashion. With the Gore device, the external carotid artery is accessed as above and a balloon-tipped sheath is advanced over the 0.035-in. stiff wire into the CCA.

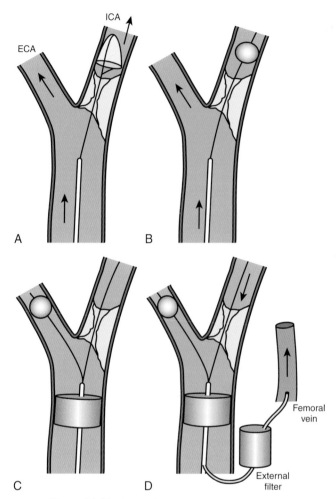

Figure 16.14 Types of embolic protection devices.

This sheath has a port for an occlusion balloon to be placed in the external carotid artery. The external and common carotid balloons are inflated, arresting antegrade flow. The Mo.Ma system is similar but consists of a single sheath with two balloons: a proximal balloon in the CCA and a distal balloon in the external carotid artery. When the balloons are inflated, blood flow is arrested. In either system, once patient tolerance of balloon occlusion is confirmed, the internal carotid lesion is crossed with a 0.014-in wire, dilated, and stented as described previously. With the Mo.Ma system, blood is manually aspirated after the stenting procedure to clear the debris distal to the CCA balloon. The Gore system, however, provides continuous flow reversal by having the arterial sheath connected to a venous sheath. Although experience with these devices is limited, data indicate that they can provide excellent results. A 1300-patient single-center prospective registry reported 99.7% procedural success with the Mo.Ma device and a 30-day death and stroke rate of 1.38%.

After the procedure, if a filter-type EPD is used, the EPD is retrieved, and a final carotid and cerebral angiography is performed. If a proximal protection device is used, the balloons are deflated and final angiography is performed. It is important to confirm that the CCA is free of dissection and that the cerebral vasculature is intact. Before removal of equipment, a neurologic exam assessing speech, movement, and mental status should be performed. If a neurologic deficit is found, a culprit lesion is sought and neurovascular rescue attempted.

Aorto-Ostial and Common Carotid Interventions

Femoral access is obtained with a 6F to 9F sheath depending on the diameter of the balloon and the stent that will be used. After anticoagulation (activated clotting time [ACT] $\geq$ 250 sec) and appropriate diagnostic imaging of the target lesion, a 5F diagnostic catheter is advanced through a guide catheter (i.e., JR 4 or multipurpose guide) to the ostium of the target CCA. The ostial lesion is crossed with a steerable 0.035-in hydrophilic glidewire. The diagnostic catheter is then advanced across the lesion into the distal vessel. The glidewire is exchanged for a stiff 0.035-in Amplatz wire, and the guide catheter is carefully advanced over the diagnostic catheter until it engages the ostium of the CCA. The diagnostic catheter is then slowly removed (Fig. 16.15).

The lesion is predilated with a balloon sized 1:1 with the CCA. As the balloon deflates, the guide is gently advanced or "telescoped" over the balloon and across the lesion. This will protect the stent as it is delivered to the lesion. The predilation balloon is removed, and a balloon-expandable stent is placed (in arteries protected by the axial skeleton, balloon-expandable stents are more often used). After positioning the stent at the target lesion, the guide catheter is withdrawn, uncovering the stent and placing it in contact with the target lesion. The proximal stent should protrude

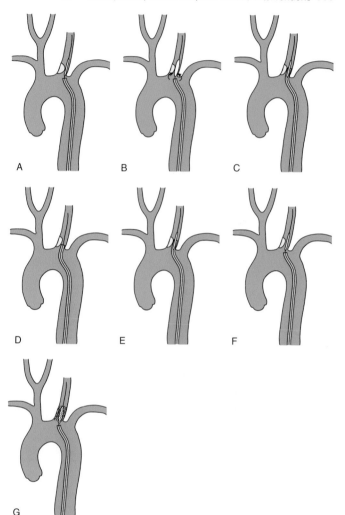

Figure 16.15 Common carotid intervention, step by step.

very slightly into the aorta (≤ 1 mm) to ensure lesion coverage. After verifying adequate placement with contrast injections through the guide catheter, the stent is deployed at nominal pressure. As the balloon deflates, the guide is again gently telescoped over the balloon to allow further stents to be delivered distally

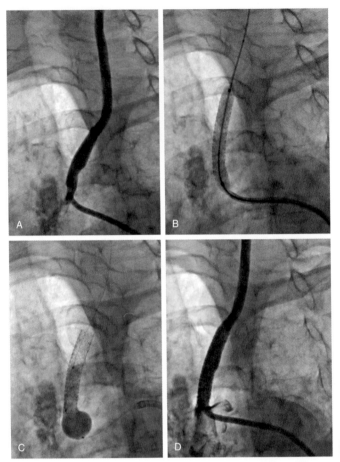

Figure 16.16 Angiography of the common carotid intervention.

if needed. A larger semicompliant balloon may be used to flare the protruding portion of the stent to facilitate future angiography. Final angiography and neurologic assessment are performed (Fig. 16.16). The access site is managed similarly to other interventional procedures. Sheath removal is performed when the ACT is less than or equal to 170 seconds if a closure device is not used.

Bilateral Carotid Stenosis

A staged approach, rather than simultaneous CAS, is preferred for bilateral CAS. There is theoretically an increased risk for cerebral hyperperfusion syndrome, bradycardia, or hypotension related to bilateral baroreceptor irritation with simultaneous CAS.

Complications and Troubleshooting

Stroke

In a review of over 54,000 patients, the 30-day risk of stroke during or after CAS was 3.9%. Most events occurred within 24 hours of the procedure. If the patient develops a focal neurologic deficit *during* the procedure, an embolic event is assumed. The main strategies used to reduce the risk of thromboembolic complications during and after CAS are appropriate patient selection, perioperative treatment with optimal medical therapy (including dual antiplatelet therapy [DAPT; aspirin and clopidogrel] and statin), optimal intraoperative anticoagulation, strict postprocedural blood pressure control, and possibly choice of approach (TCAR vs. TF-CAS) and choice of embolic protection.

Immediate cerebral angiography should be performed, and rescue intervention should be attempted. Typically, these emboli are plaque elements and not amenable to thrombolytic agents. Attempts at revascularization with angioplasty and stenting and/or thrombectomy are recommended. Mental status changes *after* the procedure warrant CT evaluation to rule out intracranial bleeding or hyperperfusion syndrome (see later).

Hemodynamic Instability

Stimulation of the carotid sinus baroreceptor is common during carotid interventions and can cause hypotension and bradycardia. Atropine (0.4–1 mg) may be used to treat acute bradycardia. A prophylactic dose may be considered before stent deployment if the patient was sensitive to predilation, but there is a risk of urinary retention in men. Aggressive fluid administration is important in treating hypotension. If vasopressor medications are needed to maintain a systolic blood pressure of at least 100 mm Hg, we use repeated boluses, as needed, of 25 mcg to 50 mcg of phenylephrine. A continuous infusion may be required if hypotension persists. In most patients, however, phenylephrine can be weaned within several hours of the procedure, and the patient can ambulate in preparation for discharge the next day. Midodrine 2.5 to 10 mg three times daily (and then titrated downward as tolerated) can be useful to support blood pressure in the setting of prolonged hypotension. Adjusting the patient's antihypertensive regimen will be necessary over the short term. Keep in mind that access site bleeding is a common cause of hypotension and should be ruled out in these patients.

Hyperperfusion Syndrome and Intracranial Hemorrhage

The opening of a stenotic carotid artery can lead to significant increases in cerebral blood flow, sometimes to levels more than twice the preprocedure flow and can lead to cerebral edema or, worse, intracranial hemorrhage. Hyperperfusion syndrome occurs in less than 1% of carotid stent patients and is defined clinically by the presence of an ipsilateral throbbing headache, a seizure, or a focal neurologic deficit.

Neurologic symptoms from cerebral edema are usually transient but must be addressed. A neurology consultation and head CT should be obtained if this diagnosis is entertained. When diagnosed, strict control of blood pressure is critical, and consideration of mannitol, diuretics, or antiepileptic medications (depending on presentation) is warranted. Medications that cause cerebral arterial vasodilation (i.e., hydralazine) should theoretically be avoided. Intracranial bleeding is life-threatening. If it occurs, antiplatelet medications should be stopped and a neurosurgical team consulted. Strict blood pressure control (goal systolic pressure of 120–140 mm Hg) may decrease the risk of hyperperfusion syndrome and intracranial bleeding.

Follow-Up

After intervention, patients should be followed to ensure the continuation of best medical therapy, monitoring the patency of the stent with DUS, and for the development of focal neurologic symptoms. DAPT with aspirin (75–325 mg daily) and clopidogrel (75 mg daily) is continued for approximately 4 to 6 weeks after the procedure and aspirin indefinitely.

After carotid artery revascularization, it is recommended to obtain DUS studies at baseline (within 1 month of intervention), 6 months, 12 months, and yearly thereafter. It is important to remember that carotid DUS velocities are altered after stenting and that overestimation of stenosis is very common.

Key References

Aronow HD, Collins TJ, Gray WA, et al. SCAI/SVM expert consensus statement on carotid stenting: training and credentialing for carotid stenting. *Catheter Cardiovasc Interv.* 2016;87:188-199.

Bates ER, Babb JD, Casey Jr DE, et al. ACCF/SCAI/SVMB/SIR/ASITN 2007 clinical expert consensus document on carotid stenting: a report of the American College of Cardiology Foundation Task Force on Clinical Expert Consensus Documents (ACCF/SCAI/SVMB/SIR/ASITN Clinical Expert Consensus Document Committee on Carotid Stenting). *J Am Coll Cardiol.* 2007;49:126-170.

Debono S, Nash J, Tambyraja AL, Newby DE, Forsythe RO. Endovascular repair for abdominal aortic aneurysms. *Heart.* 2021;107(22):1783-1789. doi:10.1136/heartjnl-2020-318288.

Ochoa VM, Yeghiazarians Y. Subclavian artery stenosis: a review for the vascular medicine practitioner. *Vasc Med.* 2011;16(1):29-34. doi:10.1177/1358863X10384174.

Prince M, Tafur JD, White CJ. When and how should we revascularize patients with atherosclerotic renal artery stenosis? *JACC Cardiovasc Interv.* 2019;12(6):505-517.

References

Antoniou GA, Antoniou SA, Torella F. Interval specific meta-analysis of endovascular vs. open repair of abdominal aortic aneurysm. *Eur J Vasc Endovasc Surg.* 2020; 60:485-487.

Bailey SR, Beckman JA, Dao TD, et al. ACC/AHA/SCAI/SIR/SVM 2018 appropriate use criteria for peripheral artery intervention: a report of the American College of Cardiology Appropriate Use Criteria Task Force, American Heart Association, Society for Cardiovascular Angiography and Interventions, Society of Interventional Radiology, and Society for Vascular Medicine. *J Am Coll Cardiol.* 2019;73(2):214-237.

Beckman JA, Ansel GM, Lyden SP, Das TS. Carotid artery stenting in asymptomatic carotid artery stenosis: JACC review topic of the week. *J Am Coll Cardiol.* 2020; 75(6):648-656.

Brott TG, Howard G, Roubin GS, et al. Long-term results of stenting versus endarterectomy for carotid-artery stenosis. *N Engl J Med.* 2016;374(11):1021-1031.

Hirsch AT, Haskal ZJ, Hertzer NR, et al. ACC/AHA 2005 guidelines for the management of patients with peripheral arterial disease (lower extremity, renal, mesenteric, and abdominal aortic): executive summary a collaborative report from the American Association for Vascular Surgery/Society for Vascular Surgery, Society for Cardiovascular Angiography and Interventions, Society for Vascular Medicine and Biology, Society of Interventional Radiology, and the ACC/AHA Task Force on Practice Guidelines (Writing Committee to Develop Guidelines for the Management of Patients With Peripheral Arterial Disease) endorsed by the American Association of Cardiovascular and Pulmonary Rehabilitation; National Heart, Lung, and Blood Institute; Society for Vascular Nursing; TransAtlantic Inter-Society Consensus; and Vascular Disease Foundation. *J Am Coll Cardiol.* 2006;47:1239-1312.

Kwolek CJ, Jaff MR, Leal JI, et al. Results of the ROADSTER multicenter trial of transcarotid stenting with dynamic flow reversal. *J Vasc Surg.* 2015;62(5):1227-1234.

Prince M, Tafur JD, White CJ. When and how should we revascularize patients with atherosclerotic renal artery stenosis? *JACC Cardiovasc Interv.* 2019;12(6):505-517.

Rosenfield K, Matsumura JS, Chaturvedi S, et al. Randomized trial of stent versus surgery for asymptomatic carotid stenosis. *N Engl J Med.* 2016;374(11):1011-1120.

Overview of Structural Heart Disease Interventions

PAUL SORAJJA • EMMANOUIL S. BRILAKIS

KEY POINTS

- Structural heart procedures include percutaneous valve replacement (or repair), left atrial appendage occlusion (or ligation), placement of devices across the intra-atrial or intra-ventricular septum, and placing plugs across spaces with perivalvular blood flow.

- Heart teams inclusive of interventional cardiologists and cardiac surgeons are central to structural procedures, particularly those involving valve replacement.

- Structural procedures require a unique integration of fluoroscopy and ultrasound guidance—often requiring expertise in two-dimensional and three-dimensional transesophageal echocardiography.

Introduction

Catheter-based structural heart interventional therapy has rapidly emerged and evolved over the past 15 years, with these treatments now established as the standard of care for many patient subsets. This chapter provides an overview of commercially available therapies and a glimpse into the future of the field.

General Considerations

For patients being considered for transcatheter valve interventions, evaluation by a multidisciplinary heart team (i.e., clinical cardiologist, imaging specialist, interventional cardiologist, and cardiac surgeon) for determination of indications and the procedural plan is strongly recommended. The purpose of the heart team is to determine the optimal therapy, particularly when multiple or complex options are available. Preoperative dental clearance is recommended to reduce likelihood of endocarditis. For all procedures, we also prepare the subxiphoid area in the event that emergent pericardiocentesis is needed and have perfusionists on call in case there is a need for peripheral support (i.e., extracorporeal membrane oxygenation).

Transcatheter Aortic Valve Replacement and Balloon Aortic Valvuloplasty

For patients with severe symptomatic aortic stenosis, transcatheter aortic valve replacement (TAVR) is a life-saving procedure. Success rates for TAVR are greater than 95%, with procedural risks of mortality in 1% to 2%, stroke in 2% to 3%, and bleeding in 5% to 7%. The need for a permanent pacemaker varies according to underlying conduction disease, as well as type and implant depth of the TAVR prosthesis, ranging from 5% to 25%. The two principal TAVR prostheses types are balloon-expandable (e.g., Sapien 3 Ultra) and self-expanding (e.g., Evolut R Pro, Portico, Acurate Neo-2, Jena-Valve) (Fig. 17.1). Transfemoral arterial access is used for TAVR in more than 95% of cases, although vessel requirements vary according to prosthesis type, size, and whether the device is to be placed with or without a sheath. TAVR can be performed for either native aortic stenosis or degenerative aortic valve prostheses. Balloon aortic valvuloplasty (BAV), although in practice since the 1980s, is now mainly used to facilitate TAVR placement when needed. In other cases, BAV can be used as standalone therapy for bridging, such as for a patient in cardiogenic shock or for the temporary relief of heart failure caused by aortic stenosis. Standalone BAV is palliative and not shown to improve survival because of the high rate of restenosis that occurs within approximately 6 months of the procedure.

Once the diagnosis of severe aortic stenosis and indications for TAVR have been established, gated contrast-enhanced computed tomography (CT) of the cardiovascular anatomy is needed to assess suitability for the procedure. The aortic valve is examined for area (primarily for balloon-expandable) and perimeter (primarily for self-expanding), with sizing calculations that are then matched to device manufacturer recommendations. Typical ranges covered by balloon-expandable prostheses (i.e., 20–29 mm Sapien Ultra) are

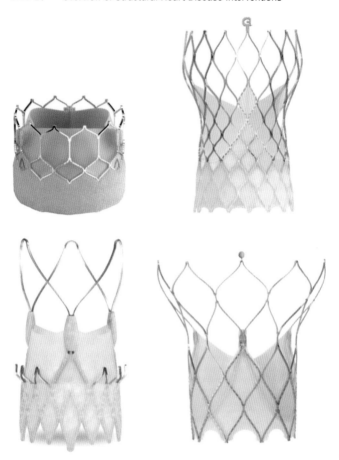

Figure 17.1 Common Prostheses for Transcatheter Aortic Valve Replacement. Left to right, Sapien 3 Ultra, Evolut R Pro, Acurate Neo-2, and Portico.

273 mm² to 680 mm². For self-expanding protheses (i.e., 23–34 mm Evolut R Pro), the typical ranges are 56 mm to 94 mm. Other, less commonly used valves have sizes within these ranges. Clearance to the coronary arteries is important, not just for native aortic stenosis but especially for valve-in-valve therapy where the degenerated leaflets are permanently fixed and could impair flow. The peripheral arteries are studied for minimal lumen diameter (MLD), tortuosity,

and disease to assess suitability for passage of the sheaths and delivery catheters. Typically, dimensions for MLD are 5.0 mm to 6.5 mm, with variation according to size and type of TAVR prosthesis. Vascular sheaths for TAVR include expandable 14 French (F) to 16F versions and ones with fixed diameters up to 22F, and some devices contain a built-in sheath (e.g., InLine for Evolut R Pro).

The TAVR procedure is frequently performed with conscious sedation, although some cases may require general anesthesia for patient comfort or transesophageal imaging. Ultrasound-guided vascular puncture facilitates percutaneous transfemoral procedures, with the preclose technique commonly employed for the large bore access site. A standard pigtail catheter placed in the contralateral access is used for aortography and to guide implant depth of the TAVR prosthesis (Figs. 17.2–17.4). A cerebral protection device (i.e., Sentinel) for potential prevention of stroke may be used via the right radial artery. For deployment of balloon-expandable prostheses, a temporary venous pacemaker is used to create temporary ventricular standstill by pacing at rates of 160 to 180 beats per minute. A temporary pacemaker is also often used to create regular rhythm at 120 beats per minute for deployment of self-expanding prostheses.

After implantation of the TAVR prosthesis, routine monitoring on telemetry is advised. The temporary pacemaker may be removed or left indwelling according to electrocardiogram (ECG) disturbances and the patient's risk for complete heart block. Most patients are discharged on postoperative day one with either single- or dual-antiplatelet therapy.

Transcatheter Mitral Valve Repair and Replacement

As a relatively less invasive therapy, percutaneous treatment for mitral regurgitation (MR), either as a repair or valve replacement, is an attractive option that may help address unmet clinical needs for patients with MR. The field of percutaneous MR treatment is highly active, with several options commercially available in clinical practice and dozens of technologies under development developed. To have outcomes comparable to surgery, percutaneous therapy requires proper patient selection through comprehensive preoperative imaging and implantation in partnership with an expert interventional imager.

Transcatheter Mitral Valve Repair

Transcatheter repair approaches can be grouped broadly into treatments that target the leaflets (e.g., MitraClip [Abbott Vascular, Santa

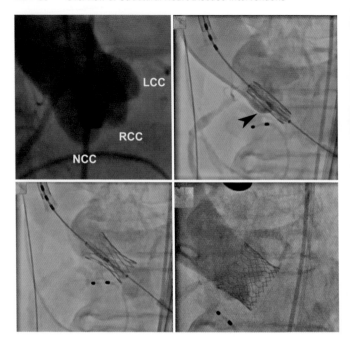

Figure 17.2 Deployment of a Balloon-Expandable Prosthesis (Sapien 3 Ultra) for Transcatheter Aortic Valve Replacement. *Top left,* Aortography is used to delineate the three cusps, which are aligned in a planar view, based on cardiac computed tomography. *Top right,* The middle marker of the deployment balloon is positioned at the aortic side of the native annulus. *Bottom left,* Under rapid ventricular pacing and with aortography, the balloon is deployed slowly to allow for positioning over 5 to 7 seconds as needed. *Bottom right,* Fully deployed prosthesis. *LCC,* Left coronary cusp; *NCC,* noncoronary cusp; *RCC,* right coronary cusp.

Clara, CA]; Pascal [Edwards Lifesciences, Irvine, CA]), mitral annulus (e.g., Cardioband [Edwards Lifesciences, Irvine, CA]; Millipede [Boston Scientific, Maple Grove, MN]), chords (e.g., Neochord [St. Louis Park, MN], Harpoon [Edwards Lifesciences, Irvine, CA]), or left ventricle (e.g., Accucinch [Ancora Heart, Santa Clara, CA]).

MitraClip is the most widely available percutaneous therapy for native MR, with over 125,000 patients treated worldwide thus far. Using a 24F transvenous, transseptal system, one or more clips are used to permanently appose the anterior and posterior leaflets to recreate and promote coaptation reserve. The MitraClip device comes in four sizes (NT, NTW, XT, and XTW) with device choice based on

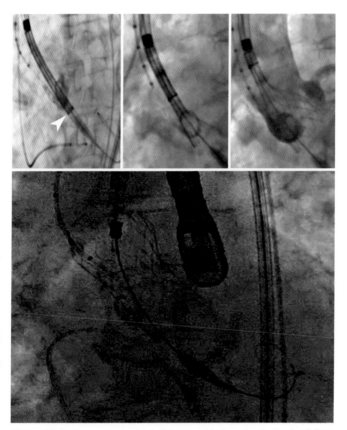

Figure 17.3 Deployment of a Self-Expandable Prosthesis (Evolut R Pro) for Transcatheter Aortic Valve Replacement. *Top left*, The marker band and inflow portion of the prosthesis is positioned 3 to 5 mm below the native aortic annulus, which has been delineated in the noncoronary cusp by contralateral aortography. *Top middle*, The valve is slowly deployed with monitoring of the marker band which indicates the capsule end, while maintaining the inflow slightly beneath the native aortic annulus. *Top right*, The valve is deployed two-thirds and assessment of final depth is determined. The prosthesis can be fully retrieved at this point. *Bottom*, Fully deployed prosthesis.

leaflet length, jet width, location of regurgitation, and size of the mitral valve. Frictional elements (i.e., "grippers") are implanted on the atrial side of the mitral leaflets after insertion into the device arms (Fig. 17.5), with verification of adequate insertion using multiple views on transesophageal echocardiogram (TEE). Overall,

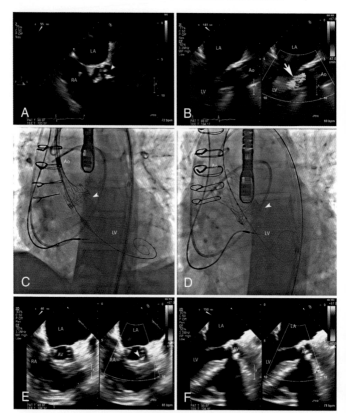

Figure 17.4 Self-Expanding Prosthesis Placement for Valve-in-Valve. The patient was a 77-year-old woman with prior placement of a 23 mm Edwards Magna prosthesis for severe aortic stenosis. (A) Preprocedural imaging with transesophageal echocardiography (*TEE*) shows the degenerated prosthesis (*arrowhead*), which was associated with a mean gradient of 74 mm Hg. (B) There also was a moderate degree of aortic insufficiency (*arrow*). (C) A 23-mm Evolut R (Medtronic, Dublin, IE) was chosen for the procedure (*arrowhead*) and placed using a retrograde approach from the right femoral artery. (D) The prosthesis was implanted at a depth of 2 to 3 mm (*arrowhead*), thereby maximizing the supra-annular position and effective orifice area. On TEE, there was a trivial degree of aortic insufficiency on the short-axis view (E, *arrow*), and none evident on long-axis imaging (F). Invasive hemodynamics showed a significant drop in the mean gradient from 82 mm Hg at baseline

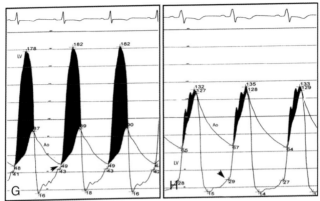

Figure 17.4, cont'd (G) to only 5 mm Hg after valve implantation (H). *AV*, Aortic valve; *LA*, left atrium; *LV*, left ventricle; *RA*, right atrium. (From Sorajja P, Pederson WA, Lesser JR, Bae R, Brilakis E. *Structural Heart Cases: A Color Atlas of Pearls and Pitfalls.* 1st ed. Elsevier; 2018.)

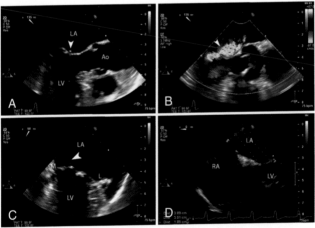

Figure 17.5   Transcatheter Mitral Valve Repair with MitraClip. (A) On transesophageal echocardiography (*TEE*), there was degenerative mitral regurgitation (*MR*) with a small flail segment (*arrowhead*). (B) Severe MR was present on color flow imaging. (C) On the TEE bicommissural view, the flail segment arose slightly medial (*arrowhead*). (D) Transseptal puncture is performed at a height of 3.9 cm to the mitral coaptation point. For the classic MitraClip system, a transseptal height of approximately 4.0 cm was sufficient, but a height of approximately 4.5 cm typically is used for MitraClip NT. *Continued*

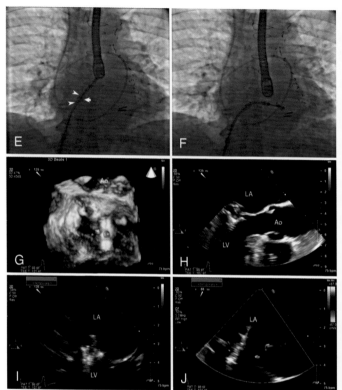

Figure 17.5, cont'd (E) The clip delivery system (*CDS*) is inserted into the steerable guide catheter (*SGC*) and straddled. Arrowheads indicate straddle markers; the arrow indicates the SGC tip. (F) The CDS is steered toward the mitral valve using the M knob and posterior torque of the SGC, followed by opening of the clip arms. (G) TEE with three-dimensional imaging allows the clip arms to be centered over the target of pathology; the arms are positioned perpendicular to the coaptation plane of the mitral valve. (H) The CDS crosses the mitral valve, followed by closure of the arms to 120 degrees to enable cupping of the leaflets. (I) Once the leaflets fall into the arms, the grippers are dropped and the arms are closed to 60 degrees. Leaflet insertion is confirmed in multiple views. (J) The clip then is completely closed, followed by an assessment for MR reduction. This closure is preferably done in the bicommissural view with simultaneous color imaging to show the location of the clip and effect on MR reduction.

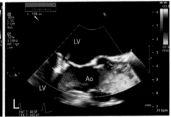

Figure 17.5, cont'd (K) The mitral gradient is checked for possible stenosis. (L) TEE imaging shows trivial residual MR after final clip deployment. *Ao*, Ascending aorta; *L*, lateral; *LA*, left atrium; *LV*, left ventricle; *M*, medial; *P*, posterior; *RA*, right atrium; *RV*, right ventricle; *S*, septal. (From Sorajja P, Pederson WA, Lesser JR, Bae R, Brilakis E. *Structural Heart Cases: A Color Atlas of Pearls and Pitfalls.* 1st ed. Elsevier; 2018.)

procedural success with reduction in MR to less than or equal to 2+ occurs in approximately 90% of selected patients, with approximately 65% of patients having residual MR less than or up to 1+, in association with an in-hospital mortality of 2% to 3%. Although single-leaflet device attachment was an early concern, the rate of this adverse event is now 1% to 2%, with embolization being rare. A learning for the procedure is present, with greater achievement of optimal reduction in MR occurring with operator experience of more than 50 cases. In the most recent experience with the MitraClip G4 system, optimal MR reduction was achieved in 90% of patients.

The PASCAL device is a 22F steerable, transvenous, transseptal system with 10-mm clasps and spring-loaded paddles that span 25 mm when open. Similar to MitraClip G4, the PASCAL device enables the operator to independently grasp each mitral valve leaflet. PASCAL also contains a 10-mm central spacer to reduce MR. PASCAL has been found to be effective in more than 95% of patients with low procedural mortality. PASCAL is the subject of ongoing trials with randomization to MitraClip in degenerative MR (CLASP IID) and versus medical therapy in functional MR (CLASP IIF). Presently, other devices for transcatheter repair also remain under investigation in the United States.

Transcatheter Mitral Valve Replacement

Transcatheter mitral valve replacement is a rapidly emerging therapy that is approved for commercial use in Europe and is under investigation in the United States. Typically, these prostheses consist of a self-expanding, double nitinol frame, with housing of the pros- thetic leaflets in a tri-leaflet, circular configuration (Fig. 17.6). Gated cardiac CT with contrast is used to size the mitral valve and to predict the risk of left ventricular outflow tract (LVOT) obstruc- tion through measurement of the neo-LVOT area. Notable factors to consider are specific to the profile of the device and also in- clude certain patient characteristics, such as angulation of the aortic-mitral curtain, size of the LVOT, left ventricular dilatation, and elongation or tethering of the mitral leaflets. In general, a neo-LVOT area of more than 250 mm^2 is favorable for implantation.

The methods for anchoring transcatheter mitral valve implan- tation (TMVI) prostheses vary and include an epicardial tether (Tendyne), radial force via a "champagne cork" effect (Intrepid, Medtronic Inc., Mounds View, MN), and engagement of the leaflets and/or subvalvular apparatus (Evoque [Edwards Lifesciences, Ir- vine, CA]; Tiara [Neovasc Inc., Richmond, BC]; Cephea, [Abbott Vascular, Chicago, IL]). These prostheses also differ in shape, with some exhibiting symmetry (Intrepid, Evoque, and Cephea) and others more closely resembling the irregular, D-shape configura- tion of the native mitral valve annulus (Tendyne and Tiara). Some others also anchor in two-step processes, whereby an anchor is placed followed by valve insertion (HighLife [Highlife Technolo- gies, Paris, FR]; M3 [Edwards Lifesciences, Irvine, CA]). Although the majority of implantations are currently performed with a trans- ventricular approach, transseptal placements are now being pur- sued. A major potential benefit of transcatheter mitral valve re- placement is complete elimination of MR.

Mitral Valve-in-Valve and Valve-in-Ring

Transcatheter mitral valve-in-valve and valve-in-ring procedures are performed typically using a femoral venous approach with transseptal placement of a Sapien prosthesis (Edwards Lifescience [Irvine, CA]). The neo-LVOT is assessed with cardiac CT for prepro- cedural risk of obstruction, with measurement to the anticipated location of the skirt of the device with implantation. Risk of LVOT obstruction is higher with valve-in-ring implantation, with variation in risk related to size, shape, and type of the surgical ring to be treated (i.e., complete vs. incomplete, rigid vs. semirigid).

After transseptal puncture, a steerable catheter (e.g., 8.5F Agi- lis) is used to place a super stiff guide (e.g., Safari) in the left ven- tricle (Fig. 17.7). A septostomy is performed with a 12- to 14-mm peripheral balloon, which may also be used to dilate the degener- ated mitral prosthesis if needed. The commander delivery is in- serted with the flexion toward the mitral valve ("upside-down E") and assembly of the Sapien valve onto the delivery balloon is

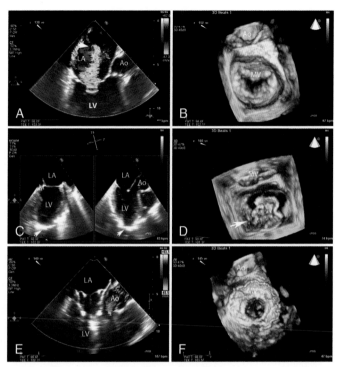

Figure 17.6 Transcatheter Mitral Valve Replacement. (A) Baseline transesophageal echocardiogram (*TEE*) with apical long-axis imaging demonstrates severe mitral regurgitation (*arrow*). The left ventricular ejection fraction was 35%. (B) TEE with three-dimensional (3D) imaging from the left atrium (i.e., surgeon's view) shows the mitral valve before intervention. (C) After a surgical cut-down, the operator chooses a site on the left ventricle that bisects the mitral valve in both the commissural (*left*) and septal-lateral planes (*right*). This site is confirmed with indentation of the left ventricle and simultaneous echocardiography (*arrows*). (D) Using a transapical approach, the Tendyne prosthesis (*arrow*) is extruded slowly and then rotated to fit in the anatomic shape of the native mitral valve. Anchoring is achieved through the use of tether connected to an epicardial pad, which also provides hemostasis. (E) After placement, Doppler color-flow imaging demonstrates no residual mitral regurgitation. (F) TEE with 3D imaging with a left atrial view shows the prosthesis in place.

Continued

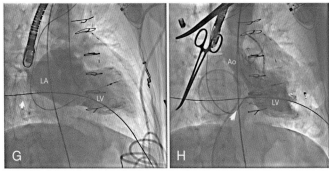

Figure 17.6, cont'd (G) Preprocedural left ventriculography demonstrates severe mitral regurgitation, with contrast opacifying the entire left atrium and several of the pulmonary veins (*arrow*). (H) After placement of the Tendyne prosthesis (*arrow*), there is no residual mitral regurgitation on left ventriculography. *Ao*, Ascending aorta; *LA*, left atrium; *LV*, left ventricle; *MV*, mitral valve prosthesis. (From Sorajja P, Pederson WA, Lesser JR, Bae R, Brilakis E. *Structural Heart Cases: A Color Atlas of Pearls and Pitfalls*. 1st ed. Elsevier; 2018.)

performed in the inferior vena cava. The Sapien prosthesis is deployed to ensure sealing by its skirt; positioning that is too atrial leads to paravalvular regurgitation and can also increase the risk for embolization. Commonly, the ventricular aspect of the Sapien prosthesis is postdilated to flare the outflow and increase device stability.

Percutaneous Paravalvular Leak Repair

Percutaneous repair of paravalvular prosthetic regurgitation is a highly effective therapy when performed in experienced centers, with procedural success in 90% of patients. Because of the complex nature of the techniques, there is a significant learning curve with a high potential for prolonged procedures (~2.5 hours) and complications (~5%), although death is rare (~0.5%). All patients should be evaluated for both active endocarditis and hemolytic anemia. Active endocarditis is a contraindication to the procedure. The presence of hemolytic anemia necessitates a high degree of closure (ideally complete) and should be known when considering therapeutic options.

Echocardiography is the primary imaging modality for the evaluation, although acoustic shadowing can pose challenges for

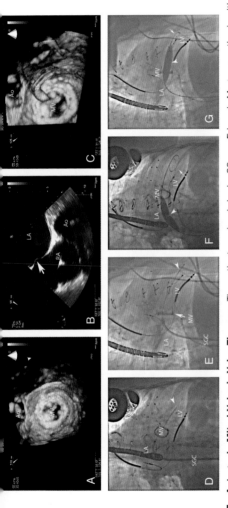

Figure 17.7 **Antegrade Mitral Valve-in-Valve Therapy.** The patient previously had a 29-mm Edwards Magna prosthesis with now severe stenosis (mean gradient of 12 mm Hg at a heart rate of 62 beats per minute on Doppler imaging). (A) End-diastolic image from transesophageal echocardiography (*TEE*) with three-dimensional (*3D*) imaging from the left atrium (i.e., surgeon's view) shows a degenerated mitral valve (*MV*) prosthesis with severe stenosis. (B) On TEE, care is taken to perform the transseptal puncture with a posterior orientation (*arrowhead*), thereby minimizing the flexion needed to turn past the septum to the mitral valve with the delivery catheter. (C) An 8.5 French (*F*), medium-curve St. Jude Agilis steerable catheter (St. Jude Medical, Fridley, MN) is placed in the left atrium and directed toward the MV prosthesis. (D) A balloon wedge catheter (*arrow*) is floated from the left atrium (*LA*) into the left ventricle (*LV*). (E) An extra-small curve Safari-2, preshaped guidewire (Boston Scientific, Maple Grove, MN) is placed in the left ventricle (*arrow*), followed by alignment of the coaxial plane of the MV prosthesis on fluoroscopy (*arrowheads*). (F–G) An 18-mm True balloon (Bard Peripheral Vascular, Tempe, AZ) is used to gently dilate the septum with partial inflation and then the MV prosthesis over the Safari-2 guidewire (*arrows*).

Continued

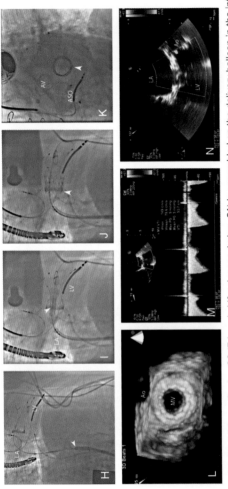

Figure 17.7, cont'd (H) A 29-mm Sapien S3 (Edwards Lifesciences, Irvine, CA) is assembled on the delivery balloon in the inferior vena cava (*arrowhead*), followed by flexion and advancement to the MV prosthesis. (I) The marker of the S3 prosthesis (*arrowhead*) is placed on the surgical valve, recognizing that shortening of the S3 will occur in the ventricular direction, and deployed with rapid ventricular pacing. The S3 prosthesis is not coaxial, but one can see the entire atrial portion located in the left atrium. (J) Final positioning shows the atrial portion of the S3 on the atrial side of the surgical prosthesis (*arrow*) with flaring of the ventricular portion to facilitate a cork-like anchoring effect. (K) The atrial septum is closed with a 32-mm Amplatzer Septal Occluder (ASO, St. Jude Medical, Fridley, MN). (L) End-diastolic image on TEE with 3D imaging showing full opening of the newly placed S3 prosthesis. The final gradient across the newly placed S3 prosthesis was only 3 mm Hg (M), and there was no evidence of mitral regurgitation on color-flow imaging with TEE (N). Ao, Ascending aorta; ASO, Amplatzer Septal Occluder; LA, left atrium; LV, left ventricle; MV, mitral valve; RA, right atrium; RV, right ventricle; RVOT, right ventricular outflow tract; SGC, steerable guide catheter. (From Sorajja P, Pederson WA, Lesser JR, Bae R, Brilakis E. *Structural Heart Cases: A Color Atlas of Pearls and Pitfalls*, 1st ed. Elsevier; 2018.)

visualizing paravalvular regurgitation in some patients. Cardiac CT is helpful for providing information regarding camera set-up in the catheterization laboratory and thus can help facilitate the success of percutaneous closure. The imaging examination determines the location and severity of the paravalvular regurgitation (including size and distance of the defect from the prosthesis annulus) and excludes central valvular involvement.

Presently, the procedure requires the off-label use of occluders, with the most commonly used devices being the AVP-2 and AVP-4 plugs (St. Jude Medical, Fridley, MN). These devices are made of self-expanding nitinol, deliverable through small caliber catheters (e.g., 4F), and have retention disks to help reduce the risk of embolization after deployment. The AVP-3 is available in Europe and currently under investigation in the United States. Other commonly used devices include the Amplatzer muscular ventricular septal defect and ductal occluders. Both of these latter occluders require relatively larger sheaths for delivery but have been successfully employed in select cases. In many instances, placement of the delivery catheters requires the use of transcatheter rails (e.g., venous-arterial, arterial-arterial, or veno-apical), which entail snaring and exteriorization to create necessary support.

Aortic Paravalvular Leak Repair

For patients with aortic paravalvular regurgitation, the most common approach for percutaneous repair is retrograde via the femoral artery (Fig. 17.8). The procedure can be performed with TEE, transthoracic echocardiogram (TTE), or intracardiac echocardiography (ICE). The image intensifier should be positioned with no overlap between the defect and the aortic prosthesis. The positioning can be approximated (e.g., left anterior oblique cranial for posterior defects; right anterior oblique caudal for anterior defects) but is best determined accurately from CT-imaging. Without such positioning, it is difficult to determine whether the guidewire is being passed into the defect external to the prosthesis.

The defect is approached with a steerable coronary catheter depending on which native cusp is involved (e.g., 6F Amplatz left or multipurpose catheter). An angled-tip, exchange-length (260 cm) hydrophilic wire (Glidewire, Terumo) is placed through the defect and often passed antegrade through the aortic valve in the event that snaring for a rail is required. Once the wire is across, a guide catheter is advanced into the left ventricle. Selection of the guide is dependent on (1) the size and number of device occluders that are needed; (2) the difficulty encountered in passing the catheter across the defect; and (3) the need for an anchor wire. With the guide catheter in the left ventricle, the device occluder is

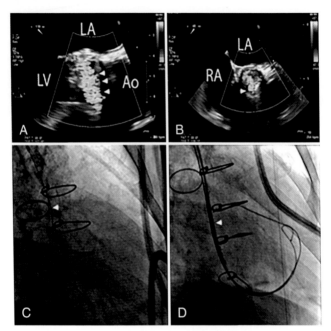

Figure 17.8 Percutaneous Repair of Aortic Paravalvular Prosthetic Regurgitation. The patient had previously underwent aortic valve replacement with a 27-mm bileaflet mechanical prosthesis (St. Jude Medical, St. Paul, MN). Transesophageal echocardiography demonstrates severe anterior paravalvular regurgitation (*arrowheads*) in a long-axis (A) and short-axis view (B). (C) An AL-1 diagnostic catheter, placed from the right femoral artery, is steered toward the defect, which is then crossed with a 260-cm, angle-tipped, extra-stiff Glidewire (*arrowhead*; Terumo, Ann Arbor, MI). (D) Over the glidewire, a 90-cm, 8 French (*F*) Flexor Shuttle (*arrowhead*; Cook Medical, Bloomington, IN) is passed into the left ventricle, followed by placement of two 0.032-inch extra-stiff Amplatz wires. (D) Over these two wires, two separate 6F Flexor Shuttle sheaths are advanced into the left ventricle. The distal retention discs of two 10-mm AVP-2 plugs (St. Jude Medical, St. Paul, MN) are extruded in the left ventricle, followed by retraction and apposition against the left ventricular side

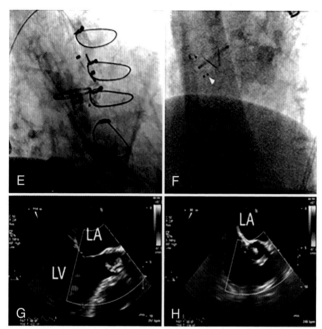

Figure 17.8, cont'd (E) and deployed (F, *arrowhead*). The final view is chosen to demonstrate normal prosthetic leaflet motion. Postprocedural transesophageal echocardiography in long-axis (G) and short-axis views (H) demonstrates mild residual regurgitation. (From Sorajja P, Pederson WA, Lesser JR, Bae R, Brilakis E. *Structural Heart Cases: A Color Atlas of Pearls and Pitfalls.* 1st ed. Elsevier; 2018.)

extruded with retention disks positioned on the ventricular and aortic sides of the defect or, as frequently with AVP-4 plugs, wholly within the defect. The final assessment must include an evaluation for prosthetic leaflet impingement and residual regurgitation. Angiography should also be considered to exclude arterial occlusion for patients requiring large device occluders and those with small aortic sinuses, low coronary height, or defects located near the coronary ostia. Once the final assessment is satisfactory, the device occluders are released.

Mitral Paravalvular Leak Repair

For patients with mitral paravalvular regurgitation, the most commonly used approach is transseptal femoral venous access and antegrade cannulation of the defects from the left atrium. Alternatively, direct transapical puncture or a retrograde approach (via the femoral artery) with retrograde cannulation from the left ventricle also can be successful.

For the antegrade approach, standard transseptal techniques with guidance from fluoroscopy and echocardiography are used to access the left atrium, with a posterior or superior position favored for medial defects (Fig. 17.9). A steerable 8.5F guide (Agilis catheter, [St. Jude, Fridley, MN]) is loaded with a telescoped catheter system, consisting of a 6F 100-cm multipurpose guide and a 5F 125-cm multipurpose diagnostic catheter. The system is steered toward the defect, which is crossed with the Glidewire (Terumo). Fluoroscopy should demonstrate positioning of the steerable guide and guidewires external to the prosthesis. The multipurpose catheters can be used to place the devices or exchanged for larger delivery catheters (e.g., 90 cm, 6–8F Cook Flexor Shuttle) that enable multiple device placements or anchor wiring. Similar to treatment of aortic defects, the distal retention disk of the occluder is extruded from the guide into the left ventricle, followed by straddling of the defect with the retention disks on both sides. Once leaflet impingement has been excluded on both echocardiography and fluoroscopy, the device occluder(s) is released.

Alcohol Septal Ablation

First described by Ulrich Sigwart in 1994, alcohol septal ablation entails percutaneous injection of alcohol into one or more septal perforator arteries, leading to a controlled myocardial infarction (MI) of the ventricular septum and relief of the dynamic LVOT obstruction. The success of alcohol septal ablation is dependent on appropriate patient selection, operator experience, and clinical expertise, with care delivered in the setting of a center dedicated to the comprehensive and longitudinal care of the hypertrophic cardiomyopathy (HCM) patient.

The therapeutic goal of alcohol septal ablation is to treat symptoms by reducing the systolic thickening of the ventricular septum that is responsible for dynamic LVOT obstruction and associated MR. Patients who may be candidates for the procedure therefore are those with: (1) severe, drug-refractory cardiovascular symptoms; (2) *dynamic* LVOT obstruction because of systolic anterior motion of the mitral valve (gradient ≥30 mm Hg at rest or ≥50 mm Hg with provocation); (3) ventricular septal thickness of 15 mm or higher; (4) no significant intrinsic mitral valve disease; (5) absence of need for concomitant cardiac surgical procedure (e.g., valve replacement, bypass grafting); and (6) suitable coronary anatomy.

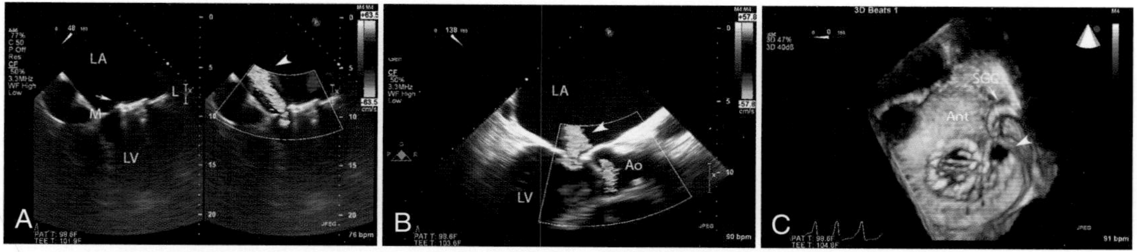

Figure 17.9 Percutaneous Repair of Mitral Paravalvular Regurgitation. A 68-year-old woman presented with exertional dyspnea and evidence of severe paravalvular regurgitation involving a previously placed bileaflet, mechanical mitral prosthesis. (A–B) Transesophageal echocardiography (*TEE*) demonstrates paravalvular regurgitation (*arrowhead*) arising medial to the mitral prosthesis (*arrow*) and anterior, close to the aortic valve annulus. (C) TEE with three-dimensional (3D) imaging from the left atrium (i.e., surgeon's view) shows the surgical prosthesis and the large paravalvular defect (*arrow*).

Continued

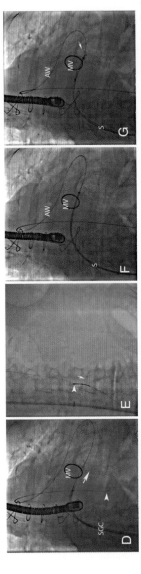

Figure 17.9 cont'd (D) An 0.035-inch, angle-tipped Glidewire (Terumo, Somerset, NJ) is passed through the defect (*arrow*) into the left ventricle and then into the descending aorta (*arrowhead*). (E) The wire is snared with a 15-mm gooseneck, which had been advanced from the left femoral artery and then exteriorized to create a rail (*arrow*). (F) This exteriorized rail both supports passage of delivery sheaths and serves as an anchor wire (AW). A 90-cm, 8F Flexor Shuttle sheath (S, Cook Medical, Bloomington, IN) is advanced over the wire into the left ventricle, followed by extrusion of the distal portion of a 10-mm, type II Amplatzer Vascular Plug (*arrow*; St. Jude Medical, St. Paul, MN) alongside the wire. (G) The fluoroscopic angles are rotated to an angle perpendicular to the plane of the MV prosthesis to facilitate examine of the prosthetic leaflets during deployment.

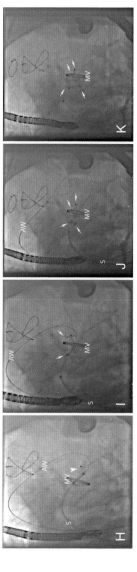

Figure 17.9 cont'd (I) The vascular plug and sheath are retracted together to position the distal portion of the plug on the left ventricular side of the MV prosthesis, followed by unsheathing of the plug across the defect (arrows). (J) With the plug still connected to its delivery cable, the sheath is removed and then reinserted over only the anchor wire. A second 10-mm plug is then deployed in similar fashion. (K) Once effectiveness has been established and there is no evidence of prosthetic leaflet impingement, the anchor wire is removed. Both plugs are then decoupled from their delivery catheters. Imaging with TEE in commissural *Continued*

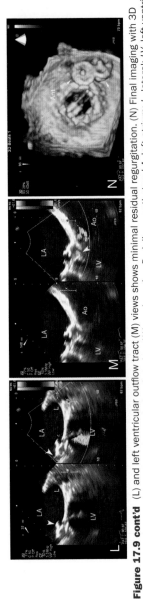

Figure 17.9 cont'd (L) and left ventricular outflow tract (M) views shows minimal residual regurgitation. (N) Final imaging with 3D TEE shows the two plugs in place (*arrows*). *Ant*, Anterior; *AW*, anchor wire; *D*, delivery catheter; *L*, lateral; *LV*, left ventricle; *M*, medial; *MV*, mitral valve; *RA*, right atrial; *S*, Shuttle sheath; *SGC*, steerable guide catheter. (From Sorajja P, Pederson WA, Lesser JR, Bae R, Brilakis E. *Structural Heart Cases: A Color Atlas of Pearls and Pitfalls.* 1st ed. Elsevier; 2018.)

The operator should be cognizant of the load-dependent sensitivity of LVOT obstruction in HCM when examining hemodynamic data from both the echocardiogram and invasive catheterization. For the most accurate intraprocedural measurement of LVOT gradients, transseptal catheterization is recommended. Retrograde assessments can also be performed with particular attention paid to the potential for catheter entrapment and to ensuring side-holes of pigtail catheters, if used, are placed below the level of subaortic obstruction. For patients without prior pacemaker placement, temporary pacemaker implantation should be performed because of the risk for high-grade atrioventricular block. The risk for pacemaker dependency from alcohol septal ablation varies according to the baseline conduction abnormalities with high rates for those with prior left bundle branch block or wide QRS duration.

Coronary angiography is used to determine the most appropriate septal artery for the procedure with examination of the angulation of the origin and length of the vessel (Fig. 17.10). Conventional 6F or 7F guide catheters are used to engage the left coronary artery with standard procedural anticoagulation (e.g., heparin 70–100 units/kg). A well-seated coaxial guide is needed to facilitate contrast injections that definitively demonstrate no communication between the septal artery and epicardial vessel after balloon occlusion. A standard-length, 0.014-inch guidewire is carried considerably distal to ensure the stiff portion is at the occlusion site followed by placement of a slightly oversized (e.g., 2.0-mm balloon for a 1.5-mm vessel), short-length (e.g., 6–9 mm), over-the-wire balloon. Oversizing of the balloon allows for occlusion of the septal artery at low pressures (3–4 atm), which permit injection of material through the wire lumen of the catheter. Coronary angiography then is performed to demonstrate no communication between the septal perforator and left anterior descending artery during balloon inflation. Next, the guidewire is removed and a septal artery angiogram via the balloon catheter confirms patency of the vessel for ablation and localization (i.e., no untoward collateralization). Angiographic contrast can be visible on echocardiography for identification of the perfusion bed, although many operators also prefer to additionally inject dedicated echocardiographic contrast (e.g., 0.5 mL Definity or Optison). Multiple echocardiographic views are used to confirm enhancement of the septal hypertrophy intimately related to LVOT obstruction and the absence of undesirable locations. After delineation of the targeted myocardium, desiccated ethanol with a total amount of approximately 0.8 mL per 10 mm thickness is infused slowly over a period of 3 to 5 minutes followed by approximately 1.0 cc of slow normal saline flush to eliminate any remaining alcohol in the balloon catheter lumen. For patients

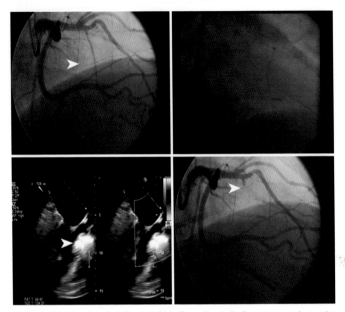

Figure 17.10 Alcohol Septal Ablation. *Top left*, Coronary angiography identifies the candidate septal artery (*arrowhead*). *Top right*, An over-the-wire balloon is inserted followed by inflation and septal angiography. Echocardiographic contrast is then administered. *Bottom left*, Comprehensive echocardiography confirms the location of the perfusion bed to be related to left ventricular outflow tract obstruction (*arrowhead*) and no other locations. *Bottom right*, After alcohol infusion, septal angiography confirms thrombosis of the vessel and territory (*arrowhead*).

without significant reduction of either the resting or provoked LVOT gradient, other septal perforator arteries can be targeted and treated in similar fashion. In general, residual peak gradients of less than 30 mm Hg and preferably less than 10 mm Hg are desired, prompting termination of the procedure.

Overall, alcohol septal ablation typically results in a 60% to 80% reduction in the LVOT gradient. These results are similar to surgery for acute procedural success, when defined as a 80% reduction or higher in the peak resting or provoked LVOT gradient with a final residual resting gradient of up to 10 mm Hg, which occurs in 80% to 85% of patients. Factors associated with higher likelihood of acute hemodynamic success include relatively less septal hypertrophy, lower LVOT gradients, and greater operator experience. Ventricular remodeling and basal septal thinning lead to further reduction in the LVOT gradient over a period of 3 to 6 months after the procedure. Procedural failure most frequently results from the lack of an appropriate septal artery, which may be absent in up to 20% of patients.

Balloon Mitral Valvuloplasty

Balloon mitral valvuloplasty was first introduced in 1984 as a therapy splitting of fused valve commissures in patients with rheumatic mitral stenosis. With improvement in techniques and equipment, balloon mitral valvuloplasty now is the procedure of choice for selected patients with severe mitral stenosis. In general, balloon mitral valvuloplasty leads to a doubling of the valve area and a 50% to 60% reduction in the transmitral gradient. Complications include acute severe MR (2%–10%), ventricular perforation (0.5%–4%), large atrial septal defect (<5%; larger of double balloon system used), MI (0.3%–0.5%), systemic embolization (0.5%–3.0%), and death (<2%). Overall, in patients with favorable valve morphology, the success rate of balloon valvuloplasty for mitral stenosis is greater than 90%, with a complication rate of less than 3% when performed by experienced hands.

Patient Selection

Procedural success, therefore, is heavily dependent on the mechanism of commissural fusion, the pliability of valve, and the state of the subvalvular apparatus. Significant retraction and fusion of the chordae papillary and muscles may prevent a satisfactory result. One method is the Abascal (or Wilkins) score in which points (1–4) are assigned according to the physical characteristics of the mitral valve and summated (Table 17.1). Because commissural splitting is the dominant mechanism for the effectiveness of valvuloplasty, presence or absence of commissural calcification also should be determined. Calcification of the commissures increases the risk of valve leaflet tearing because of the differential stress effects of the inflated balloon. Patients with a high Abascal score can still be considered for balloon valvuloplasty if there is not significant calcification of the mitral commissures. Conditions that preclude candidacy for balloon valvuloplasty are left atrial thrombus and moderate or severe MR.

   Patients with symptoms caused by severe mitral stenosis (valve area <1.5 cm^2) or high inducible gradients (>15 mm Hg) with a suitable, pliable valve may be considered for balloon valvuloplasty. Asymptomatic patients with significant stenosis also may be considered if there is favorable valve morphology, particularly

Table 17.1

Wilkins or Abascal Score for Determining Eligibility for Mitral Balloon Valvuloplasty				
Score	Leaflet mobility	Valve thickness	Subvalvular thickening	Calcification
1	Highly mobile	Normal (4–5 mm)	Minimal thickening	Single area
2	Decreased in midportion and base	Midleaflet/ marginal thickening	Chordal thickening up to 1/3 of chordal length	Confined to leaflet margins
3	Forward movement in diastole	5–8 mm	Chordal thickening up to 2/3 of chordal length	Up to mid leaflet
4	No or minimal Forward movement in diastole	Severe (≥8 mm)	Complete to papillary muscle	Throughout most of valve leaflets

in the presence of significant pulmonary hypertension or new atrial fibrillation. Balloon mitral valvuloplasty also has been used successfully to treat increasing symptoms of heart failure in pregnant patients.

Procedure

The most common technique for balloon mitral valvuloplasty is a transvenous, antegrade approach with a transseptal puncture through the fossa ovalis and placement of an Inoue balloon. Punctures superior or inferior to the fossa ovalis can lead to difficulty in crossing the mitral valve with the balloon catheter. Through the transseptal sheath, a heavy-duty spring coil guidewire is placed into the left atrium. The transseptal sheath is then exchanged for a 14F long dilator, which is used to dilate the femoral access site and the interatrial septum.

The size of the Inoue balloon catheter is determined by the patient's height (size in mm = [height in cm ÷ 10] + 10]). Each

Inoue balloon catheter is examined for accuracy of inflation size before insertion. The Inoue balloon is elongated, passed over the guidewire into the left atrium, and then shortened. The spring coil guidewire is exchanged for a J-tipped stylet, which is then used to guide the balloon through the valve orifice with care to avoid entanglement with the subvalvular apparatus. The Inoue balloon is constructed with different compliances, so that increasing inflation pressures first inflate the distal end in the left ventricle, followed by the proximal end in the left atrium. The stylet is withdrawn slightly to fix the balloon crossing the mitral valve (Fig. 17.11). The balloon is then fully inflated to inflate its center, facilitating commissural splitting and valve dilatation. Repeat dilatation with increasing inflation sizes can be performed in a stepwise fashion (1–2 mm increments) until satisfactory hemodynamic results are achieved. After successful dilatation, the balloon is elongated in the left atrium to prevent atrial septal defects during withdrawal of the balloon into the right atrium. An oxygen saturation run then is performed to exclude significant left-to-right shunting, and residual MR is assessed by either echocardiography or left ventriculography.

Left Atrial Appendage Closure

Percutaneous closure of left atrial appendage (LAAC) is indicated for patients with atrial fibrillation who cannot take oral anticoagulation chronically for stroke prevention. The determination is best made with validated methods for assessment of indications for oral anticoagulation with the $CHADS_2$ or CHA_2DS_2VASc score and the risk of bleeding with the HAS-BLED scoring systems (Tables 17.2–17.3).

The procedure is performed most commonly with TEE, although ICE with conscious sedation is also used. Often, a preoperative cardiac CT is used to gain knowledge of the shape, size, and orientation of the appendage for choice of catheter and device. These imaging assessments are essential because of considerable variation in anatomy of the LAA, which has been described as windsock, chicken wing, cactus, and cauliflower (Fig. 17.12).

The most commonly implanted device is the nitinol-based Watchman, whose current version is the FLX. The Watchman FLX (20–35 mm diameters) has a rounded ball configuration during deployment to enhance safety and is fully retrievable and repositionable. In the PINNACLE study, procedure success rates with Watchman FLX were 98.8%, with no procedural mortality, no pericardial effusion requiring surgery, and the only adverse event being ischemic stroke (0.5%). The Amulet is an LAAC device under

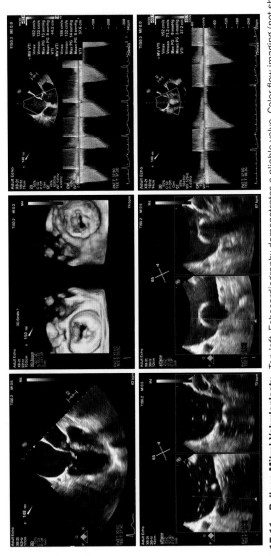

Figure 17.11 **Balloon Mitral Valvuloplasty.** *Top left,* Echocardiography demonstrates a pliable valve. Color flow imaging (not shown) indicates mild mitral regurgitation. *Top middle,* Fusion of both commissures is present. *Top right,* Doppler echocardiography shows severe mitral stenosis. *Bottom left,* The distal balloon is inflated and retracted to the mitral valve under echocardiographic guidance. *Bottom middle,* After confirmation of positioning within the chord-free zone, the proximal balloon and then waist is fully inflated. *Bottom right,* The postprocedural mitral gradient is significantly reduced.

Table 17.2

Thromboembolic Risk Scores for Patient Selection Before Left Atrial Appendage (LAA) Closure	
CHADS$_2$	
Characteristic	**Points**
Congestive heart failure	1
Hypertension	1
Age $\geq$75 years	1
Diabetes mellitus	1
Stroke, transient ischemic attack, or thromboembolism	2
Maximum score	6
CHA$_2$DS$_2$VASc	
Characteristic	**Points**
Congestive heart failure	1
Hypertension	1
Age $\geq$75 years	2
Diabetes mellitus	1
Stroke, transient ischemic attack, or thromboembolism	2
Vascular disease (prior MI, PAD, or aortic plaque)	1
Age 65–74 years	1
Sex category = female	1
Maximum score	9

MI, Myocardial infarction; *PAD,* peripheral arterial disease.
(From January CT, Wann LS, Alpert JS, et al. 2014 AHA/ACC/HRS guideline for the management of patients with atrial fibrillation: A report of the American College of Cardiology/American Heart Association Task Force on Practice Guidelines and the Heart Rhythm Society. *J Am Coll Cardiol.* 2014;64[21]:e1–e76.)

investigation with coming availability for use in the United States. This device, also fully retrievable, is a nitinol occluder with a polyester covering, consisting of a 16- to 34-mm lobe and disc connected by a flexible waist.

A key part is transseptal puncture that is localized to the inferior-posterior part of the atrial septum to establish a favorable trajectory to the LAA with the delivery sheath. The procedure should be performed with left atrial pressure greater than 10 mm Hg to ensure expansion of the LAA for echocardiography, which involves meticulously conducted measurements of the ostium and depth. Device selection is 10% to 20% greater than the maximum width, with assurance that depth is sufficient (i.e., avoiding implants for a relatively shallow and wide LAA).

The Watchman delivery sheath comes in three configurations: double-curve (majority of cases), single (for predominant posterior

Table 17.3

HAS-BLED Bleeding Risk Score	
Characteristic	Points
Hypertension (uncontrolled systolic blood pressure >160 mm Hg)	1
Abnormal liver or renal function[a]	1 each, maximum 2
Stroke (previous history)	1
Bleeding history or disposition (e.g., anemia)	1
Labile international normalized ratio (INR; i.e., time in therapeutic range <60%)	1
Elderly age (>65 years)	1
Drugs that promote bleeding or excess alcohol consumption (>7 units per week)	1 each, maximum 2
Maximum score	9

[a]Abnormal liver function was defined as cirrhosis or biochemical evidence of significant hepatic derangement; abnormal renal function was defined as serum creatinine > 200 μmol/L (2.26 mg/dL).
(From Pisters R, Lane DA, Nieuwlaat R, de Vos CB, Crijns HJGM, Lip GYH. A novel user-friendly score [HAS-BLED] to assess 1-year risk of major bleeding in patients with atrial fibrillation: The Euro Heart Survey. *Chest.* 2010;138[5]:1093–1100.)

lobe), and anterior (for anterior lobe). A pigtail catheter is inserted into the delivery sheath and used to intubate the LAA (Fig. 17.13). Angiography of the LAA is performed with a hand injection using a right anterior oblique-caudal (30/30 degrees) projection, similar to a TEE 135-degree view. The operator then advances the delivery sheath into the LAA, often with a gentle counterclockwise (anterior) rotation, with depth markers according to size of implant desired. A delivery system with the attached device is then inserted and deployed through careful self-expansion and positioning within the LAA. Determination for final release of the device is made with the PASS criteria (Fig. 17.14):

Position: Proximal shoulders of the device are at or just distal to and span the entire LAA ostium.

Anchor: Gently pull back and release the deployment knob to visualize the movement of the device and LAA together.

Size: The maximum diameter of device by TEE is consistent with adequate device compression.

Seal: Ensure all lobes are distal to the shoulders of the device and sealed (≤5 mm jet on TEE).

After deployment, aspirin and warfarin are initiated, without bridging heparin therapy, for an international normalized ratio (INR) goal of 2.0 to 3.0 until the 45-day visit. If TEE shows an LAA seal (5-mm peri-device flow), warfarin is discontinued and the

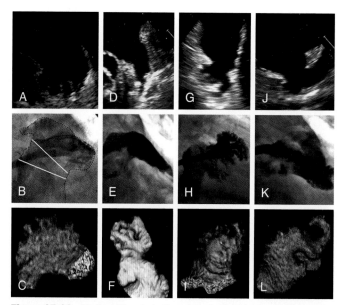

Figure 17.12 **Various Morphologies of the Left Atrial Appendage.** The four proposed classifications of left atrial appendage morphologies as shown by transesophageal echocardiography (*top*), cine angiography (*middle*), and three-dimensional computed tomography (*bottom*). (A–C) Cauliflower. (D–F) Windsock. (G–I) Cactus. (J–L) Chicken wing. (From Biegel R, Wunderlich NC, Ho SY, Arsanjani R, Siegel RJ. The left atrial appendage: Anatomy, function, and noninvasive evaluation. *JACC Cardiovasc Imaging.* 2014;7[12]:1251–1265.)

patient is placed on dual-antiplatelet therapy with the addition of clopidogrel 75 mg/day. At 6 months, the patient is placed on monotherapy with continuation of aspirin and stoppage of clopidogrel.

Atrial Septal Defect and Patent Foramen Ovale Closure

Atrial septal defects (ASDs) and patent foramen ovale (PFO) both represent communications across the atrial septum and have similar techniques for closure but with different clinical indications. For ASDs, key indications for closure are the presence of a large, *secundum* defect greater than 5 mm, evidence of volume overload from shunting (typically with a Qp/Qs >1.5), and anatomy (i.e., rims) suitable for closure. In these patients, anomalous pulmonary

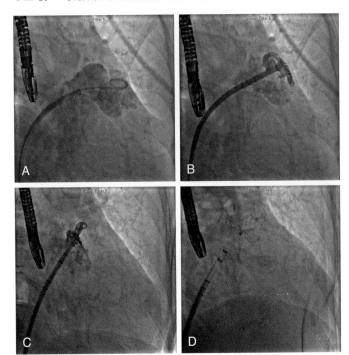

Figure 17.13 Fluoroscopic Guidance of Watchman Left Atrial Appendage (LAA) Closure. Baseline transesophageal echocardiogram demonstrated a maximal LAA ostium width of 25 mm; therefore a 30-mm occluder represents the smallest acceptable device size to provide the minimum allowable compression (at least 8%). (A) LAA angiography is performed in the right anterior oblique-caudal projection through a 6 French (*F*) diagnostic pigtail catheter that has been advanced through the dedicated 14F access sheath. The distalmost marker delineates the tip of the access sheath, which is at the LAA ostium. (B) The access sheath is advanced deeply into the LAA over the pigtail catheter while applying counterclockwise rotation to orient the sheath coaxially with the LAA ostium. The first (most proximal) and second markers are nearly straddling the plane of the LAA ostium (*arrows*), consistent with sufficient depth for a 30-mm device. (C) LAA after device deployment. Contrast can enter the LAA through the perforated cap of the device, which endothelializes in the weeks after implantation. The proximal shoulders of the device arrows rest at the level of the LAA predicted by the fluoroscopic markers before delivery. According to TEE, the widest diameter of the device was 24.5 mm consistent with adequate compression (14.7%). (D) Fluoroscopy of the device after release from the delivery cable. (From Price MJ, Holmes, DR. Mechanical closure devices for atrial fibrillation. *Trends Cardiovasc Med.* 2014;24[6]:225–231.)

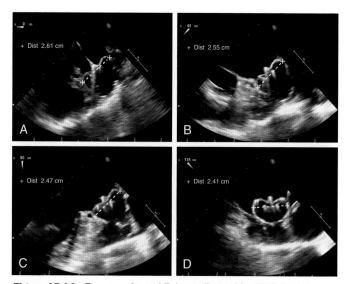

Figure 17.14   Transesophageal Echocardiographic (TEE) Assessment of Watchman Device Implantation. After deployment of a Watchman 30-mm device, the left atrial appendage (*LAA*) is assessed at 0, 45, 90, and 135 degrees (Panels A, B, and C, respectively). Compression is determined by measuring the distance across the shoulders of the device in the plane of the threaded insert. In this case, the device diameter ranges from 24.1 mm to 26.1 mm (13%–20% compression), is well-positioned, there is no color flow around the device into the LAA, and the LAA moved with the device as a unit when the delivery cable was tugged gently. Therefore the device was released from the cable with successful LAA occlusion. (From Price MJ, Holmes, DR. Mechanical closure devices for atrial fibrillation. *Trends Cardiovasc Med.* 2014;24[6]:225–231.)

venous connections, sinus venosus defect, mitral valve disease, and severe, irreversible pulmonary artery hypertension should be excluded. For patients being considered for PFO closure, the key clinical indication for closure is cryptogenic stroke because of paradoxical embolism in a relatively young patient (i.e., <55 years of age), with exclusion of atrial arrhythmias, hypercoagulable disorder, and cerebrovascular disease as potential causes. Older patients may be considered for PFO closure, but the risk of recurrent stroke to age-related disease should be considered. In this context, calculation of the risk of paradoxical embolism (RoPE) score may be useful.

The techniques for closure of ASD and PFO share similar general principles (Figs. 17.15–17.16). The procedures may be performed with TEE or ICE guidance. Such imaging is used to assess the rims in all directions (bicaval for superior-inferior; short-axis for anterior-posterior), with greater than 5 mm being ideal, as well as landing zones relative to caval flow and the posterior wall of the aorta. After femoral venous access and placement of a 6F sheath, the defects are wired from the inferior vena cava with a straight or j-tipped standard wire loaded inside a steerable catheter, such as a diagnostic multipurpose. In some instances, a glide-wire facilitates crossing, which is confirmed on echocardiography. The diagnostic catheter is advanced into the left atrium, followed by exchange for a supportive wire (e.g., superstiff, extrastiff, or Safari). The defect can be sized with a sizing balloon, followed by a device choice that is typically 10% greater than the waist. In other instances, especially for PFO defects, the device size is chosen based on an assessment of the rims and without balloon sizing. The delivery sheath is placed, followed by insertion of the occluder. The left atrial side of the occluder is exposed in the left atrium and retraction of the entire assembly is perform to juxtapose it onto the atrial septum. The right atrial side of the occluder is then exposed. Sealing and stabilization are assessed on both echocardiography and fluoroscopy before full release. If closure is inadequate, the device can be retrieved in the delivery sheath and either exchanged or redeployed.

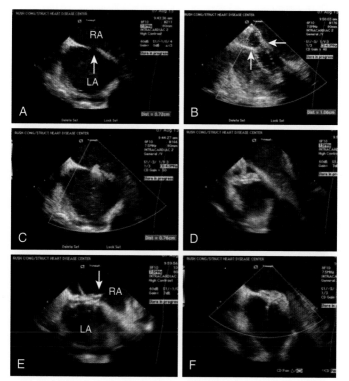

Figure 17.15 Intracardiac Echocardiography in a Patient With a Small Secundum Atrial Septal Defect (ASD). (A, C) Septal view, demonstrating the ASD (*arrow*) without and with color Doppler, the right and left atria, and the superior and inferior rims. (B) The left atrial disc (*arrow*) deployed in the left atrium; balloon sizing of the defect, measuring the stop flow diameter, between the two arrows. (D) The left atrial disc is well seen in the left atrium. (E) The right atrial disc (*arrow*) is deployed in the right atrium. (F) After the device has been released, demonstrating good device position and no residual flow by color Doppler.

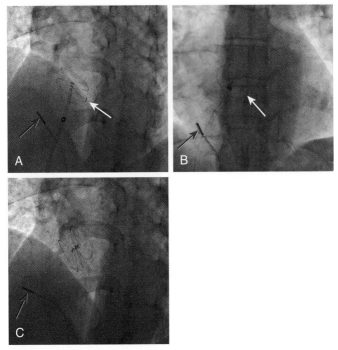

Figure 17.16 Cineangiographic Images of a Patient for Patent Foramen Closure. (A) The left atrial disc (*white arrow*) deployed in the left atrium. (B) The right atrial disc deployed in the right atrium. (C) The device released, demonstrating good position. Red arrow shows position of the intracardiac echo transducer.

Key References

Bavaria JE, Tommaso CL, Brindis RG, et al. 2018 AATS/ ACC/SCAI/STS Expert Consensus Systems of Care Document: operator and institutional recommendations and requirements for transcatheter aortic valve replacement. *J Am Coll Cardiol.* 2019;73:340-374.

Bonow RO, O'Gara PT, Adams DH, et al. 2019 AATS/ACC/SCAI/STS expert consensus systems of care document: operator and institutional recommendations and requirements for transcatheter mitral valve intervention: a joint report of the American Association for Thoracic Surgery, the American College of Cardiology, the Society for Cardiovascular Angiography and Interventions, and The Society of Thoracic Surgeons. *J Am Coll Cardiol.* 2020;76:96-117.

Horlick E, Kavinsky CJ, Amin A, et al. SCAI expert consensus statement on operator and institutional requirements for PFO closure for secondary prevention of paradoxical embolic stroke. *Catheter Cardiovasc Interv.* 2019;93:859-874. https://doi.org/10.1002/ccd.28111.

Kavinsky CJ, Kumamoto FM, Barry AA, et al. SCAI/ACC/HRS institutional and operator requirements for left atrial appendage occlusion. *J Am Coll Cardiol*. 2016;67: 2295-2305.

Otto CM, Kumbhani DJ, Alexander KP, et al. 2017 ACC expert consensus decision pathway for transcatheter aortic valve replacement in the management of adults with aortic stenosis: a report of the American College of Cardiology Task Force on Clinical Expert Consensus Documents. *J Am Coll Cardiol*. 2017;69:1313-1346.

References

Arora S, Misenheimer JA, Ramaraj R. Transcatheter aortic valve replacement: comprehensive review and present status. *Tex Heart Inst J*. 2018;45:122.

Joseph TA, Lane CE, Fender EA, Zack CJ, Rihal CS. Catheter-based closure of aortic and mitral paravalvular leaks: existing techniques and new frontiers. *Expert Rev Med Devices*. 2018;15(9):653-663.

Masoudi FA, Calkins H, Kavinsky CJ, et al. 2015 ACC/HRS/SCAI left atrial appendage occlusion device societal overview: a professional society overview from the American College of Cardiology, Heart Rhythm Society, and Society for Cardiovascular Angiography and Interventions. *J Am Coll Cardiol*. 2015;66:1497-1513.

Rigopoulos AG, Sakellaropoulos S, Ali M, et al. Transcatheter septal ablation in hypertrophic obstructive cardiomyopathy: a technical guide and review of published results. *Heart Fail Rev*. 2018;23(6):907-917.

Index

Page numbers followed by *'f'* indicate figures, *'t'* indicate tables, *'b'* indicate boxes.